Computer Applications in Radiation Oncology

Associate Editors
Peter Neurath, Bengt E. Bjarngard, Frances B. Dobrowolski,
Lionel Cohen, D. John Wright, Frank W. Lane, Pavel V. Houdek,
and John R. Cunningham

COMPUTER APPLICATIONS IN RADIATION ONCOLOGY

Edward S. Sternick, Editor

PROCEEDINGS OF THE FIFTH INTERNATIONAL CONFERENCE ON THE USE OF COMPUTERS IN RADIATION THERAPY

Distributed by The University Press of New England
Hanover, New Hampshire, 1976

Library of Congress Catalogue Card Number 75-44904
International Standard Book Number 0-87451-126-7

Printed in the United States of America.

The Fifth International Conference on the Use of Computers in Radiation Therapy was held at Dartmouth College, Hanover, New Hampshire, August 18-23, 1974. It was funded under Public Health Service Grant Number 1 R13 CA 16888-01.

OFFICERS OF THE CONFERENCE

Chairman: Edward S. Sternick

Organizing Committee:

U.S.A.

Bengt E. Bjarngard
Lionel Cohen
Lawrence Davis
Frances Dobrowolski
Harvey Frey
Frederick W. George III
J. Garrett Holt
Peter W. Neurath
Carol Newton
William Siler
Marilyn Stovall
D. John Wright

United Kingdom

John S. Clifton
Montague Cohen

Canada

John R. Cunningham
Theodor Sterling

Germany

Ulf Rosenow

France

Andree Dutreix

The Netherlands

Jan Van de Geijn

Sweden

Jan Cederlund

Administrative Assistant: Sylvia Driscoll
Treasurer: B. Joan Lester
Editorial Assistants: Eleanor McQuade, Sylvia Driscoll
Local Arrangements: Farideh Bagne, Bruce Curran, Evan Douple, Roger Howes, Michael Hughes, Molly McQuade, Katherine Shapleigh, William Sigward, Joseph Ting

Preface

The importance of computer technology to clinical radiation therapy has been increasingly recognized since the mid-1950's, when it was first proposed that isodose curves be calculated electronically rather than by hand. For the past decade, a number of physicists, computer specialists, and radiotherapists have met periodically at relatively small international gatherings to exchange ideas with the intent of putting into immediate practice the new computer techniques and hardware being developed in various parts of the world.

The latest meeting in this series, the Fifth International Conference on the Use of Computers in Radiation Therapy, convened at Dartmouth College during the week of August 18-23, 1974, and adopted as its general theme "Preparing for the Next Five Years." It was anticipated that major technological advances in the state of the art which had become available in recent years would allow the participants in the Conference to conceptualize a comprehensive, computer-based system or systems that could provide all of the computing facilities needed in a modern department of radiation oncology. These requirements, broadly defined, include:

(1) Control of Patient Flow and Records
(2) Automation, Verification, and Control of Therapy Equipment
(3) Treatment Planning
(4) Biological Modeling
(5) Tumor Registries

There were two major questions to be addressed by the conferees: (1) What should the computer package consist of in terms of both hardware and software? (2) What should the priorities be in different stages of development?

It was recognized that active participation both prior to and during the meeting was the sine qua non for success. Thus membership at the Conference was by invitation to scientists around the world who were known to be involved with computer technology as applied to radiation therapy. Registrants included 140 physicists, radiotherapists, computer scientists, and manufacturers' representatives from eighteen different countries. Several months prior to the meeting, conferees were encouraged to submit abstracts of their current activity for distribution to the entire membership. These abstracts served as the foundation on which the structure of the Conference was fabricated. Response to the request for material was enthusiastic and prolific. Unfortunately, limitations of time made it impossible to allow oral presentation of each of the submitted papers, but they are reproduced in these Proceedings together with a complete set of abstracts.

The meeting was recorded in its entirety, and transcripts of discussions and comments are also included here. Where editing was done in the interest of economy of space and comprehension, a strong effort was made to preserve the intent and idiomatic flavor of the speaker.

The Associate Editors labored diligently, and they have my unreserved appreciation for their generous assistance in the creation of this volume. The members of the Organizing Committee deserve highest commendation for their unfailing candor and constructive recommendations concerning the format and content of the Conference. Those who served on the Local Arrangements Committee must be congratulated for their dedication to the principles of hospitality and cordiality during the week of the meeting. I especially thank Sylvia Driscoll for her outstanding administrative efforts to ensure the success of the Conference, Joan Lester for efficient management of Conference funds, and Eleanor McQuade for assuming responsibility for the preparation of the manuscript.

The Organizing Committee gratefully acknowledges the financial support provided by the following sponsors: National Cancer Institute; Mary Hitchcock Memorial Hospital; American Association of Physicists in Medicine; New Hampshire Chapter, American College of Radiology; Artronix Instrumentation; Brown Boveri Corporation; Atomic Energy of Canada Ltd.; CGR Medical Corporation; Siemens Corporation; Varian Radiation Division; SHM Nuclear Corporation; Lester Chevrolet/Volvo.

Edward S. Sternick

Hanover, New Hampshire
April 1976

Contents

Welcoming Addresses

On behalf of the faculty of the Dartmouth Medical School it is my privilege to welcome the Fifth International Conference on the Use of Computers in Radiation Therapy. You have picked a good time to visit us in Hanover—the month of August. I say this because we have long, cold winters in northern New England and ofttimes very short summers—so much so that the natives hereabouts say that New Hampshire and Vermont have but two seasons, winter and August.

The program for this Conference looks extremely interesting and appears to be of very high caliber. To an outsider such as myself, who knows little about either computers or modern radiation therapy, the topics that you will discuss in themselves symbolize the startling advances of modern technology. All of us are acutely aware of these advances, termed by many a knowledge explosion in the biomedical sciences. This dramatic increase in knowledge makes urgent the need for better communications of the type that this Conference should provide. Because the Dartmouth Medical School, like others, is itself vitally concerned with the acquisition and transmission of knowledge, we count it an honor to sponsor a program such as yours.

I can tell you nothing about radiation therapy. My greatest service to you this morning will be to be brief. But before closing you might like to know just a tiny bit about your sponsoring institution, Dartmouth. Dartmouth College is by American standards an old one, by standards elsewhere in the world, relatively new. It was founded in 1769, just before the American Revolution. The medical school followed almost thirty years later, in 1797, just before the turn of the century. The Medical School offered a complete curriculum leading to the M.D. degree until the 1900's and then for almost sixty years —that is, until just recently—offered training in only the preclinical sciences. Now the School is in an exciting new phase as we return to a complete M.D. program for all our students. In fact, this Conference is being held in the very month when we admit the first class, since 1914, that will in its entirety receive the Dartmouth M.D. degree.

There is a great deal more that I would like to tell you about the school—but time does not permit. I have said enough. I know you are anxious to get on with the business at hand. Thank you for visiting us in Hanover. Best wishes for a pleasant stay and a stimulating conference.

James C. Strickler, M.D.
Dean, Dartmouth Medical School

This is one of my first opportunities to extend a formal welcome to a conference convening in Hanover. In some respects a conference addressed to the subject of computers in radiation therapy is singularly appropriate for such a welcome.

Thayer School is now involved in developing a graduate program in biomedical engineering. As a small school it is impossible for us to emphasize the full range of problems and opportunities that exist in that field. Hence we have decided to emphasize those areas based on the strengths that exist within the Hanover area. A major computer center, a first-rate medical school, a major hospital complex with a cancer center intimately involved in development and application of the latest information related to improved patient care made the choice of the area of radiation therapy as part of our biomedical engineering program a simple one. The convening of the Fifth International Conference on the Use of Computers in Radiation Therapy at Dartmouth gives support and encouragement to me and the Thayer School in this decision.

On a personal note, my first research involvement as a graduate student, more years ago now than I wish to recount, was in backfiguring the size of the atomic weapons detonated over Hiroshima and Nagasaki from damage data collected by field observation. Our concern was primarily with blast damage, but information on radiation effects was also part of the data available. It is extremely gratifying now, even in this minor way, to be associated with you, whose concern with radiation is its application to the needs and aid of man.

A college is the traditional forum for the open and free dissemination of knowledge. I hope this forum serves you well these next few days. I applaud your concern with the generation of knowledge, and even more I support and applaud your efforts to make your work and knowledge available to all whose concern is with an improved level of care. In behalf of the Thayer School, welcome to Hanover. Have a productive week.

Carl F. Long, D.Eng.
Dean, Thayer School of Engineering

Affiliations

ABEDIN-ZADEH, R.
International Atomic Energy Agency
Vienna, Austria

AGOSTINELLI, A.
Yale University
New Haven, Connecticut

AHTEN, E. R.
USC Medical Center
Los Angeles, California

ANDERSON, D. P.
USC Medical Center
Los Angeles, California

APELES, P.
USC Medical Center
Los Angeles, California

BAKER, R. J.
USC Medical Center
Los Angeles, California

BALTER, J. A.
USC Medical Center
Los Angeles, California

BARRAL, J-C.
Centre D'Etudes et de Recherches de Toulouse, Toulouse, France

BENTLEY, R. E.
The Royal Marsden Hospital
Sutton, Surrey, U.K.

BJARNGARD, B.
Harvard Medical School
Boston, Massachusetts

BLINICK, J.
Maine Medical Center
Portland, Maine

BOUSQUET, L.
Centre D'Etudes et de Recherches de Toulouse, Toulouse, France

BOYER, A. L.
Harvard Medical School
Boston, Massachusetts

BRAHMAVAR, S. M.
Springfield Hospital Medical Center
Springfield, Massachusetts

BRASCHO, D. J.
University of Alabama School of Medicine, Birmingham, Alabama

BROWN, D.
Tufts-New England Medical Center
Boston, Massachusetts

BUSCH, M.
Medizinische Poliklinik der Universität
Marburg, Federal Republic of Germany

CEDERLUND, J.
Akademiska Sjukhuset
Uppsala, Sweden

CHAPMAN, D.
UCLA Center for the Health Sciences
Los Angeles, California

CHRISPENS, J. E.
Loma Linda University School of Medicine, Loma Linda, California

CHU, W. T.
Loma Linda University School of Medicine, Loma Linda, California

CHUI, C. S.
Mt. Sinai School of Medicine
New York, New York

CHUNG-BIN, A.
Rush College of Medicine
Chicago, Illinois

CLAMPITT, S.
University of California Medical Center
San Francisco, California

CLARKE, P. Z.
Case Western Reserve University Hospitals, Cleveland, Ohio

CLEMENS, J.
Harvard Medical School
Boston, Massachusetts

CLIFTON, J. S.
University College Hospital
London, U.K.

COHEN, L.
Michael Reese Medical Center
Chicago, Illinois

COHEN, M.
The London Hospital
London, U.K.

COLLINS, V.
Rosewood General Hospital
Houston, Texas

CROSSLAND, P.
Middlesex Hospital Medical School
London, U.K.

CUNNINGHAM, J. R.
Ontario Cancer Institute
Toronto, Canada

CURRAN, B.
Dartmouth-Hitchcock Medical Center
Hanover, New Hampshire

DADE, M.
Siemens
Erlangen, Federal Republic of Germany

DAHLIN, H.
Uppsala University
Uppsala, Sweden

DAVIS, H.
Jet Propulsion Laboratory
Pasadena, California

DAVIS, L.
University of Pennsylvania
Philadelphia, Pennsylvania

DAWSON, D. J.
Ontario Cancer Treatment and Research Foundation, London, Ontario, Canada

DENK, M. W.
Cooper Hospital
Camden, New Jersey

DOBROWOLSKI, F.
University of New Mexico School of Medicine, Albuquerque, New Mexico

DOUPLE, E. B.
Dartmouth-Hitchcock Medical Center
Hanover, New Hampshire

DREW, J. F.
Ontario Cancer Treatment and Research Foundation, London, Ontario, Canada

EISENLOHR, H. H.
International Atomic Energy Agency
Vienna, Austria

ELLIS, F.
Memorial Hospital for Cancer and Allied Diseases, New York, New York

FEHRENTZ, D.
Universitäs-Strahlenklinik
Heidelberg, Federal Republic of Germany

FOLLAND, R. E.
Tufts-New England Medical Center
Boston, Massachusetts

FREIDA, D.
UCLA Center for the Health Sciences
Los Angeles, California

FREY, H.
UCLA Center for the Health Sciences
Los Angeles, California

FRIDH, L.
Sahlgrenska Sjukhuset
Goteborg, Sweden

FURUSHIMA, N.
Nippon Electric Co. Ltd.
Tokyo, Japan

GARCES, R. M.
Evanston Hospital
Evanston, Illinois

GARY-BOBO, J.
Clinique St.-Eloi
Montpellier, France

GELL, G.
Univ.-Klink für Radiologie
Graz, Austria

GEORGE, F. W. III
USC Medical Center
Los Angeles, California

GHILEZAN, N.
Institutul Oncologie
Cluj, Romania

GLICKSMAN, A.
Brown University
Providence, Rhode Island

GOITEIN, M.
Harvard Medical School
Boston, Massachusetts

GRAFFMAN, S.
Uppsala University Hospital
Uppsala, Sweden

GRIEM, M. L.
University of Chicago
Chicago, Illinois

GUSTAFSSON, T.
University of Lund
Lund, Sweden

HAHN, J.
Mt. Sinai School of Medicine
New York, New York

HANSEN, G.
World Health Organization
Washington, D.C.

HAYBITTLE, J. L.
Addenbrooke Hospital
Cambridge, U.K.

HAYMOND, H. R.
USC Medical Center
Los Angeles, California

HENDERSON, C. I.
M.E.L. Equip. Co. Ltd.
Crawley, Sussex, U.K.

HENDRICKSON, F.
Rush College of Medicine
Chicago, Illinois

HENRY, J. A.
Universite De Bruxelles
Brussels, Belgium

HESSELIUS, I.
Uppsala University Hospital
Uppsala, Sweden

HOLT, J. G.
Memorial Hospital for Cancer and
Allied Diseases, New York, New York

HOUDEK, P. V.
University of Miami School of Medicine
Miami, Florida

HUGHES, M.
Dartmouth-Hitchcock Medical Center
Hanover, New Hampshire

INAMURA, K.
Nippon Electric Co. Ltd.
Tokyo, Japan

INGRAM, D.
University College Hospital
London, U.K.

JACOBSON, D. M.
Loma Linda University School of
Medicine, Loma Linda, California

JAMESON, D. G.
Middlesex Hospital Medical School
London, U.K.

JOHANSSON, K-A.
Sahlgrenska Sjukhuset
Goteborg, Sweden

JOHNSON, J. W.
UCLA Center for the Health Sciences
Los Angeles, California

JOHNSSON, J. E.
University of Lund,
Lund, Sweden

JONES, D.
University of Washington
Seattle, Washington

JUNG, B.
Akademiska Sjukhus
Uppsala, Sweden

KARLSSON, P. O.
Uppsala University
Uppsala, Sweden

KARTHA, P.
Rush College of Medicine
Chicago, Illinois

KARZMARK, C. J.
Stanford University School of Medicine
Stanford, California

KIJEWSKI, P.
Harvard Medical School
Boston, Massachusetts

KIPPING, D.
Varian Associates
Palo Alto, California

KIRK, J.
West of Scotland Health Boards
Glasgow, Scotland

KORZENIEWSKI, F.
Rush College of Medicine
Chicago, Illinois

KUBO, Y.
Nippon Electric Co. Ltd.
Tokyo, Japan

KUROHARA, S. S.
USC Medical Center
Los Angeles, California

LANE, F. W.
Dartmouth-Hitchcock Medical Center
Hanover, New Hampshire

LANSU, M. J.
Cooper Hospital
Camden, New Jersey

LANZL, L. H.
University of Chicago
Chicago, Illinois

LARSEN, R.
Harvard Medical School
Boston, Massachusetts

LERCH, I. A.
International Atomic Energy Agency
Vienna, Austria

LESTER, J.
Dartmouth-Hitchcock Medical Center
Hanover, New Hampshire

LIDEN, K.
University of Lund
Lund, Sweden

LIDOFSKY, L. J.
Columbia University
New York, New York

LILLICRAP, S. C.
Royal Marsden Hospital
Sutton, Surrey, U.K.

LINDSKOUG, B.
Sahlgrenska Sjukhusset
Goteborg, Sweden

LOFROTH, P-O
Akademiska Sjukhuset
Uppsala, Sweden

LUNDY, A.
University of California-Los Alamos Scientific Laboratory, Los Alamos, New Mexico

MACDONALD, J. C. F.
Ontario Cancer Treatment and Research Foundation, London, Ontario, Canada

MACKINNEY, J. G.
USC Medical Center
Los Angeles, California

MAMPEY, R.
Centre D'Etudes et de Recherches de Toulouse, Toulouse, France

MANSFIELD, C.
Thomas Jefferson University
Philadelphia, Pennsylvania

MARCHANT, D. J.
Tufts-New England Medical Center
Boston, Massachusetts

MATSUOKA, A.
Nippon Electric Co. Ltd.
Tokyo, Japan

MAYHEW, D.
University College Hospital
London, U.K.

MCKIERNAN, F.
Yale University
New Haven, Connecticut

MILAN, J.
Royal Marsden Hospital
Sutton, Surrey, U.K.

MILLER, A.
UCLA Center for the Health Sciences
Los Angeles, California

MINOR, M.
University of California-Los Alamos Scientific Laboratory, Los Alamos, New Mexico

MOLLER, T. R.
University of Lund
Lund, Sweden

MULVEY, P. J.
University College Hospital
London, U.K.

NEBLETT, D. L.
USC Medical Center
Los Angeles, California

NEILSEN, I. R.
Loma Linda School of Medicine
Loma Linda, California

NELSON, R. F.
Cooper Hospital
Camden, New Jersey

NEURATH, P. W.
Tufts-New England Medical Center
Boston, Massachusetts

NEWTON, C. M.
UCLA Center for the Health Sciences
Los Angeles, California

NORDBERG, U-B
University of Lund
Lund, Sweden

NOTTER, G.
Sahlgrenska Sjukhusset
Goteborg, Sweden

OLSEN, B.
Uppsala University
Uppsala, Sweden

OTANI, S.
Nippon Electric Co. Ltd.
Tokyo, Japan

PENGILLEY, R. E.
Hammersmith Hospital
London, U.K.

PERRY, H.
Sinai Hospital of Detroit
Detroit, Michigan

POTENZA, R.
Varian Associates
Palo Alto, California

POWELL, W. T.
Tufts-New England Medical Center
Boston, Massachusetts

PRASAD, S. G.
Evanston Hospital
Evanston, Illinois

PREWITT, J. M. S.
National Institute of Health
Bethesda, Maryland

RAGAN, D. P.
Mallinckrodt Institute of Radiology
St. Louis, Missouri

RAGNHULT, I
Sahlgrenska Sjukhuset
Goteborg, Sweden

REGIS, H.
Centre D'Etudes et de Recherches de Toulouse, Toulouse, France

RENN, R. A.
Evanston Hospital
Evanston, Illinois

RENNER, W. D.
West Virginia University Medical Center
Morgantown, West Virginia

ROEDER, D. L.
University of California-Los Alamos Scientific Laboratory, Los Alamos, New Mexico

ROSENBLOOM, M. E.
The Royal Marsden Hospital
Sutton, Surrey, U.K.

ROSENOW, U.
Universitäts-Frauenklinik
Göttingen, Federal Republic of Germany

ROTHMEIER, J.
University of Massachusetts Medical School, Worcester, Massachusetts

ROZENFELD, M.
University of Chicago
Chicago, Illinois

RUST, D. C.
Stanford University School of Medicine
Stanford, California

SCHAEFLEIN, J. W.
USC Medical Center
Los Angeles, California

SCHILLACI, M. E.
University of California-Los Alamos Scientific Laboratory, Los Alamos, New Mexico

SCHNEIDER, W.
Uppsala University
Uppsala, Sweden

SCHULZ, R. J.
Yale University
New Haven, Connecticut

SEYMOUR, R. M.
Tufts-New England Medical Center
Boston, Massachusetts

SHALEK, R. J.
University of Texas Medical Center
Houston, Texas

SHERWOOD, P.
Tufts-New England Medical Center
Boston, Massachusetts

SHLAER, S.
University of California-Los Alamos Scientific Laboratory, Los Alamos, New Mexico

SHRIVASTAVA, P. N.
Allegheny General Hospital
Pittsburgh, Pennsylvania

SILER, W.
University of Alabama
Birmingham, Alabama

SLATER, J. M.
Loma Linda University School of Medicine, Loma Linda, California

SMITH, A. R.
University of Texas Medical Center
Houston, Texas

SMITH, V.
University of California Medical Center
San Francisco, California

SNELL, J. E.
Siemens
Solna, Sweden

STEBEN, J. D.
Thomas Jefferson University
Philadelphia, Pennsylvania

STERNICK, E. S.
Dartmouth-Hitchcock Medical Center
Hanover, New Hampshire

STOVALL, M.
University of Texas Medical Center
Houston, Texas

SUNDSTROM, A.
University of Lund
Lund, Sweden

SUNTHARALINGAM, N.
Thomas Jefferson University
Philadelphia, Pennsylvania

SVENSSON, G. K.
Harvard Medical School
Boston, Massachusetts

THELIN, A. M.
Akademiska Sjukhus
Uppsala, Sweden

TING, J.
Dartmouth-Hitchcock Medical Center
Hanover, New Hampshire

TODD-POKROPEK, A.
University College Hospital
London, U.K.

TURNIER, H.
University of Miami School of Medicine, Miami, Florida

UEDA, Y.
Nippon Electric Co. Ltd.
Tokyo, Japan

VOKOFF, R.
UCLA Center for the Health Sciences
Los Angeles, California

WACHTOR, T.
Rush College of Medicine
Chicago, Illinois

WASHINGTON, J.
University of Washington
Seattle, Washington

WEBB, E.
USC Medical Center
Los Angeles, California

WHELDON, T. E.
West of Scotland Health Boards
Glasgow, Scotland

WILKINSON, J. M.
Christie Hospital
Manchester, U.K.

WRIGHT, D. J.
Geisinger Medical Center
Danville, Pennsylvania

WU, R.
Thomas Jefferson University
Philadelphia, Pennsylvania

YU, S-N
Mt. Sinai School of Medicine
New York, New York

ZETTERLUND, S.
Akademiska Sjukhuset
Uppsala, Sweden

1 — Coding #1 In patient

2 — Coding #1 Out patient, office

3 — Coding #2 Define disease treatment prescription

4 — Treatment planning interactive

5 — Enter treatment information

6 — First treatment parameters

7 — Subsequent treatment parameters

8 — Completion of treatment

9 — Coding #3 Patient treatment response

10 — Transfer to disk for storage

11 — Coding #4 Follow-up

12 — Statistic analysis

Fig. 1. Time Sequence of Computer Interaction with Clinical Activity.

physician's office or the departmental registration desk. At this point all patients are assigned a physics number for future reference. The first character of the number indicates the institution, since more than one institution is currently using our system; the second character indicates the year, followed by two numerical digits indicating the month, followed by a three-digit number assigned to the patient, chronologically, starting from January 1 of that year. By intersection 3 the physician has examined the patient and completed the evaluation, and the coding form, containing the definition of the disease and the proposed treatment prescription is complete. At intersection 4 the physics dosimetry section performs the treatment-planning activities required for this particular patient. At intersection 5 the patient is ready for treatment. The technologist in charge of the treatment room will enter the pertinent information concerning the patient's treatment. All of the physical parameters for the first treatment of all ports will be recorded at intersection 6 for future verification of treatment. At intersection 7 the physical-treatment parameters for all subsequent treatments will be recorded. By intersection 8 treatment is completed. The technologists will inform the computer of the completion of treatment and a summary of the treatment parameters can be obtained. At intersection 9 the physician will evaluate the response of the treatment and complete a coding form. At this time all information acquired by the computer concerning this patient will be transferred to a back-up mass storage device (disk or tape). At intersection 10 follow-up information is acquired by the computer and later merged with the previous information of the patient. At intersection 11 the stored patient records can be periodically scanned by the computer to generate address labels for patients prior to their follow-up date. It will also generate a list of patients for follow-up during a particular week or month which can be used by the staff to review and take the appropriate action for patients who don't appear for their scheduled follow-up visit. By telephoning, or sending an additional letter to the patient, we can, by this procedure, drastically improve the follow-up. A statistical analysis can also be performed by scanning the stored patient follow-up records to generate the survival table for a particular site and staging.

Since the patient information is stored on a disk throughout from the beginning to the end of treatment (our current practice is three months), all this information can be retrieved at any time from a remote terminal.

We are aware that there is still controversy and lack of consensus on what information should be in the patient information system. It is difficult to enforce rules or policies on physicians in a department. Instead, the system of information retrieval must be made attractive to them, for without their cooperation it will have little chance of success.

Our current coding forms evolved from this philosophy. In 1965, when we had all the patient's information contained in one coding form, we were faced with numerous incompleted forms, because the information required became available at different times. In order to complete it, physicians had to search for the coding form three times. With their busy schedules, this was almost impossible. Consequently, we have separated it into four forms, and each is completed at a different time. This system seems to be reasonably successful.

As for content, we believe that both the content of the coding form and the training of the person filling it out determines the usefulness and reliability of the information. If the coding forms are designed so that trained clerical staffs can complete them by referring to the information available in ordinary patient records, the information obtained in this manner is likely to lose the reliability and specificity required by radiotherapists, and its usefulness is therefore greatly limited. Our coding form is designed so that it must be coded by a qualified radiotherapist. The physician completing it will most likely feel comfortable using this information, while being fully aware of its limitations. It is still questionable whether the same information will be useful to physicians at other institutions. The content of a coding form very much depends on what kind of questions are to be answered. If one doesn't know the questions, it is unlikely that a good coding form can be designed. Therefore, the form should be very simple and short. Also, there should be forms for special studies when we know the questions being asked. They should be comprehensive and long, but with specific objectives.

The acceptance and cooperation of the staff is based on the benefits that are generated from the procedures. For example, if the physician fills out the information retrieval form, he does not have to complete a form for a hospital registry, which is tedious and, in general, not pertinent to radiation therapy. The information, when recorded automatically by the machine, verifies the treatment which the technologists have found to be valuable, especially when working alone. Acceptance is therefore conditional on the immediate benefits to individuals involved in the task. In a busy clinical environment the staffs in general usually do not appreciate the long-range ones.

The cost of the hardware of this computer is $63,000. Based on 2.2 percent monthly leasing cost for a five-year period, it would cost $1.50 per treatment. This cost is not unreasonable, since it covers multiple functions. The developmental cost of the entire computer system is about five man years. Only one fourth of a programmer's time to maintain the system routinely and to perform all of the clinical functions is required.

We freely admit that the present Rush system for a departmental data management scheme was built upon the ashes of several past failures. There is no guarantee that this system will be a success, but we have made many improvements over previous systems. The value of future analysis of the data being collected will determine its worth.

In conclusion, from our experiences, we consider the information system required for a radiation therapy department as not merely a task of clerical, technical, administrative, and programming efforts, but a scientific task involving the consideration of human engineering. To assure its implementability the system should be developed in a clinical environment, definitely not under isolated laboratory conditions. The acceptance by the staff should be through the process of education and influence rather than by enforcement of the procedures as a matter of policy. The concepts of cost and objective should always be realistic.

REFERENCES

1. T. Wachtor, A. Chung-Bin, and F. Hendrickson, "Rush Radiation Oncology Computer System," *Computer Applications in Radiation Oncology*, Proceedings of the Fifth International Conference on the Use of Computers in Radiation Therapy (August 1974).
2. A. Chung-Bin, T. Wachtor, P. Kartha, and F. Hendrickson, "Development and Experience in Computer Monitoring and the Verification of Daily Patient Treatment Parameters," *Computer Applications in Radiation Oncology*, Proceedings of the Fifth International Conference on the Use of Computers in Radiation Therapy (August 1974).

QUESTIONS

RENNER: What kind of backup do you use to store information in case your discs should be wiped out by accident?

CHUNG-BIN: We have two discs. We always have a backup disc for the records. The reliability of the records is very important.

2. Computer-Assisted Patient Management

J. G. Mackinney
F. W. George, III
H. R. Haymond
S. S. Kurohara
D. L. Neblett
J. A. Balter

Introduction

At Los Angeles County - U.S.C. Medical Center an automation project for radiation medicine has been pursued intensively during the past three years. This paper presents the context and the goals of our project at the level of a general system analysis. One of these goals is to create a system that can be used at other treatment centers. Before you can adopt or adapt our work, at the system level, we will have to agree on many definitions and procedures.

We need to examine each automated function as a tool and we need to agree on priorities, both for our center and at the national level. Synergistic effects may result if the complete system has been carefully designed to meet its goals in the real environment. Faulty design will only waste time and money, with damaging repercussions in the larger organization.

1. Dramatis Personae

We have considered local use of the automated system by persons in twelve different roles:

Administrator	Patient	Resident
Clerk	Physician	Secretary
Dosimetrist	Recorder	Student
Nurse	Researcher	Technologist

Their functions must be carefully examined in each department so that the computer system helps them to perform it more effectively.

2. Computer System

For a number of reasons it seemed best to design around a local minicomputer. We wanted it to control the linear accelerator, which requires a set of inputs and outputs, at least ten, and preferably twenty times per second; that kind of service is simply not possible from a central data-processing computer. We felt it made economic sense to expand the control computer into a departmental information system, since we anticipated doing a lot of programming and since a relatively small increase in price ($40,000 out of a total $200,000 for the automated accelerator) would buy information handling power.

We now have a larger system on order, but it still appears that our original system had the size and speed to satisfy many of our aims. The main limitation from the clinical viewpoint is that there was and will be no back-up capacity. The system has 48 kilobytes core storage, 2.4 megabytes disc memory, 6 CRT terminals, 1 remote telephone link, 1 page printer (60 lines per minute), 1 magnetic tape unit, and 1 TTY.

3. Patient Data Files

A decision was made early in the project to concentrate on current patients to a maximum of two hundred in treatment and about ten times that in follow-up. This is possible within the confines of a small disc memory if only enough data is kept on follow-ups to ensure proper filing of new information. Patient histories, treatment summaries, and examination results are collected on the system but do not stay there. Conceptually, the system transmits that kind of data to a data-processing center as soon as each record is completed, or perhaps at the close of each treatment day.

For patients in treatment, or in a consultation status that could lead to treatment, information is divided among several files. These are: Master, History, Diagnosis, Treatment, Site, and Test. This division is intended to save both disc space and the number of disc references made by various programs. Copies of the forms can be obtained from the authors.

The Master file contains the addresses of the other records. It also shows how to reach the patient, when he was last seen, the date of his next appointment, and so forth. The History record content would ideally depend on diagnosis, so that it could be limited to factors known or suspected of being disease-relevant; more development is needed here. The Diagnosis record also includes a checklist of items in the patient's chart, such as pathology reports and specific consent forms, showing whether each one is required in the particular case, and if required, the date it was added to the chart.

The Treatment record contains summary data, but its main function is to serve as the top node or reference for the site and test files and, when teletherapy is involved, the field and plan records. Each site record refers to a location in the body where the dosage must be specifically estimated, so that the "site" concept includes both tumors and sensitive organs. The Test file is used to specify and record monitoring tests, such as red cell count, whose results may determine changes in the treatment plan.

4. Other Files and Functions

This includes a phone list of our own staff and all our most frequently called numbers, including the other departments and institutions that are responsible for most of our referrals. We can use index references to the phone list to make patient data records more compact while they are in the current file. In general, the name of, for instance, the referring physician is not something to be kept on records used for statistical purposes when even the patient's name should be removed; so the fact that our phone list is constantly being updated does not prevent us from taking advantage of indexing. It does mean that we must allocate enough space for the current list plus about one year's changes.

Scheduling is a tedious and error-prone task that the computer can handle well, so a set of schedule files is an important part of the system. After some thought we came up with a general format that a single program can maintain to schedule both facilities and people.

Once a patient's treatment is prescribed, it is possible to set up a complete schedule for all procedures, tests, examinations, and so on. Naturally this must be done in terms of available facilities and urgency. An important current objective is to create computerized files of the treatment protocols approved by our staff physicians that cover the bulk of the patients. Once a protocol is agreed on for a particular case, the patient's schedule can be created automatically. At first the system will contain only part of the needed information, and its schedules will need much changing and completion; this handwork should be no more onerous than the appointment-book method. As we get into the habit of keeping the system informed—for example, that Dr. X is taking a vacation or that most of the staff are attending a meeting after lunch next Wednesday—the amount of confusion should decrease noticeably. Also, to the extent that protocols are defined in the system, our patterns of patient care can be monitored. In particular, deviations from protocol can be brought to light at once, and justification for them can be requested while the matter is timely.

In the past, our department has not been responsible for billing in any way, so that function has been neglected in our planning. We are now, however, under increasing pressure to provide accurate records of each procedure for each patient. Such transaction records form another transient file, which is transferred to the main hospital system at the close of each day.

We do need to keep accounts of budgets, expenditures, and current balances for grant funds. It has been our hope that someone else would develop a package that we could adopt with little change. At any rate, the files for this small-scale accounting also belong in the system.

The last function that needs to be mentioned here is computer-assisted instruction. The immediate goal is to document the system itself in this manner, so that a user's guide is available for each part of the system. Beyond this, we want to take advantage of the large body of programmed instruction now available for training in cancer diagnosis and treatment.

5. A Scenario for Clinical Decisions

One of our concerns has been to promote the use of standard protocols, to the point of enforcement. Another has been to make sure that the clinically relevant factors of the patient's disease and condition became part of the computer record. Last June, EMI published a report called "Patterns of Clinical and Research Radiation Therapy in Cancer Care"; some of you took part in it. We feel that the kind of procedure shown in that study answers both the concerns just mentioned. We envision it being used by a resident in radiation therapy or by a staff physician refreshing his memory. In our scenario, the physician at the computer terminal enters the patient's name and one or two terms or stock phrases denoting the tumor type and site. These terms would be sufficient to enable the system to select a decision tree from its library, and a question-and-answer sequence would begin.

The two chief obstacles to this plan are, first, the amount of sheer detail work required to generate trees and protocols for a useful fraction of the caseload, and, second, the difficulty of reaching expert consensus on proper treatment over the same range. If the initial stage covers fewer than half the cases in a given area, such as lung or gynecological cancers, we cannot expect physicians to use it.

6. In Retrospect

The thinking that led to this project can be summarized in the form of six hypotheses:

(1) Good practice requires plotting the estimated dose distribution for most patients.

(2) Beam treatment machine setup under computer control will be fast, reliable, and precise.
(3) A computerized information system can significantly improve patient management.
(4) Private industry will not develop adequate systems by itself; research institutions using public funds must carry a large share of the effort.
(5) Off-the-shelf computer equipment can meet our needs in terms of speed, reliability, and cost.
(6) The system will be most cost-effective if it maximizes the use of a single minicomputer.

7. Design Principles

We have been following several design principles which deserve mention now and which should be discussed.

(1) Responsibility always rests with the human operator.
(2) The system can be overridden, in almost every case, by anyone who registers an authorized identity code. The event will be logged in detail and reported to the proper authority for review.
(3) Physicians, nurses, and clerks should not have to learn standard operating systems, and in most situations they should not even have access to the operating system.
(4) If the person at the terminal enters something ridiculous, he should be warned immediately and given a second chance.

8. Clinic Management

When we move away from machine control and mathematical calculations into the world of clinical routine and patient management, we are tackling a more complex job. We are at once involved in the ways in which groups of people interact with each other. This branch of cybernetics is being explored in all areas of our society, under various names and guises, as the growth of technology and population forces us to develop new ways of working together. There have already been a number of costly failures, and rather few cases of limited success. The key is to make the computer work for people. It is all too easy for the system designer to play God and declare, "We're all going to do it *my* way." The fact is, every step must be agreed on before it can be accepted. There is not much room for dictators in this development—not if we want to assert our humanity. In the field of radiotherapy we are really fortunate in having potential system users who are basically people-oriented. They may be hard to satisfy, but their humanistic prejudices may save us from the kind of control we associate with 1984.

3. The Tufts Therapeutic Radiology Department Information System

P. W. Neurath
D. Brown
P. Sherwood

Introduction

A computer based information system (1) can be described on several levels. One level concerns the objectives for collecting, displaying, and recording the information and those for retrieving and analyzing it. A second level describes the kinds of information which need to be collected. The third level deals with the technical aspects by which the computer performs these functions. The fourth important level is concerned with the economic impact of the system.

Definition of Organization and Criteria

As a starting point it is probably best to consider the overall purposes or objectives of a departmental computer-based information system for radiotherapy. Let us assume that we are dealing with a large, academic, radiation-oncology department which treats and later follows 1000 or more new patients per year, trains several radiation oncologists, each for two or more years, and has an active radiation therapy research program. Such a department may wish to justify a computer system on the basis of two criteria. One is the saving of professional time, its most expensive resource. The second is the ability to improve the performance of the department qualitatively; i.e. to do research or manage patients better in ways that cannot be done without the use of the computer as a tool.

Objectives of Information Systems

One can define the ideal objectives of the ultimate radiation therapy department information system as follows:

---

* Supported by National Cancer Institute, CA12178.

1. Keep one single, complete, unified record of the patient (medical and administrative).
2. Enter data by having doctors, nurses, receptionists, and others dictate in normal English or automatically by machines.
3. Be able to review any selected portion of the record from numerous locations which have terminals.
4. Be able to retrieve any group of patients who meet any combination of defined criteria.
5. Have the computer print all necessary paper work automatically (bills, appointment schedules, letters to referring physicians, progress notes, discharge summaries, follow-up reminders, tumor registry reports, PSRO reports).
6. Flag patients who fall into established protocols, indicate the prescribed tests and treatment sequence; and indicate exceptions from protocol.

Meeting these specific objectives would save a large mount of professional time that is now needed to hunt for needed data, arrange these data, search for relevant items in the record, and generate routine communications that reflect various pieces of the data already in the record.

Unfortunately, present-day computer systems as well as the ones that can be foreseen in the next few years do not allow all these objectives to be met even technically, and economic factors add further limits.

The most serious technical problem is that a computer is not only unable to understand spoken English but cannot even understand typewritten natural English sentences. For information to be retrievable it must be highly structured; every term must be uniquely defined, properly spelled, and entered in a prescribed sequence.

The computer must, for example, be given the Name (last, first initial), Date of Birth (month/day/year), Sex, Race (White, Black, Oriental, Other), Site of Tumor (e.g., left female breast, upper inner quadrant), Pathology (Adenocarcinoma), Size of Lesion (maximum diameter in cms), Date of Diagnosis (month/year), where Diagnosis was made (hospital code No.), and how Pathology, etc. was confirmed. If this procedure is followed, the computer can use this unambiguous, *quantified* information in many different contexts.

The way in which it returns (outputs) this information is also similarly circumscribed. For example, the format for tables of results or of patients' treatment must be very carefully specified. A holiday in a series of dates, a term with too many letters to fit a column are both easy to handle if the report is made out with paper and pencil but must be programmed in great detail before the computer can produce a legible output table.

In consideration of these limitations, current objectives have been to:

1. Create one unified computerized data base to contain all items needed for *most* administrative functions and all *basic* medical data;
2. Permit random retrieval of that data;
3. Have these data on line for "instant" editing and review with comprehensive searches and reports available in a matter of minutes to hours;
4. Perform data entry into the computer by the use of trained personnel with paper forms as the primary interface for input of medical data from physicians;
5. Avoid any duplication of data entry by physicians and others;
6. Have the data serve multiple functions, viz.:
   a. Data entry results in summaries for insertion into the patient's chart:
      i. at admission
      ii. after initial work-up and treatment planning
      iii. at the completion of a course of radiation therapy
      iv. cumulatively at each follow-up
      v. at a second or retreatment;
   b. Printing of daily schedules of each treatment on each machine and of new and follow-up appointments;
   c. Automatic preparation of:
      i. an itemized bill for each patient at end of treatment
      ii. up-dated statistics of all procedures and dollar income categories for the department on a monthly, year-to-date, and annual basis;
   d. Weekly checklists of all patients under treatment for use in departmental chart rounds;
   e. Weekly alphabetized summaries of:
      i. all new patients
      ii. all patients completing treatment;
   f. Statistical routines allow the retrieval of:
      i. lists of patients (name and/or hospital number, age, sex etc.) meeting various inclusive and/or exclusive criteria that are easily specified, with independently specifiable data output
      ii. numerical tabulations giving labelled rows and columns of numbers of patients in various categories
      iii. survival tables and other cross tabulations of any selected groups of patients.

All of these functions are to be based on patient data entry at terminals by as few operators as possible working from patient forms and from the modified and annotated schedules and appointment lists and from charge slips.

Two further departmental information objectives which involve the creation of two additional separate data bases are the following:

7. To set up a simple financial grants management system which allows an approximate up-to-date look at all expenditures. Desired outputs are to be organized on a monthly basis for each category by each account with personnel cross-referenced as well. Editing of any item at random is to be possible at any time within a year or two.
8. To create a bibliographic file of all reprints, books, etc. kept in the departmental files, which is retrievable by every word or combination of (exclusive or inclusive) words in the title as well as by author(s), added key words, etc. There are currently over 4000 such items in the Department.

Finally, it is desired to have

9. The patient data interface with a hospital-wide tumor registry. Details of this registry are described in a separate paper to be presented at this conference (2). The Tumor Registry uses the same but it is otherwise separate. A set of programs which transfers selected data items from the department data base to the hospital tumor registry on a monthly basis is therefore desired.

All nine of these objectives have been implemented and are working routinely.

Additional aims, implementation of which are planned for and partially working, are the automatic acquisition of patient treatment data from one ^{60}Co machine, as well as the preparation of a complete detailed radiation treatment plan for the whole planned course of treatment (i.e. typically covering 35 or more calendar days) for a patient, listing all fields, all sites, all treatments, and resulting radiation doses daily, and obtainable by entering the plan(s) for each field.

In addition to the end uses described, there are functions required by the computer system to make these results possible. It must, for instance, keep accounts of usage and store a number of code libraries such as the applicable part of the Systematized Nomenclature of Pathology (3), the American Cancer Society Tumor Nomenclature (4), a coded list of all physicians, hospitals, and clinics, and their addresses. All of these and many more internal functions meet the overall objective of making the system work.

Data Content of System

The data that make up the substance of the information system come from a variety of sources. A patient's identifying data are obtained during an interview, with an operator typing in the data at the terminal. These interview data are nearly 100 percent complete and accurate, and they are almost always entered on time.

The date a patient starts treatment, the date and type of every treatment, whether he is an in or out patient, and the date of his last treatment are furnished by the radiotherapy technician using the daily machine schedules. Because these data serve to treat the patient and are used for billing purposes, this information too tends to be complete and accurate.

The specifically medical information presents the greatest difficulty. Conceptually, it can be thought of as serving two somewhat disparate medical uses. One is that of the present and future care of an isolated particular patient. As such it needs to be detailed, specific, and relevant to that patient's condition. The second medical use is to review comparable cases for quality control, teaching, and research. That requires the medical information to be clearly categorized, and a common set of data answered for every patient.

Combining these requirements and embodying them in forms has been a difficult task. Its implementation has, however, improved the quality of our medical records for all patients. By forcing a structured approach to recording data, it ensures that the initial paper record is more complete and that important items are not overlooked when working up a patient or evaluating a patient during follow-up.

The information asked for is minimal and structured; multiple choice answers are provided wherever possible. An interesting problem is that of coding the diagnosis. The doctor simply writes in the pathology and site in detail. The computer operator finds the corresponding SNOP[3] code and enters that. For a summary the computer prints the SNOP code description that is in its dictionary file. In addition it determines the major, minor, and sub category into which a patient with the combination of site and pathology codes falls. The major and minor categories are adapted from End Results in Cancer (5) while the subcategories are those from the Manual of Tumor Nomenclature (4).

An optimal set of data small enough so as not to take an appreciable time to record and comprehensive enough to be useful is difficult to define. The information to be recorded must consequently differ for different classes of patients; each recording form should fit one sheet of paper. Many physicians must agree to use the same forms, and all of them must be comfortable with them. To achieve this without being rigid and authoritarian has been a major task. Currently we have forms (data structures) adapted to GYN, BREAST, and certain LYMPHOMA patients, and one for all others (GENERAL).

Looking toward the future, additional specialized forms are under preparation, but it will probably take several more years to have the ten or more most prevalent disease categories adequately covered.

Also under revision and scheduled for implementation in October 1974 is the automatic entry of treatment plan and treatment data.

Access to the data stored currently is almost as flexible as any user has required to date. The most serious problems in terms of DATA CONTENT which have been encountered are:

1. Errors in the Data: A few errors arise from clerical mistakes; others arise from misinterpretation of questions. We have been trying to devise programs that will reject or flag contradictory or inappropriate answers.
2. Missing Data Items: These cause as many or more problems than the incorrect data. Constant vigilance is required to maintain quality on a routine, daily, year-in-and-year-out basis.

We are constantly analyzing our data, and such analyses often reveal errors and omissions in the data base. These are then searched for systematically, and corrected wherever possible by reference to the complete patient chart.

The MUMPS DEC PDP 11/20 computer system used to implement the information system has been described previously (1) and its more recent up-dated specifications are given in the paper by Seymour et al. to be presented at this conference (6). The computer is kept running to serve the departmental and other MUMPS system users from 8 A.M. to 5:30 P.M. Monday through Friday with a 98 percent plus availability factor. Usually the system is also available on a twenty-four-hour basis, but from 5:30 to 9 P.M. or later, programming or other computer system work may require cutting off all MUMPS users. This schedule, by implication, requires that the highly skilled professional programmers and engineers must be willing to work evenings.

Our biggest problem has been to find reliable printing terminals that put out good legible copy. Computer hardware problems are also so frequent that redundancy of such vulnerable items as computer power supplies, memory boards, terminal controllers, etc., as well as expert, in-house, on the spot engineering help, is necessary to maintain uninterrupted service.

Costs

Computer costs are notoriously difficult to specify; competition is fierce; and many prices have declined as much as 20 percent per year for several years. To duplicate our information system today would probably cost approximately $40,000 to $50,000 for the computer, including tapes, discs, and terminal interfaces; $5,000 to $10,000 for the basic software; and $25,000 to $30,000 for the terminals. This is a total capital investment of $70,000 to $90,000, representing an annual cost of perhaps $20,000 to $30,000 amortized over five years and including interest charges. Maintenance will cost about $5,000 to $10,000 per year.

The minimal operating personnel required are two secretarial people, one with billing and accounting skills, the other with knowledge of medical terminology; and one fulltime systems programmer who can also identify major hardware problems and fix minor ones. The first two people replace more than two who would do similar work where there is no computer to provide assistance in preparing billing information, transcribing dictation, etc. Because no such departmental information system is static, an additional programmer to make changes, add features, etc. is probably essential as well. The costs for these four people are approximately $50,000 per year, with an offsetting personnel cost of perhaps $30,000, making a net personnel cost of $20,000 per year.

Thus the total of amortization, maintenance, and net personnel cost would run between $45,000 and $60,000 per year, with about half of this for operating and maintenance personnel. In a department treating 1000 or more new patients per year, this runs at about $50.00 per patient, less in a larger department. If the increased effectiveness in patient care, teaching, and research is equivalent to adding just one extra staff member, this kind of system would pay for itself.

Our own costs have included the development of all the programs and hardware described here and in References 2 and 6 which required the efforts of an additional programmer and an engineer over three years, as well as a research fellow for one year. The latter helped structure the medical data. Considerable summer work by students has also been done. This investment of $100,000 would not need to be duplicated if other departments find our approaches useful. Our programs are available either for use as they stand or for the concepts they embody.

Conclusions and Discussion

The ideal computerized information system that would have the computer do all the work and make no demands on the persons using it is not yet in sight. The actual system described here requires that the users change their behavior. To the extent that they can learn to do so, the system rapidly becomes a tool which not only saves time but allows them to perform tasks that would be difficult or impossible to do without it. Because of the extent and diversity of specifically medical information, as compared to medical service delivery and administrative information, a great deal of programming and data-base building must be invested to obtain the potentially high payoffs in this area. We are at a stage where the current benefits of our system about equal the operating costs inclusive of a modest amortization of the equipment. Additional research and development is needed to decrease the cost/benefits ratio.

Because of the lack of experience in the use of such systems worldwide, the exploration of ideas and approaches other than our own is needed as well. In countries where medical service records *must* be kept in an elaborate, prescribed, structured manner as part and parcel of, for instance, a national insurance scheme, the "costs" of educating staff to perform the same procedures—while simultaneously capturing this information in a departmentally useful computer system—may be much reduced, thus easing the introduction of such systems.

Judging from our experience, the computerized information system has been workable with present-day technology. It has helped us improve our patient records by forcing us to think harder about the records and it has made a great deal of information about our patients and our department's efforts available which we simply could not get at before. If further work in progress is successful, we expect to make use of the developing capabilities to improve our teaching and our abilities to perform investigations for improved radiotherapy.

REFERENCES

1. P. W. Neurath, F. G. Bloedorn, J. E. Munzenrider, and M. G. Pedrazzi, "A Selective Patient Information System," *Cancer* 33, 1653 (1974).
2. R. E. Folland, P. W. Neurath, and W. H. Powell, "The Tufts-New England Medical Center Computer Based Tumor Registry," presented at The Fifth International Conference on Computers, Hanover, New Hampshire (August 1974).
3. "Systematized Nomenclature of Pathology," College of American Pathologists (1969).
4. "Manual of Tumor Nomenclature and Coding," American Cancer Society (1968).
5. End Results in Cancer, Report No. 4, L. M. Axtell, S. J. Cutler, and M. H. Myers, ed. U.S. Dept. of HEW, Pub. No. (NIH) 73-272 (1972).
6. P. W. Neurath and R. S. Seymour, "The Hardware and Software Used in the Automation of a Theratron 80 Cobalt Machine," presented at the Fifth International Conference on Computers, Hanover, New Hampshire (August 1974).

QUESTIONS

MANSFIELD: One of the weak points in all of this is the form that the physician (resident or staff person) has to fill out. What do you do about a form that is incomplete or a form that may have been incompletely filled out?

NEURATH: We have questions that must be answered. Other questions don't have to be answered at the time of entry. The computer summary is sent to the physician for signature, just as in a dictated note. Just as with a typed note, you are going to have to check it and approve it. Not everybody does, but in theory your signature indicates you have read it. All information is on disc file for a period of five years and can be edited at any time, so if you don't know something now you can enter it later and it will be recorded. I am not excluding physicists and other people from criticisms I made. They equally want the impossible from the computer.

FREY: It sounds as though your department is extremely dependent on this computer. What prevents your department from being paralyzed in the event of hardware failure?

NEURATH: The summaries are all on paper so nothing happens if the computer goes down. However, we like to keep the computer up all the time. We have only one computer, but many parts are duplicated, and our up-time is well over 98 percent.

4. Diversified Radiotherapy Department Computer Support

D. P. Ragan

Mallinckrodt Institute of Radiology has been involved in computer applications in radiation therapy for the past eight years. Our most successful endeavor was the development of the PC radiotherapy Treatment Planning System in conjunction with the Biomedical Computer Labs. A much less successful effort was the development of a Tumor Registry System on a conventional time-sharing system. Two and a half years ago a review of this system was launched; the following stems from the results of that review.

Rationale

The implementation of a tumor registry is anything but straightforward. It is difficult to justify in three particular ways: the cost and effort involved in maintaining even the most rudimentary lists of patients, site, and diagnosis; the lack of any immediate rewards from such a system; and a rather dismal performance record of past tumor registries.

It was felt that our tumor registry was very lacking in several respects. It was inconvenient and inflexible both in data accession and entry and in data retrieval. Even those questions the computer system could answer required a great deal of patience from the requesting staff member. And finally, despite this lack of capability, costs continued to soar. The acquisition of new data when added to the continued burden of system maintenance was impractical. In order to reduce the cost, to increase the system response, and to increase flexibility, the possibility of establishing our own in-house computer capability was considered.

It was apparent from the outset that the financial expense of a small mini-computer system for the purpose of the tumor registry alone could not be justified. Therefore other applications were sought which would require similar computer capability within the department. Many areas were found which could possibly benefit from computer assistance. These ranged from billing and scheduling to administrative summaries. All the possible applications had one thing in common, however: they were all marginal applications. An example of this is patient billing, which, although a straightforward application, is in most radiotherapy departments such a low-volume operation that automating the system results in a more costly overall system.

Sufficient applications were ultimately found to justify the anticipated cost of an in-house mini-computer system. Four factors were identified which would be specifically enhanced. It was felt that the credibility of computers had been severely damaged among personnel by the failure of previous computerized tumor registry efforts. Multiple applications would allow spreading the cost of a computer system and associated personnel over more functions. It was believed that the existence of an in-house computing facility would allow for the implementation of more speculative applications than might otherwise be attempted. And finally, the possibility of communication between applications within the department offered the promise of solving some redundant data acquisition problems and intergroup communications problems. An application which exemplifies these features is the field set-up calculation. This involves calculating the given dose or tumor dose from a physician's prescription. The four points involved are (1) *credibility* (field setup is a simple application used several times a day; it is always there and always works); (2) *cost* (the task could never be self-supporting, since it saves a negligible amount of personnel time and the added accuracy obtained is difficult to put a high price on); (3) *speculative* (although one implementation of a similar automatic calculator solution to this problem has been reported (1), it is hard to imagine a cost effective stand-alone solution); and (4) *communication* (most information needed for the tumor registry dosimetry section is effortlessly obtained by the daily operation of this routine by dosimetry staff).

System Functions

Two basic functions coupled with the tumor registry tasks form the basis of our initial system (2). The first of these must, of course, be billing, which in any modern American hospital is of some importance. The second application is patient scheduling. The computer hardware necessary to perform these basic functions could easily be expanded to perform more marginal ancillary functions. The data gathered in the process of scheduling and billing would enhance the accuracy and detail of our tumor registry data. For these purposes a four-user MUMPS PC system was purchased in January 1974. Within six months, billing and scheduling were implemented and the PC was being used as a remote terminal to the Washington University campus tumor registry data base. In the year that followed a significant number of additional functions have been implemented. These are detailed as follows:

I. Patient Flow
   a) Therapy Machine Schedules
   b) Doctors Schedules
   c) In Patient Dispatch Schedule
   d) Real Time Patient Queue

II. Records
   a) Active individual patient information retrieval
   b) Tumor Registry
   c) Chart Library System

III. Administration
   a) Automatic Generation of Patient Charges
   b) Administrative Summaries
   c) Bookkeeping and Financial Management

IV. Physics
   a) Therapy Machine Verification
   b) Chart Checking Scheduling
   c) Field Setup Calculation
   d) Physics Calibration Tables

V. General Aids
   a) Remote Terminal to IBM 360
   b) Table and Text Editing

The patient flow programs utilize the active patients' records, of which there are about two hundred at any one time. The primary source of current information for this file is the therapy machine schedules. Machine schedules, doctor schedules, in-patient dispatch schedules, lists of patients finished, charts due for dosimetry, lists of active patients, etc. are all selective sorts for different department functions and staff. The different schedules serve as worksheets for the personnel during a day's activities. At the end of the day files are edited and new schedules are produced in a batch file operation. With the acquisition of dedicated terminals for the therapy machine technicians, the batch file operation will be phased out.

Augmenting the hard-copy therapy machine schedule is a real-time patient queue. This consists of TV monitors scattered throughout the department which are driven by a centralized character generator. It operates in much the same fashion as flight information monitors at airports. Patients are entered by the receptionist or nursing personnel. This provides a time-ordered queue of patients sorted by therapy machine. It is available for patient review so that they can be sure they are not being forgotten and is available for review by the physicians so that they can see if any of their patients are presently being treated.

The execution of the daily scheduling and patient-flow functions provides a large data base that is available for inquiry. Additional data such as tumor registry information are added to these basic data to provide a complete patient profile. Somewhat simpler but in the same area of record-keeping is a chart library system to keep track of the parallel paper chart system.

A large amount of data of administrative importance is accumulated in the process of daily scheduling. These data are collected and printed out daily, weekly, and yearly in a variety of administrative summaries. In addition, the patient's daily charges are automatically computed from the therapy machine schedules. This provides both a savings in personnel time and a decrease in lost charges.

As a totally separate administrative function, the system also keeps a complete financial accounting system. All financial transactions, both clinical and grant supported, are entered. Budgeted amount, encumbrances, and actual cash outlays are recorded. Periodic summaries are generated for individual requisitions, for groups by class/department, and for current grant status. This portion of the system is relied upon to keep track of approximately two million dollars worth of transactions each year.

The physics group is another important user of the system. Chart checking, which must be done on a ten-day schedule, is automatically queued and monitored by the therapy machine scheduling modules. Dosimetry is given a list of charts to be checked, and the patients are flagged on the therapy machine schedules. In addition, the computer terminal is available to the dosimetry section for field setup and calculation. Information entered in order to calculate the tumor dose, for instance, is contributed to the tumor registry system.

In addition, ancillary physics tasks are performed. Calibration charts for Cobalt 60 therapy machines at outlying hospitals are automatically generated from empirical data. This saves large amounts of personnel time and improves accuracy. There is also a therapy machine verification system for our Clinac 35 currently being built which will operate at the MUMPS language level.

Miscellaneous general aids are also provided by the computer system. The computer is available as a remote batch terminal to the campus IBM 360 during those times when the MUMPS system itself is not up. It is hoped that eventually consult notes will be typed on the computer system, simulating the IBM MTST system.

Several functions are purposely not performed on our information processing system. These include treatment planning, biological modeling, and development of "heavy" physics applications. The rationale for this approach is that, first, there now exists sufficient application to justify a small information-processing computer system, and, second, that a system designed for information processing is most efficiently used for that purpose and not to be stretched to other applications. Another application considered and rejected was a reprint library system similar to MEDLINE. It was felt that this particular application required a large amount of data entry with minimal returns, and would duplicate commercially available time-sharing systems.

Systems Description

The system chosen to perform these functions was an in-house mini-computer MUMPS system. It had the advantage of low cost, sophisticated string-handling capabilities, multi-terminal capabilities, and moderate terminal response. The major criticism leveled against MUMPS was its ability to respond within less than a second for menu-style question and answer routines. Since rapid interaction with physicians was not a primary concern, this was not considered a severe handicap.

A PC (Program Console) manufactured by Artronix (at the time developmental) was selected for hardware. The choice was made for the following reasons: (1) the system was, and is, the least expensive MUMPS system commercially available; (2) it was felt that we could influence the direction in which implementation would proceed on the MUMPS PC system; (3) since the PC was already the most commonly exploited computer in the radiotherapy world, cost advantages to small departments capable of doing treatment-planning in the morning and information-system processing in the afternoon made development on the PC attractive; and (4) if information processing did not prove as valuable for the PC as originally hoped, the system could be converted, at small loss, to treatment-planning. All except the last are still convincing reasons to proceed with MUMPS PC development.

Currently we are operating a six-user 32K core PC 12/7 MUMPS system. Applications worked thus far have been extremely promising, and shortly this current arrangement will be expanded into a 48K system with multiple small partitions, or effectively sixteen to twenty users. It must be pointed out that of these twenty most are what could be classified as constant but infrequent users. That is, small amounts of data are entered periodically throughout the day, causing a minimal load on the system and therefore minimal degradation from the large number of users.

At present fourteen terminals are in use. An increase is expected concurrent with the increase in available partitions. It is interesting to note that at St. John's Hospital a single terminal connected to the Mallinckrodt system provides all of the scheduling and tumor registry functions for an entire hospital therapy department. The cost of this "whole department system" is between $300 and $500 per month depending on how many extras are included in the costing.

Cost Justification

Realistic cost justification for a system like this is extremely difficult. The cost of a six-user system with six terminals, tapes, disks, etc. comes to approximately $75,000. The annual cost amortized over five years, plus software and hardware service contract, plus one $10,000 a year salaried programmer comes to about $30,000 per year. If five production terminals are assumed, that yields about $500 per month, per terminal.

If this is calculated on a per-patient basis, the following rough figures are generated: For the patient flow and information system approximately three terminals are required at $18,000 per year. For 2,000 new patients per year this results in $9.00 per patient. Maintenance of the tumor registry requires approximately two terminals or about $12,000 per year. Again, for 2,000 new patients per year this is $6.00 per patient or, if we include all patients in the data base (which is over 10,000 patients), $1.00 per patient per year.

The principal problem in cost justification involves the evaluation of the cost of services performed. It is felt that the savings in personnel time for billing and scheduling plus the improved accuracy of billing (approximately $3,000 per month in saved billing charges) is sufficient justification for the costs involved. The additional functions (patient queue, tumor registry, financial management system, letter writing system, etc.) certainly add to the cost effectiveness of the system.

System Acceptance

Acceptance among the medical and paramedical staff has been remarkably positive. There was an initial period of overexpectation and a second period of disillusionment. Currently we are in a reevaluation period and constructive change. A primary objective—enhancing the credibility of computer operations within the therapy department—has been accomplished very effectively. A recent meeting of medical staff to discuss problems of general clinical operation identified no problems with presently implemented computer systems but generated interest among the medical staff for new areas of computer assistance (as the charting of patient progress through the course of treatment). Acceptance of systems among the paramedical personnel was mixed but generally favorable after a reasonable break-in period.

Future Plans

It is felt that this work as well as the similar work of Neurath (3) demonstrates the value of a small in-house MUMPS system for medium to large-size radiotherapy departments. Small departments that cannot rationalize the cost of either the treatment-planning system or an information-handling system may be able to afford a PC system capable of working half time at each task. A six-user system with similar software can be effectively utilized in a production environment (rather than a research environment) in both of the above instances.

Like most academic institutions, however, we cannot leave well enough alone. As mentioned previously, there are plans to expand the existing hardware system to provide soft-copy therapy machine schedules that will eliminate the need for most therapy technician interaction with the patient's paper chart. The use of the computer for medical transcription and preparation of scientific papers provides a far more versatile and less costly system than an IBM MTST system. Automated submission of insurance for patients as well as numerous small administrative functions need to be incorporated. The computer-assisted follow-up protocols will be established. And finally, the tumor registry efforts, which were our main reason for existence, will be expanded and improved wherever possible.

It is believed that the improved performance of modern hardware-software combinations such as MUMPS-PC provide a unique opportunity for radiation therapy departments. A great deal can be contributed to the delivery of health care through the use of information systems to provide scheduling communications and quality control functions. Institutions active in the development of such software can best serve the radiotherapy community by developing systems of sufficient value to be picked up and marketed by firms such as Artronix, Varian, and Meditech.

REFERENCES

1. Fitzgerald, Mauderli, and Schulman, "CO^{60} Dosimetry With a Desk Top Calculator," *Radiology* 110, 677 (March 1974).
2. F. Domke, F. A. Jones, W. E. Powers, and D. Ragan, "A Radiation Therapy Department Information System," Proceedings of the 1973 MUMPS Users' Group Meeting (1973).
3. P. W. Neurath, F. G. Bloedorn, J. E. Munzenrider, and M. G. Pedrazzi, "A Selective Patient Information System," *Cancer* (to be published).

Session IIa: Contributed Short Papers on Specific Aspects of Information Systems

1. Computer-Based Patient Record and Follow-Up System for Radiotherapy

T. R. Moller
J. E. Johnsson
A. Sundstrom
T. Gustafsson

1. Introduction

We started in 1967 with a system in which medical and physical information was collected on specifically designed forms and punched on paper tape. We soon found this system too rigid and time-consuming and therefore started to develop a more direct data-collection technique.

Our philosophy in developing the present computerized information system at our department has been to integrate all pertinent information on diagnosis and the different types of treatment as well as long-term follow-up data in the registers, enabling retrieval and statistical analysis of the parameters.

2.1 Data Collection

The system of data acquisition should fulfill the following requirements:

(a) the existing medical record should be preserved;
(b) the results of different investigations as well as progress notes should be entered in the record;
(c) double registration should be avoided;
(d) information should be given in plain language, and coding should be kept to a minimum;
(e) information should be collected as close to its site of origin as possible, i.e. unnecessary data transfer between different media should be avoided.

Medical information is entered in the record according to the doctor's dictation. The dictation must have a special structure—giving the exact headlines and sub-headlines to be used and following a certain order. Only the appropriate information may be given under each heading, in special cases as a choice between given alternative expressions in plain language. The secretary types the dictation on a magnetic-tape encoder, IBM MT72, which is an IBM Selectric typewriter equipped with two tape cassettes. On one tape, called the "master" tape, all headings and sub-headings as well as certain expressions to be used are stored. These are divided into logical subgroups, each describing a special piece of information, for example operation-narrative, description of microscopic biopsy examination, etc. There are altogether about thirty different subgroups, which can be selected in arbitrary order by means of a rotation-knob (a push-button selector would have been preferable). The doctor's dictation should correspond to the master tape; for each new heading the secretary pushes the start button on the MT72, and the appropriate word is typed out in the correct position. Then, the secretary has only to enter the dictated text and, when this is finished, proceed to the next heading.

As the record in this way is typed on the paper, all information is simultaneously recorded on the second tape cassette, called the "slave" tape. Every time the secretary pushes the start button, the heading is not only typed out but also transferred to the slave tape, together with an internal code number, identifying the item. On the hard copy the automatically written headings are in black and the variable text typed by the secretary appears blue if it is accepted for recording on the slave tape by the hardware checks.

The cassette-tapes are then converted to standard 9-track half-inch computer-compatible tape in an IBM 2495. This file forms the input to a special program, which decodes the information and generates transactions, which update the main register. Data punched on cards or paper tape can be fed directly to this program.

2.2 Main Registers

The main register is sequentially organized in variable-length format. Record-linking is based on the ten-digit census or civic registration number, which unambiguously identifies every Swedish citizen.

Since the register contains information on more than 10,000 patients, the search for and sorting of information may be rather time-consuming. Therefore, a special register containing some often-used variables in fixed format is generated. This register, stored on disk, is frequently used for statistical purposes. In addition, an up-to-date list of patients is produced for administrative use.

2.3 Direct-Access Routine

To facilitate corrections in the main register, the decoded information is transferred from the sequential files to a disk file in a form suitable for direct-access purposes. An alphanumerical CRT display operates on this file. Search for a specific record can be performed on the ten-digit census number or fourteen characters of the name of the patient. The record is displayed on the screen, one line for each decoded information. The commands that can be executed include entering of new data, exchange of incorrect data, and deletion of data and even the record as a whole. The corrections are accumulated in a special file that updates the main register at certain intervals. The same data can thus be corrected several times during this time interval.

Programs enabling generation of specific statistics directly from the VDU are presently under development.

2.4 Follow-up Routine

Most of our patients will be followed by personal check-ups in the outpatient department of our clinic. After five years of recurrence-free observation, some of the patients are followed by a mailing routine. At predetermined intervals, a questionnaire is printed out and sent to the patient. It is printed on a Data-mailer, and the contents of the questionnaire depend on the diagnosis. Similar forms may also be sent to other clinics or institutions, and to the registrar's office in the area the patient resides in.

Upon reception of the answers from the patients, the answers are sorted in two categories: one free of symptoms and one with new symptoms. Patients belonging to the latter category will usually be called for a personal check-up. This routine will include about 6,000 patient records.

2.5 Documentation of External Beam Therapy

A special program has been developed for documentation of external beam therapy. For this purpose a special record form has been designed. After completion of treatment, certain variables are punched on cards directly from this record form. These variables include a description of target volume, critical organs, and absorbed dose to different parts of the target volume. Field data, such as quality of radiation, peak absorbed dose, filters, patient-positioning, and beam geometry as well as dose-planning data are also recorded. For each patient, a treatment report is printed out and this is included in the patient's case notes (1).

This system (BEKO) forms a link between the record system

(RUFS) and the treatment-planning system (DIDOS) (2, 3), and data may be exchanged between the systems. Thus it is possible to obtain very detailed information on external treatment of a specific patient as well as, for example, survival time of a group of patients treated with the same technique.

3. Operational Characteristics

The system is run on a UNIVAC 1108. Updating of the register is done in batch mode, usually every second week. At each updating, a new statistical file is generated, as well as a new register in demand mode for direct access. Various types of listings can be done on request.

From a remote terminal—UNIVAC 9200/II, located at the clinic—various statistical programs and listings can be executed. Corrections are entered via the UNISCOPE 100 or on the MT72 by the secretaries.

The follow-up routine is run once or twice a month.

4. Concluding Remarks

The main objectives in designing the present system have been:

(a) to create an up-to-date patient register for administrative use;
(b) to automate the follow-up mailing routine;
(c) to generate print-outs of different types of reports;
(d) to keep a constant surveillance on cure rate, morbidity, and mortality of different groups of patients;
(e) to set up an integrated data base with easy access to facilitate special statistics.

Since the start of the project, most of these goals have been achieved. At present the system is running smoothly and giving valuable information. The integration of medical, physical, and technical data has proven to be of importance in evaluation of various treatment techniques.

The system is also intended to form the base of a future regional cancer registry.

One of the main obstacles has been the MT72. The price for rental ($5,000 per year) is too high to allow the number of machines needed, and therefore we are searching for a substitute. We hope to be able to exchange this equipment in the near future.

cathode ray tube (CRT) terminals were used to record the events; one was placed inside the treatment room and the other outside. The list displayed on the CRTs, comprised fourteen time events, an entry to a mode to enter patient data, and a command to switch control to the other terminal. Each of these events or selections on the list had a specific keyboard key associated with it. For example, the number 2 key indicated that the technologist entered the treatment room. The observer followed the technologist, monitored the technologist's and patient's actions, and recorded these events by making single-key selections on the CRT keyboard. The computer in turn recorded these event codes along with the time and any other important parameters. When the technologist and observer left or entered the treatment room, a single key depressure allowed the observer to transfer control to the other terminal. With just one terminal being active or ready to accept entries at a time, the possibility of extraneous entries was greatly reduced.

A second computer program was running simultaneously with the program that serviced the CRTs. The second program continuously monitored the linear accelerator's motor controllers and the beam-on condition. At the completion of any movement the program recorded the time the movement started, the time the movement stopped, and the positions of all eight axes of movement at the completion of movement. After the treatment beam had been turned off, the second program recorded the times the treatment beam was turned on and off, plus the total dose delivered as determined by the linear accelerator control-console dose meter. This data collected by the second program was merged automatically and instantaneously with the data collected by the observer with the first program.

Events

The fourteen event times recorded are listed below:

(1) *Technologist starts preparation.* This signifies the first action the technician takes in the treatment of a patient, locating the patient chart or checking for the next name on the treatment schedule.

(2) *Technologist enters treatment.*

(3) *Patient enters treatment room.*

(4) *Patient undresses.*

(5) *Patient positioned on treatment couch.* This does not include the time to install any accessories, just the time to get the proper position on the treatment stretcher.

(6) *Skin marks refurbished.*

(7) *Accessories in position.* This marks the point in time when all of the treatment accessories have been correctly installed and

positioned for treatment. This would include such devices as blocks, regular and shaped; bolus; methane molds; litecast; wedges; etc.

(8) *Port film.* Normally the observer would make this entry at the beginning and end of the port sequence, thereby identifying that block of time required for the procedure.

(9) *Technologist exits from treatment room.*

(10) *Treatment accessories disassembled.*

(11) *Patient off treatment stretcher.*

(12) *Patient dresses.*

(13) *Patient exits from treatment room.*

(14) *Technologist finished.* This implies that the technologist has finished with all the related activites for a given patient.

The above list of events are merely *recorded* as they are entered by the computer. The *separation* and *analysis* is done later. In the case of a patient's treatment which entails several ports, there could possibly be two sets of accessory times, and positively two sets of technician entry or exits and treatment times, since the technician would enter the room after treating the first port, in order to set up and treat the second. It is also possible, and sometimes common, to have an *overlap* between a new patient entering and an old patient exiting—that is, a period of time when the next patient enters the treatment room before the exit of the old or last patient treated. With the current programs, these events are recorded as they happen and the analysis done later.

The *patient identification mode* is entered by selecting the appropriate key when all sixteen choices (the fourteen time events, I.D. modes, and terminal transfer as previously discussed) are displayed. As an aid in analysis, the following information items are entered for each patient:

(1) *Patient hospital identification number*

(2) *Patient mobility status*

  (a) *Ambulatory*

  (b) *Slow*

  (c) *Stretcher*

  (d) *Wheelchair*

(3) *Number of fields.* This is the number of fields or portals to be treated during this period.

(4) *Treatment site.* A list of common treatment sites is presented alphabetically with its associated Standard Nomenclature of Pathology (SNOP) code, and the observer makes the appropriate selection.

(5) *Treatment immobilization device*

  (a) None

  (b) Litecast only

(c) Urethane mold only
(d) Litecast and urethane mold

The above series of questions is presented on the CRT after the observer selects the patient identification keyboard key. This information can be entered at any time, but normally it is entered during the "beam on" time for the convenience of the observer.

Programming and File Handling

The programming for the data collection consists of two FORTRAN programs running under VORTEX (Varian's real-time, multi-tasking operating system). This operating system allows both the FORTRAN observer's program and FORTRAN automatic "movement" and "beam-on" surveillance program to be run simultaneously. These two programs are totally independent in their data collection but share the same disc file for the recording of the collected data. A third program is used to read the disc file created by the first two programs, reorganize the data, and write it out on 9-track IBM compatible tape. The data are reorganized into single patient blocks, with the patient identification coming first, followed by the sequence of times and events codes. An overlap code is added to the patient identification information, signaling if a patient exit-entrance overlap has occurred. Also certain general information is added to the patient record, such as the date the data were collected, the number of technologists, and their initials. In this way, each patient record is a complete entry, with all the pertinent data included. Patients with overlaps will have all their transactions or events recorded plus the other patient's entrance and/or exit event. By this means, total information for that treatment can be obtained.

Hardware

The equipment used in this study was a Varian 620/f computer operation under VORTEX (Varian's real-time, multi-tasking operating system). The specific computer peripherals used were two CRT terminals to collect data, one outside the treatment room and one inside. A data disc for temporary storage of data and a 9-track IBM compatible magnetic tape were also available. The magnetic tape provided the means of storing a large data base in a form that is a suitable vehicle for analysis of the data on a larger computer system—namely the hospital's IBM 360-50 computer system.

Data Collection Conditions

The data were collected on 17 randomly chosen days over a period of 59 days. The total observation time was 38 hours 35 minutes, and the observations were generally made in the morning between 8:00 and 11:00 A.M., which represents the peak in the treatment load. The treatment equipment normally delivers a dose rate of 200 rads to a point 1.2 cm depth at 80 SSD for a 10 × 10 field.

These treatments were normally administered by a staff radiation technologist aided by a radiation technologist student.

The study encompassed 176 patients who were treated with 362 treatment fields or ports; no rotational or moving field techniques were employed.

Results

The data were divided into a number of different ways to evaluate different categories of patients.

Since one reason for collecting the data was to provide a datum point for the effect of automatic or computer-controlled treatment-equipment setup, several motor-on and related times were collected and tabulated. The "motor move time" represents the total time that one or more of the 8 axial-drive motors was turned on. The "time between motor movements" represents the summation of times between the first "motor-on" period and the last "motor-off" period in which no motor was energized. This time could represent time in which the technologist was making a decision as to which axis to move next.

The "beam-on time"category is self-explanatory. The "technician and patient in/out time" represents the total time it takes to enter and exit the room. The "accessory time" is the time devoted to positioning blocks, compensators, bolus, etc. "Miscellaneous time" includes all other times: patient getting off the treatment unit, patient dressing, port film time, etc.

Any category with fewer than five cases was left out as not having sufficient data to be significant.

When we analyzed the data, we found that the similarities in times were more noticeable than the differences—specifically, the time difference in treating with two ports per treatment instead of one, and the lack of difference in time between treating a slow ambulatory patient and a patient in a wheelchair or on a stretcher.

3. Scheduling in External Beam Radiotherapy

H. Dahlin
B. Jung
P. O. Karlsson
A. M. Thelin

Introduction

It was more than a decade after the introduction of computers into radiotherapy before it was recognized that to take full advantage of the gains offered by the computer, its use must be integrated with the ordinary working procedures of the department. Ease of communication between users and the computer must be emphasized in all phases of the clinical work, and any duplication should be avoided.

At the beginning, the use of the computers in radiotherapy was mostly concerned with the calculation of dose plans. Results from these first attempts were good but did not solve any new problems in treatment strategy or clinical organization. Their efforts were not in that direction. Physicists, radiotherapists, and computer specialists all over the world repeated the same development for over ten years, and new dose-calculating programs are still being initiated.

Fortunately, because of the difficult economic situation during the last few years, we are forced to convince politicians and hospital administrators of the usefulness of each step taken with computers in radiotherapy. The tasks that a computer system should be able to handle can be summarized as follows:

Administration

- Listing of referrals
- Waiting lists
- Summons
- Bookings
- Patient identification and registration
- Retrieval of earlier information about the patient
- Billing

Clinical Examination and Tests
- Storage of patient-record information
- Codification of tumor type and spread
- Tests (bacteriological, chemical, cytological etc.)

Treatment Planning
- Registration of patient outline, tumor location and spread, and necessary anatomic details
- Radiation-beam parameters
- Computation of dose distributions in two or three dimensions
- Selection of best dose distribution
- Treatment time schedule

Treatment
- Patient setting-up
- Verification of set-up
- Registration of treatment data
- Treatment checks
- Updating

Follow Up
- Treatment summary
- Updating of patient state
- Summons for follow-up examinations
- Scientific evaluation of results

It can be seen that the computation of dose-plans is only a small fraction of all problems that must be solved by the computer.

In treatment planning there is one part that is of importance to the irradiation of the patients, the "Treatment time schedules." When a patient is going to be treated with external beam radiotherapy, a dose plan and information about how to deliver the dose in time must be available. There are two basic sources of information, the physicians' prescription and the simulator data.

For several years an automatic system for record-keeping in external-beam radiotherapy has been running in Uppsala. This system is one of many in radiotherapy and radiophysics at the Academic Hospital in Uppsala.

The program schedules the whole treatment series for each patient. The printout simulates the manual records and lists the dates of treatment and the corresponding field numbers, reference doses, accumulated maximum, minimum, and mean doses in the target area as well as in critical organs. The program takes Saturdays, Sundays, and holidays into account and allows for automatic contraction of the treatment series if the preliminary schedule would end immediately after a long holiday (Christmas, Easter, etc.). In case of changes in the schedule due to radiation equipment failure, the patient's absence from a scheduled treatment, or altered weekly or total-dose prescriptions, the program will automatically update the already performed treatments and print out a new list according to the new criterion.

For each day a "treatment apparatus list" is printed out, which informs the staff which patients are going to be treated, the specific day, and on which equipment. Another useful feature of the program is a daily printed patient-status list, which makes it possible for the radiotherapists to obtain a quick overview of the patient population each day.

Some data needed for the program are entered via a keyboard in the form of a dialogue, and others automatically from the dose-plan files and follow-up registers.

The radiotherapy computer applications are performed on a PDP-11 computer linked to an IBM 370/155 at the Uppsala University Datacenter. To make up these schedules, data are transmitted via a 1200 baud dial-up telephone line to the central computer, and results retransmitted to the local computer. The terminal is operated by hospital personnel; for the treatment scheduling any of the technicians enter the data.

When developing this system, the clinical staff was strongly involved. That made it possible to have a program work in the clinical routine, immediately after the debugging procedures. The contact with the clinical staff, including not only physicists and radiotherapists but also therapy technicians and nurses, was very instructive.

No computerized medical system can run clinically if the staff concerned is not convinced of and well informed about the system. Therefore, it is very important that the development be gradual and as far as possible based on the manual routines in use.

Because of this strategy we are now putting new criteria into the systems, particularly the radiobiological part, such as CRE, NSD, SHMT, etc. The advantages of such a complete system can be summarized as follows:

1. Individualized treatment schedule for the whole prescribed treatment series is prepared in advance.
2. Duplicates of individual treatment schedules are available at treatment machines and conference rooms, and updated daily.
3. Duplicates of treatment lists are at machines, conference rooms, and dose-planning desks, and updated daily.
4. Treatment delivery is optimized with respect to fractionation effects and rest periods, weekends, holidays, and scheduled equipment shut-downs.
5. The use of patient wards is optimized.
6. Treatment schedules are updated automatically after equipment failure or patients' absence from treatment.
7. The automatic transfer of basic data information for check-and-confirm interlock systems is possible.

4. The Radiation Therapy System at Sahlgrenska Sjukhuset in Goteborg

B. Lindskoug
K-A. Johansson
G. Notter
I. Ragnhult
L. Fridh

At the Fourth International Conference on the Use of Computers in Radiation Therapy (1) we learned that high priority should be given to 2-D multiplanar dose-distribution calculations. The system planned at our department is meant to facilitate the transfer of the primary anatomical patient data to the computer by using automated equipment on line with a mini-computer. Our goal is to make the procedures involved so simple and the access time for primary data so short that multiplanar calculations may be a realistic possibility.

Some of the radiotherapy procedures for which a mini-computer can be useful are demonstrated in Fig. 1. Arrows indicate the direction of information flow.

Dose Planning, Radplan

The mini-computer (PDP8/E) is part of a system (RADPLAN) dedicated for dose-planning in 2-D. The software is based on the Royal Marsden Hospital system, a program package written by Bentley and Milan (2). The program has been modified to take account of tissue heterogeneities (3). At the moment 90 percent of all plans are made using the RADPLAN system.

Patient Outlines, Scope

A 2-D multiplanar presentation of dose distribution calculations requires a number of correct transversal contours of the patient. We intend to use the instrument developed at the Newcastle General Hospital by David Thompson (4), the so-called SCOPE (Surface Contour Optical Projection Equipment). This system uses a laser beam to produce a thin sheet of light which will define the plane of cross-section through the patient. By viewing this illuminated contour from either side as well as from above the patient, using wide-angle lenses on two TV cameras, it is possible to view up to 270 degrees around the patient. Even deeply concave parts such as the neck will be covered. The SCOPE framework will be mounted over a table, so that the whole system can be moved along the body axis of the patient. The TV cameras will be on line with the computer, which enables a full contour of one transversal section of the patient to be transferred into the core within 0.2 seconds. Even if one outline is taken at every second centimeter along a 20-centimeter field, the total time will be only a few minutes, most of which will be used in positioning the patient.

The outlines of the patient will also be used for calculation of missing tissue compensators. The results of the calculation will be written out in a table indicating the thickness of material needed to compensate for missing tissue and the correction of the monitor factor.

In the computer room the necessary contours can be recalled and plotted out in life size by an x-y plotter. All the recorded reference marks will also be plotted.

Internal Topography

For required information on the internal topography of a whole body, an automatic—computerized—tomographic scanner such as the ACTA scanner (5) would be most useful, particularly if the scanner could be used in combination with the SCOPE. The contours and the tomographic scans could thus be made during the same patient set-up. The number of complete tomographic scans needed will depend on the region to be treated and the actual case.

Treatment Scheduling

We also intend to use the minicomputer for treatment scheduling. Various types of fractionation regimes are used at the clinic and will be handled. When the fractionation regime and the CRE-value have been prescribed (CRE = Cumulated Radiation Effect), the program will list the schedule for the entire treatment period—that is, the dates on which the patient will come for treatment (with holidays excluded), the absorbed dose to be given to the tumor at each treatment session, and the resulting CRE values at the end of each week. Instead of making a total dose prescription, the CRE concept is, in fact, used already in the first prescription in order to guarantee a biological-equivalent total dose. As soon as the prescribed CRE value has been reached, the treatments will be stopped. The same program will also include the option for changing or updating a schedule (that is, if the patient cannot come for treatment during one week), in which case the program will write a new schedule and calculate the corresponding new CRE value considering the unintentional pause in the treatment session.

Verification of Dose Plans

Computer calculation of dose plans will be used extensively in the future, but the risks involved in this procedure are obvious. The primary information of patient anatomy, target volume, and primary field data stored in memory, as well as the algorithms used in the software, will all be accepted in routine work without questioning the limits of validity of the resulting output from the computer. The primary information may be used for detailed calculation, and the results acknowledged as being of higher precision than they really are.

The verification will be made in three steps in our laboratory:

1. *In anatomical phantom.* In case of new treatment techniques, the dose plans are first verified in an anatomical phantom by using an automated TLD system.
2. *In vivo measurements.* The same TLD system can be used for in vivo measurements in vessels or other body cavities during radiotherapy.
3. *Routine dose checks during radiotherapy.* In each day's work, checks are made on all patients several times during the treatment sessions. The given absorbed dose is routinely checked by means of semiconductors hanging down in coils from the ceiling. These are easily applied on the patient's skin at the entrance point and the exit side. This will give a check of the dose actually delivered, including all steps in the treatment procedures.

The semiconductors will be checked in the two ways expected to give consistent results:

(a) by comparing the semiconductor reading on the surface of a phantom with the reading of a substandard ionization chamber inside the phantom at the reference depth for different field sizes.

(b) by noting the reading at the first treatment occasion for a particular patient when a physician and a physicist are present.

Ordinary field checks are also made for shaped fields, head and neck treatments, etc. by means of direct film exposure during the treatment.

More rare but very important are the TLD checks in vivo. An automated TLD system is used. The dosimeters are permanently enclosed in teflon tubes that can be introduced into body cavities or into holes two millimeters in diameter in an Alderson phantom. The dosimeters are individually calibrated by means of a standard irradiation in which the tubes pass through a radioactive source. This standard irradiation is performed in less than two minutes for a dose of 100 rads given to 100 dosimeters. The read-out data and the calibration constants are punched on paper tape. The system may also be on line with the computer.

In vivo checks of dose distributions are common in the Scandinavian countries. Experiences indicate that such checks should be recommended. In short it may be stated that the more we computerize, the greater the need to verify the computations. The correct answer to the question whether our dose calcuations are correct will only be found inside the patient himself.

Patient Flow and Records

No decision concerning a system to be used for patient records has yet been made. We hope that a national, possibly international, system will be agreed upon.

Final Remarks

A minicomputer system can be useful for many purposes at rather small cost.

Two unique systems exist today and will transfer primary patient data on line to the computer—namely the SCOPE, for the out-lines of the patients, and the ACTA or EMI scanners, for the inner topography. Both systems are extensively automated and will give rational procedures.

Frequent checks and verifications of the calculated dose plans are necessary and may be made in vivo using a semiconductor system or an automated TLD reader with computer adapted output.

We are restrictive concerning automation of treatment and computer control of treatment parameters. The history of radiotherapy includes a series of mistakes, accidents, and narrow escapes of which many have occurred recently. Before we go into complexity and sophistication like 3-D dose planning and treatment automation, we must be sure that our present technique is safe for both patients and personnel. Our striving during the last two years has been for simplicity and safety in methods and procedures, rather than complexity and sophistication.

REFERENCES

1. Proceedings, Fourth International Conference on the Use of Computers in Radiation Therapy, Uppsala, Sweden, August 7-11 (1972).
2. R. E. Bentley and J. Milan, "An interactive digital computer system for radiotherapy treatment planning," Brit. J. Radiol., 44, 826 (1971).
3. J. Milan and R. E. Bentley, "The storage and manipulation of radiation dose data in a small computer," Brit. J. Radiol., 47, 115 (1974).
4. D. J. Thompson, "Recording surface outlines of body cross sections by a PDP 8.I computer linked to television cameras," Digest of the Third International Conference on Medical Physics, including medical engineering, Goteborg, Sweden, Chalmers University of Technology (1972).
5. R. S. Ledley, G. DiChiro, A. J. Luessenhop, and H. L. Twigg, "Computerized Transaxial X-Ray Tomography of the Human Body," Science, 186, 207 (1974).

FIG. 1.

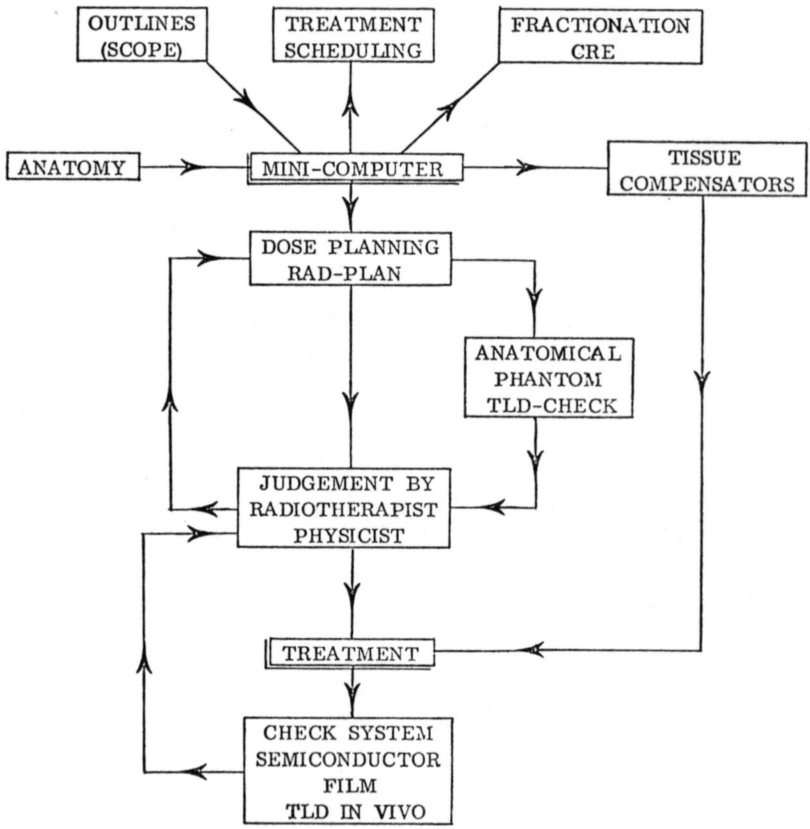
OUTLINES
(SCOPE)
TREATMENT
SCHEDULING
FRACTIONATION
CRE
ANATOMY
MINI-COMPUTER
TISSUE
COMPENSATORS
DOSE PLANNING
RAD-PLAN
ANATOMICAL
PHANTOM
TLD-CHECK
JUDGEMENT BY
RADIOTHERAPIST
PHYSICIST
TREATMENT
CHECK SYSTEM
SEMICONDUCTOR
FILM
TLD IN VIVO

Session IIb: Panel Discussion. "Should a radiotherapy department have a computer information system, and if so, what are the options?"

Chairperson	*Panelists*
J. W. Johnson	J. Cederlund
	F. W. George, III
	A. S. Glicksman
	N. Suntharalingam

JOHNSON: We've seen a number of systems this morning. The great preponderance of them seem to be small, dedicated computers with multiple functions. I think that one of the things that was left out in these discussions was the need for getting this type of technology out into the community hospitals. The type of funding support and the type of technology required to develop these systems necessarily has to develop at a major center. But I also think we have to move towards going out and dealing with the problems of the small institutions; and it is going to be the responsibility of the bigger centers to go out and look at the problems of the small hospital.

I think also in making decisions about what type of system of hardware and software we should recommend for developing centers, we must take into account the fact that each institution is of a specific type—that is, an institution involved in education, training, and research, or an institution involved in serving the community. These differences have to be considered in making decisions about the type of system that you really want to use. A small hospital may not want to have a computer system at its location; it may not want to have to support the programming staff and technical staff required. Therefore, they have to go out and seek this type of computer support either in the private sector or in larger institutions.

GLICKSMAN: I'd like to ask a series of questions. Does every department need every aspect of what computers can do in a Radiotherapy Department? Maybe we ought to enumerate the ground rules. There is traditional treatment planning which has been well done and exploited over the last decade. In addition, we can now integrate the simulator and the computer to get a more instant isodose situation, and feed the prescription out to a system for treatment verification.

The second area would be in daily scheduling, the traffic flow. The administration is to pay for all of this including the billing. Then the patient becomes a statistic, either on treatment or later for the tumor registry. The radiotherapy record is not the tumor registry and the tumor registry is not necessarily the total patient record. We have three areas which have to be distinguished.

And, finally there is the area of radiobiology and biophysics for the implementation of further advances.

With that in mind, does every department need every aspect of these computer supports? I think that one would obviously see that the answer to that is *no*. There are some departments that may want to do this as a research area. There may be some that will find it an advantage economically. But most departments in the United States do not treat 2,000 patients a year. Most departments do not treat a thousand patients a year. If you are getting one new patient a day, that amounts to five patients a week or approximately 250 patients a year. Until you reach 500 patients per year, you do not need a computer to do the treatment verification—you need a good technician. You need good radiotherapists who are concerned with the patient's care. That's where the investment should be, rather than thinking that you have to have all the toys with which the bigger departments are playing.

Another question to which the panelists might want to address themselves is: Does computer assistance improve the kind of treatment delivered? Does computer assistance improve the treatment delivery? The final corollary to that question is: What difference does it make to the patient five years hence? What's the payoff to the patient? Does the patient have a better chance of being cured because of all this?

GEORGE: The kind of arrangement I would like to have is a computer-assisted integrated radiotherapy department, where all of the functions are integrated into a so-called synectic system, which refers to a system in which the whole is much greater than the sum of its parts. An example of such a system is one that permits the accomplishment of functions which could not be accomplished by separate stand-alone programs.

You will recall that at Uppsala most of the discussions and presentations at the time were on stand-alone applications programs in the area of machine-controlled tumor registries and treatment-planning. I was impressed by the presentations this morning in which the emphasis was on the integration of many functions using a multi-tasking, multi-terminal, multi-user, more or less time-sharing system to integrate all the equipment, all the facilities, and all the functions of the department into a whole.

I was interested that Arvin Glicksman took the position then that all departments should not have a comprehensive system. He feels that they should not all have a system that has every function. My position is that yes, even a small department does need such a system. My reasons are that such a system is particularly important in a small department—the impact on the necessity of scheduling, optimal utilization, or cost effectiveness of facilities can be accomplished only by comprehensive systems where you know you can integrate the doctor's time with the clinic nurse's time with the machine's time, the time available on the simulator, etc.

In closing, I would point out that I am spending a year at the National Cancer Institute, and I feel that a very high priority area is computer development in radiotherapy. We do now have a line item in the budget for radiotherapy development. It is very important that those interested in computerized radiotherapy develop a strategic and operational plan for the development of computerization in radiotherapy, and hopefully that will be an outcome of this conference.

SUNTHARALINGAM: I resolve to give comments pertaining to the feasibility of computerized information systems from the viewpoint of a clinical radiological physicist. I come from a medium-sized department, not treating 2,000 patients a year but 800. We already have an information system that is ongoing. Do I see a need for computerizing this information system? Purely from the technical aspects, removing the physician from the scene, I can see that need in our medium-sized department. But I would take Dr. Glicksman's stand that certainly there is no need for having computerized information systems in community hospitals.

I think we can draw an analogy to treatment-planning. It was left to the larger centers to demonstrate the need for fairly precise systematic treatment-planning for some of the sophisticated techniques we use today in modern radiation therapy. I think the radiation therapy community is aware that the dose delivered must be attained within a plus or minus 5 percent precision. This had to be demonstrated by the larger centers for the medium-sized and smaller centers to follow. Now, similarly, I think the larger centers have to take the initiative in demonstrating the value of computerized information systems in overall patient care.

CEDERLUND: When you start work on a system like this, you have many ideas you want to work into it; but often it is like a house move. When we first moved from Lund, I brought a lot of things with me, and my wife asked if I really needed them. I said, "Well, sure, I'm going to use them. I've used them so far." And so we put them away in the attic, and then seven years later we moved to Uppsala, she took them out again, and said, "Well, you haven't used them this far, can we throw them away now? " I think we should be careful that we don't carry a lot of junk in our programming, and we must have some means of evaluating whether or not we need this.

The second thing I'd like to draw your attention to or rather question is the following: Do we, when we build up a system like this, think only of our local problems and how to handle them, or should we also look at what other clinics are doing and try to build a system that in the end can be compatible so that we can exchange ideas and build up an international data bank?

ELLIS: Regarding Dr. Glicksman's statement, I'd question whether any department needs a computer, because when you look at the statistics that have been published of results of cancer treatment, they come mostly from places like Manchester, Stockholm, and France, at times when they didn't have computers. It's very rare to see statistics to compare to those nowadays.

GLICKSMAN: I'm in agreement as to what the fundamental payoff has to be—does the patient really benefit? Dr. Ellis has addressed himself to that particular point. We don't have any evidence that the patient is really going to benefit from the computer applications as yet.

FREY: I find myself in the peculiar position of supporting Dr. George. I feel that practically every department that has any pretensions at all to doing modern radiotherapy needs a computer, at least for dose calculations, unless it plans on doing merely palliative large-field type of work. As long as the department has to have this capability, then all of these other things that you are talking about as unnecessary have a relatively small marginal cost. If you have the computer capability, it takes very little more to add these things, and what it does do is to share the cost of the hardware needed for the basic dose calculation among other sections that are perhaps better able to carry it. I don't think it is really a question of need, but that it is very easy and cost-effective once you have the computer.

SUNTHARALINGAM: What is the actual cost of getting a small mini-computer into a department that is trying to install accelerators and hire staff radiation therapists and appropriate medical physics support?

NEURATH: The cost of the computer is relatively trivial, but the marginal cost is not marginal—that is, if you're going to keep information on patients in a structured way and in a very complete way, it is going to demand more attention on somebody's part, whether it is a registrar, nurse, or resident. Whoever it is will have to make an effort. This effort may not appear on the books, but it's got to be made if you want to have retrievable information.

As far as not having impressive data from computer systems is concerned, I think it's generally conceded that you have to have a five-year or more accumulation before you can publish anything very significant. So perhaps it's not fair to criticize computer systems that have been in existence less than five years for not publishing a twenty-year review of data.

TING: I'm very impressed with some of the systems presented today using large dedicated computers to handle patient records and treatment-planning, but I am surprised that nobody brought up the possibility of a commercialized time-sharing system. The patient-record retrieval system definitely is a possibility for time-sharing to handle at a moderate cost. With small computers you have to worry about capital costs as well as programmer costs and hardware maintenance. Most of the centers discussed today must have several programmers plus additional hardware maintenance personnel. If you divide all these costs up on a per-capita patient basis, time-sharing systems may be more attractive.

CLIFTON: Listening to the presentation this morning, one is struck by the fact that these total systems are basically designed to automate what we do by hand. And I think this is a recipe for disaster. Now there are two points that come from this. First, if we look towards the end of this conference, we're going to be discussing what we can do for developing countries. And it strikes one in listening to the presentations this morning that one of the fundamental concepts is the question of billing and money. Now, this is not necessarily the way that all health systems operate. And I think if you're talking of a total information system, you have to consider whether this is a fundamental plank on which you build. The second one is, if we're talking about a fundamental total information system, what do you do with your current pictorial information? Are you going to be satisfied in ten years' time with a record system that records everything that you can record with a typewriter at the moment, but doesn't store your radiograph or your histology slide?

NEURATH: Let me say just one thing in conclusion. Some of us still talk about what the computer can do versus what the person can do. I think we all ought to know better. The computer is a tool, and a person has to be able to use the tool. It's that sort of approach that will get us somewhere.

II. Automation and Verification
Chairperson: B. Bjarngard

Session III: Contributed Short Papers on Record and Verify Systems

1. Development and Experience in Computer Monitoring and Verification of Daily Patient Treatment Parameters

A. Chung-Bin
P. Kartha
T. Wachtor
F. Hendrickson

The Department of Radiation Oncology of Rush - Presbyterian - St. Luke's Medical Center, Chicago, acquired a PDP 11/20 computer in March 1972. The purpose of this computer was to develop an automation package for a modified AECL Theratron 80 Teletherapy unit. After the development of some suitable software and the appropriate hardware interface, we decided to monitor the daily patient setup parameters. The purpose of this was to study human errors in treatment setups. At that time the technicians were relatively unsophisticated as to computer usage and the goals of the project. We feel that this removed some element of biasing in the study.

The technicians were instructed to enter the patient's identification into the computer at the start of every treatment. This procedure was carried out for several months. The data recorded in the computer was then printed, and analyzed according to the treatment chart for those patients.

Generally, there were two types of errors. One type we call the systematic error—inherent in the system, typically caused by analog type settings. The other type we call accidental error—caused by a gross oversight or mistake. Preliminary analysis of 253 setups revealed a systematic error whose magnitude produced one standard deviation of about 1 degree, 1 millimeter, and 1 second for parameters measured in those units. Analysis of the same data gave an accidental error rate of about 0.14 per patient setup. However, if one multiplies by the total number of parameters actually set up at the beginning of the treatment, the error rate per operation is about 2 percent. This figure of 2 percent seems to be about a human norm, and has been observed by others (1). After this study it was decided to initiate a treatment-verification scheme, even though we were not aware of the clinical effect of this error rate.

The monitoring continued, and another study involving several thousand setups was completed. (2) The accidental error rate for this study was in good agreement with the preliminary study. A study of the error rate by days of the week showed no significant difference between the days. The analysis was repeated using morning and afternoon as the separation criterion. Again no significant differences in error rate were detected. The study was again performed using individual technicians as the separation criterion. It was found that there was a difference in error rates between technicians that spanned an order of magnitude. A calibration and reliability study of the hardware was performed, which showed very good consistency, if not complete linearity in the potentiometers. All of the above seems to confirm the error rate in the order of about 2 percent.

A verification procedure was established. Since May 1974 both a Clinac 4 and Theratron 80 have been monitored and verified. It takes about one minute of technician time per patient setup. Although this verification system is carried out smoothly, we do have computer down-time due to hardware and software failures.

The procedure has received mixed acceptance by the technicians. It is interesting to note that the technician with the lowest error rate praises the system, while the one with the highest condemns it. Several technicians have requested its use on Saturdays, when the computer is normally off, while others have become sophisticated in avoiding its use.

Our experience is that it is very important for the verification method to be easily executable and not interfere with the workload of the machine. To attain this goal it is absolutely necessary to have some time-sharing computer capability, so that detailed information does not have to be entered into the computer at treatment time. Also, the system should be reliable. Frequent down-time causes adverse reactions to using the computer. In our operating system, concurrent development work causes frequent periods of down-time. We hope to alleviate this by incorporating a hardware-protected operating system at some time in the near future. If there is not development work on the computer, however, and only reliable programs are used, this form of verification can run on a PDP 11/20 computer with as little as 12K of core memory and one disk. This relatively small system can provide verification of several machines along with a modest information management package.

In conclusion, our experience shows that a computer with some time sharing ability is necessary, that system reliability is of extreme importance, and that the actual burden on the treatment technician should be kept as small as possible.

REFERENCE

1. Minor, F., and Revesman, S. L., *J. Appl. Psychology* 40, 332 (1962).

2. Kartha, P., Chung-Bin, A., Wachtor, T., and Hendrickson, F. R., *Med. Physics* 2, 331 (1975).

QUESTIONS

FREY: I have the impression that in the smaller study there were 0.14 errors per treatment, which is 14 percent, and in the later one it was closer to 3 or 4 percent.

WACHTOR: We have 0.14 errors per treatment; that is, if we had 100 treatments, 14 of them had a gross error in that treatment. However, within the treatment there are five parameters being set.

FREY: Fourteen patients out of 100 will have some error—

WACHTOR: Yes, some gross error.

FREY: Well, now in your "Total" column on the last slide it was still in the range of 3 or 4 percent.

WACHTOR: That is per parameter. There is 14 percent error, but if you divide by five parameters, it comes out around 3 percent error per parameter.

ELLIS: Fifteen degrees for the gantry angle seems to be a very big margin to allow. Also, half a minute when you have 100 rads per minute seems to be a very big error. I've wondered why you chose those values.

WACHTOR: At least on a Theratron-80—the way the scales are set for the gantry angle—the normal errors you're going to make are something on the order of 15 degrees. You rarely make 30-degree errors, it seems. You rarely see a 10-second error—it just doesn't happen. A Theratron-80 has a click-click-click for the number of minutes, and you'll either get one click too many or one click too few and it gives you a minute error.

2. An Attempt to Check Radiation Treatment Parameters with a Mini-Computer

J. Cederlund
P-O Lofroth
S. Zetterlund

As a result of a joint project between the Uppsala Data Center, the Academical Hospital and the Siemens Company, we have had a Siemens-305 computer available for development work. One of the projects was to study the feasibility of computer-controlled dynamic treatment, by interfacing the computer to a Philips Linear Accelerator type SL-75. A demonstration of the system was performed at the Fourth International Conference on the Use of Computers in Radiation Therapy (1).

The project was successful insofar as it demonstrated that the computer could control the movement of the accelerator with sufficient speed and accuracy. We were not able to convince either the administration or ourselves that in competition with other pressing needs it would, at this time, be wise to spend the necessary amount of funds or expend the brainpower needed to develop a system that could meet all clinical demands on reliability and safety. Since, however, the interface was there, and since it would be possible to run a small background program on the computer for about two months, we decided to simulate a chip-computer, with about 1 k core memory and access to adequate memory capacity on disk.

The limited core memory was utilized for a small main program that combined different program segments for the reading of digital signals, the calibration of ADC-converted analogue signals, and communication with a teletype machine. Table 1 shows the registered parameters: Section 1 contains the input of administrative information from the teletype unit, Section II the parameters read during the setup of the patient, and Section III finally the parameters read when the treatment was completed. An important parameter in this section was the reading of the dose on a microionization chamber placed on the patient's skin in the center of the field. After corrections for pressure, temperature, and build-up effects, it indicates what we term the reference dose to the patient.

The program was used for documentation and verification. It was not possible to perform the verification in real time, because several different disks were used on the available disk drive, and therefore no treatment data could be stored and no immediate comparison between prescribed and actually set-up treatment data was possible. Altogether, the parameters for about 240 treatments were read during four weeks. The information from the teletype paper tape was transferred weekly to a disk and subsequently edited and printed in suitable tables to give a survey of the treatments of each patient.

Since one of the aims of the investigation was to check the constancy of the reading, a test program was run twice weekly. The main emphasis was on the conversion and calibration of the analogue signals. For this test program a larger part of the core memory was utilized than for the patient parameter reading. Seven analogue parameters were investigated. Each was read by the computer at four different settings. From this a calibration curve was computed. Using this calibration curve, a comparison was made between the set values and the computed values. The deviation between these two values was never larger than the resolution of the ADC.

The number of recorded treatments was too small to allow statistical analyses, but the following observations were made. No obvious errors were discovered. Setup values for dose and time were correct, as well as wedge angle and sense. The gantry angle was set up with a precision better than one degree. Treatment-field dimensions were set up with deviations in the interval 1–3 mm, and on some occasions up to 5 mm. The collimator angle was shown to have a deviation of about ± 4 percent. At small field sizes it could amount to 5 percent. The size of these deviations is reasonable considering the lack of a special attachment for the patient on the treatment table.

From this trial we conclude that with a small computer (about 1 k core memory) with access to an external mass-memory, it is possible to build a Record and Verify System.

REFERENCE

1. Lofroth, P. O., and Cederlund, J., "Automation of a linear accelerator SL-75," *Proceedings of the Fourth International Conference on the Use of Computers in Radiation Therapy*, Uppsala (August 1972).

QUESTIONS

MACKINNEY: Do I understand that all the potentiometers and measuring devices were prepared by you and not by the manufacturer?

CEDERLUND: The manufacturer did install the potentiometers on the machine and gave us the interface. From there on, we took over the signal.

Table 1.
Recorded Parameters

I *Administrative Information*	*II* *Set-up Parameters*	*III* *Parameters after Completed Treatment*
Date	Kind of Radiation	Dose 1
Identification Number	Energy	Dose 2
Field Number	Dose	Time
Reference Dose	Time	Value from Micro Ionization Chamber
	Wedge Angle	
	Gantry Rotation	
	Collimator Rotation	
	Field Size x	
	Field Size y	
	Turntable Angle	
	Table Height	

3. The CART System: Automated Verification, Recording, and Controlled Accelerator Setup

D. Kipping
R. Potenza

Introduction

During the past decade, the use of computers in radiotherapy has rapidly progressed to the point where computer-based ancillary functions are standard in many treatment centers. Work in several medical research centers (1-4) and other independent studies (5) have shown that computer verification of treatment setup parameters could eliminate a significant source of potential treatment errors. In addition, computer maintenance of treatment records and computer-assisted (automatic) treatment setup could increase the efficiency of radiotherapy department operations. In response to these considerations, Varian conceived the CART (Computer Assisted Radiation Therapy) system to provide verify, record, and controlled setup capabilities with its Clinac® line of medical linear accelerators. At the present time, the CART system design is completed, and the system is in the final phase of prototype testing.

The CART system design rests on balancing a number of key controlling factors. Some are common to existing research systems, now or soon to be in daily use; some are derived from general clinical considerations; and others are derived from requirements unique to the manufacturer of radiotherapy equipment. This paper describes the fundamental design criteria for the CART system, its capabilities, its operation, and details of the CART hardware and software.

Fundamental Design Criteria

Before the detailed design of CART could proceed, four design criteria were established:

(1) Safety

(2) The flexibility of a computer
(3) Record keeping capability
(4) Commercial viability

A primary criterion is that CART shall enhance safety. The system must remain in a secondary role, with primary control always in the hands of the operator. Decisions by the system can be manually overridden at any time, and under no circumstances can the system be capable of turning on the treatment beam. Under automatic setup, while the accelerator is in motion, the system will monitor the relative positions of the couch and the gantry and avoid the possibility of a collision. System failure or an operator's manual override must immediately stop all system-controlled motion.

The second design criterion is that verify and record functions be as comprehensive and flexible as possible. The use of a computer-based system is the most practical way to implement these requirements. The controlled setup function places an even higher demand on the design. Implementation of this function falls easily within the power of a mini-computer system. Hence these requirements led naturally to the implementation of a full mini-computer based system.

Thirdly, because the verification process is comprehensive, stored data includes all parameters needed to specify a complete treatment setup. The patient record must be individualized for each patient and be in a form that can be stored with the standard patient chart and files. These criteria led to the requirement for a high capacity, removable mass-storage medium.

Finally, as a commercial product, a key design requirement is that the system must be flexible enough to use in many different institutions without reprogramming. System reliability, maintainability, and documentation should be sufficient for the manufacturer to support the equipment at the same level as the primary radiotherapy treatment unit. The system should be easy to use and not require support from additional specialized staff. Therefore, the system should be self-contained and installed on a "turnkey" basis.

These four criteria and their interplay were analyzed to establish the system design, and resulted in a system with the specific capabilities and configuration described below.

CART Capabilities and Configuration

CART is designed to assist the technologist in verifying and recording a prescribed treatment on the accelerator. The system prohibits the commencement of treatment until all accelerator settings correspond to the planned treatment. An alternate version of CART controls the motions of the accelerator such that, during patient setup, the control circuits simultaneously drive the motors in the gantry, collimator head, and treatment couch to the prescribed positions for commencement of treatment. Implementation of these basic functions in CART has resulted in a system with a specific configuration and set of capabilities, summarized as follows:

1. *Verification*
   (a) Confirms patient identification
   (b) Checks mechanical settings of the accelerator gantry, collimator system, and treatment couch
   (c) Checks treatment console settings, including dose, timer, energy, arc-therapy parameters, accessory status, and, when appropriate, modality (electron or X-ray) and energy
   (d) Checks accelerator system's safety interlocks
   (e) Confirms that the treatment fields given are those planned for each specific treatment day
2. *Stored Record*
   (a) Prescribed daily schedule for treatment fields
   (b) Prescribed settings for each treatment field
   (c) Actual dose delivered per treatment field
   (d) Cumulative dose delivered at up to eight anatomical sites of interest
   (e) Deviations taken from the planned treatment schedule
3. *Control*
   (a) All mechanical motions activated simultaneously
   (b) Anticollision monitoring during automatic setup
4. *Operational Features*
   (a) CRT and keyboard interaction with operator
   (b) Permanent individualized patient record
   (c) Facilities for entering the initial information for a new patient
   (d) Facilities for editing the record of patient currently under treatment
   (e) Free-form messages, oriented to both patient and treatment setup and stored as part of the patient record
   (f) Hard copy of daily treatment information and other aspects of treatment record
5. *Hardware Components and Configuration*
   These are shown in Figure 1.

The above capabilities and system configuration provide the basic specification of the CART system. Details of the design and implementation are described in the remaining sections of the paper.

The Patient Record

The content of the patient treatment record can best be described by first noting the terminology adopted within the system. Each treatment field (photon or electron) is called a "portal." The data base for a portal contains all of the information needed to specify the application of the accelerator treatment beam according to the physician's prescription. Each portal is designated by a single letter (A, B, X, etc.), and CART allows specifications of up to 24 distinct portals per patient. Portals are arranged into a prescribed treatment schedule by specifying the sequence of portals in order of treatment days. Up to 7 different portals can be scheduled for any one day, and up to 50 treatment days can be specified in a single treatment schedule.

The treatment record data base is maintained on an individual flexible disk for each patient and occupies about 10 percent of the total capacity of the disk. The data in the record is shown in Table 1, and includes the following:

1. The Master File, incorporating the patient's name, identification code, and other treatment status information;
2. The Treatment File, which includes the treatment sequence on a day-by-day basis and a patient-oriented message keyed to each treatment day; and
3. The Portal File, which includes the detailed specification for treatment setup for all defined portals.

An important feature of the CART record is the accumulation of dose received at each of eight anatomical sites of interest. The definition of these sites is completely specified by the user and includes a six-character name and the ratio of applied monitor units to the dose received at each site.

Operator Interaction with the System

During clinical use, communication of information to the technologist concerning the accelerator, patient records, or CART system status is by text displayed on the CRT. The text is organized into single frames on the screen, each frame corresponding to one complete function or operation of the CART system. Communication from the technologist to the system is through keyboard commands. Those most frequently used are also single key buttons.

A summary of the logic paths for operation of CART is given in Figure 2, which shows four basic paths:

1. Standard treatment
2. Data review
3. Initialization of a new patient record
4. Editing of an existing patient record

Each block in the figure represents a single CRT frame, and the lines represent a keyboard command. Entry to all but the initialization path requires specification and confirmation of patient identification code.

To administer a standard treatment the normal procedure is to insert the patient's treatment disk and type in his identification code. After this code is checked against the prestored value on the disk, the "treatment status" frame is displayed. This frame summarizes the treatment planned for the day and presents other information related to the patient. A single key command causes display of the "treatment frame" for the first scheduled portal of the day. The "planned" and "current" values of treatment parameters are shown side-by-side on the CRT and on the slave monitor in the treatment room. If these values do not agree within a specified tolerance, an asterisk appears between the two values and beam-on is disabled until agreement is reached by adjusting the appropriate treatment parameters. (System tolerances are specified by the user and apply to all patients. Minimum tolerances readable on the CRT are 1 mm for linear positions and 0.1° for angles. Operational tolerances are usually broader.) Figure 3 is an example of this treatment frame (before verification is achieved). For automatic setup the technologist must be present in the treatment room, since both the safety switch and a button on the accelerator pendant (AUTO) must be kept depressed. CART monitors the relative positions of the couch and the gantry during automatic setup to predict the possibility of collision. If a potential collision is detected, the couch and gantry are moved relative to each other so that the final prescribed position is achieved without collision. As an additional convenience, a second button on the pendant (HOME) drives the couch and other mechanical parameters to a standard position for patient loading and unloading.

Once the patient is completely set up and the beam is ready, the CART system assumes a monitoring role. Control of the accelerator is completely in the hands of the technologist. After the treatment is administered and the beam is turned off, the "chart update" frame automatically appears on the CRT. This frame presents dose information which may be entered into the patient chart. Control is then returned to the treatment status frame. Depending on the treatment schedule, another portal can be administered or the system can return to the inactive frame preparatory to treatment of another patient.

The second logic path provides review of the patient data. A complete listing of the treatment schedule is contained in one display frame. Another frame includes dose data and the accumulated dose at eight anatomical sites of interest. Finally, the details of all portals defined for treatment may be reviewed.

A third logic path allows the operator to initialize the record for a new patient (see Figure 2). The "initialize" frame allows entry of patient name, identification code, and other basic data. The "record status" frame gives a summary of the data entered so far. From there, other frames can be invoked to enter specific information:

1. The anatomical sites of interest can be named and initial dose values can be entered.
2. The portals to be treated can be defined and specific values entered.
3. The daily sequence of portals can be entered.
4. During initial patient setup with the accelerator, the eight mechanical parameters may be read directly by the computer into the Portal File and need not be entered manually.

Finally, during a typical course of therapy, it is often necessary to make changes in the treatment prescription; the edit logic path is then taken. Although editing is operationally almost identical to initialization, a major difference is that no information concerning treatments already given may be changed in any way. This ensures that an accurate historical record is preserved.

System Interface with the Accelerator

The functions of verify, record, and controlled setup require monitoring the positions of all mechanical parameters of the accelerator and couch, monitoring the control console parameters, and interrogating the accelerator system's operational status. In addition, for controlled setup, the computer must interface with the drive motor controls.

The eight mechanical motions of the accelerator and couch are monitored by potentiometers that provide an accuracy of 1 mm for linear motions of 0.1° for angles. These analog signals are converted to digital form then read by the computer. The other parameters, such as dose, are in digital form in the therapy machine and are read directly by the computer. The mechanical motions of the accelerator and couch are driven by reversible, variable-speed, direct-current motors, using Silicon Controlled Rectifier motor controls. CART controls the motor speeds by converting digital commands to analog signals that drive these motor controls. All mechanical motions have travel limits provided by either electrical limit switches or mechanical stops, coupled with mechanical slip clutches. In no case will damage result if a control signal is maintained after a limit has been reached.

Disk System

The dual flexible ("floppy") disk system was chosen because it achieves the desired balance between performance and operator convenience. CART uses two independent disk drives, each of which utilizes a removable disk with a 131,072 16-bit word capacity. Functionally, one drive contains the System Program Disk, while the other contains the current Patient Disk. A disk-based system offers several advantages over other low-cost peripheral devices or core resident software:

1. It permits system programs to be nonresident and to be brought in upon demand (typical load time is less than one second).
2. Additional software functions can be added by bringing in programs from disk with no additional core required.
3. The data for each patient are kept on his own disk, which can be removed and conveniently stored with his other records.

The choice of a dual-drive disk system offers several additional advantages:

4. It allows complete separation of operating software from patient records, thus easing software maintenance problems.
5. It provides the ability to copy disks and to easily archive patient or program data.
6. It simplifies system software, since the operating software device and the patient data device are identical.

Operating Software

The operating software is written in Varian 620/L assembly language and consists of three essentially independent parts:

1. a resident Disk-Operating System, which supports core image files and is used as the program swapping mechanism;
2. a resident Real Time Executive, which handles interrupts and performs multi-tasking;
3. the CART Application Program (CAP), which is nonresident, and segments of which are brought into core upon demand.

At the application level of CAP, there are three classes of software: command processing, frame generation, and real-time tasks. Since the system is command oriented, essentially nothing happens until a new command is received from the CRT keyboard. The command processor analyzes each new command and causes the appropriate action to be taken. Typical actions are: a new frame is generated, a new core load is brought in, the edit subroutines are called, a task is scheduled or released, core or disk data is updated, etc. If a new CRT frame is to be generated, the frame generation software first assures that all required data is in core, then makes calls on the input/output formatter and CRT driver to put up the frame. Teletype output uses the same frame generation software, except that the output is directed to the teletype driver.

The following real-time tasks may be scheduled to run on a periodic basis:

1. Verification—about every second
2. Motor control—every 50 ms
3. Collision avoidance—every 50 ms

For the verify function, the accelerator status is read and compared with the portal description previously read from the patient disk. If all parameters are verified, the beam is enabled. Motor control is activated during controlled setup to drive the accelerator to the required positions. Feedback control algorithms are implemented to run the motors at maximum speed, while minimizing friction, overshoot, and lag. Collision avoidance consists of a mathematical model of the accelerator, couch, and patient-volume geometry. The software computes the relative position of the gantry and the couch, and if a collision is impending, the control path is changed. Collision avoidance is table driven, so one program works for all models of Clinac.

Finally, CAP provides for handling errors and abnormal conditions. Operator input errors do not cause erroneous system actions. Instead, English language error messages are displayed on the CRT. Limited changes to the treatment sequence and portal definition are possible at the time of treatment, because manual treatment is always possible. Records are updated with actual dose values even if the dose required was not given for some reason. If a nonrecoverable error (either hardware or software) is detected, the procedure is to print an error message, release the accelerator from computer control, and halt the computer in an orderly fashion. In most cases a system failure will not cause loss of data, and the system can be restarted immediately if the hardware is intact.

Summary

This paper has described the design criteria, capabilities, and configuration of the CART system. In addition, specific details of system operation and system hardware and software structure have been presented. CART is in the final prototype testing phase, but clinical experience with the current system may indicate the need for further refinements. With CART this process has been anticipated. Since the software structure is basically modular, important modifications can be made while affecting a minimum of the total system software.

REFERENCES

1. Chung-Bin, A., Kartha, P., Wachtor, T., and Hendrickson, F., in Proceedings of the Fifth International Conference on the Use of Computers in Radiation Therapy, Dartmouth College, 18–23 August (1974).
2. Karzmark, C. J., and Rust, D. C., *Br. J. Radiol.*, *45*, 276 (1972).
3. Karzmark, C. J., and Rust, D. C., *Radiology*, *105*, 157 (1972).
4. Golden, R., Cundiff, J. H., Grant, W. H., III, and Shalek, R. J.,

Cancer, *29*, 1468 (1972).
5. Herring, D. F., and Compton, D. M. J., *Br. J. Radiol.*, Special Report No. 5, 51 (1971).

QUESTIONS

FREY: What is the basic cost of the linear accelerator itself, the accelerator with the record and verify, and with the control features?

POTENZA: The record and verify function provides the basic hardware for all the functions, and the price for that is approximately $35,000. An additional $10,000 is for control setup. It does not include preparation of the accelerator.

CHUNG-BIN: Is this system in standard use?

POTENZA: No, not the current CART system that I described. The University of Wisconsin CART-I was installed, and Dave Neblett is using some of the original CART software in his expanded system.

Table 1.

Treatment Record Data Base
Maintained on Each Patient Disk

Master File

Patient Name	Number of Treatments in Plan
Patient ID Code	Number of Treatments Given
Date Record Initialized	Portal Status Summary
Date Record Last Edited	Indexes to Other Files
Date Patient Last Treated	Diagnosis—199 characters of free form text

Treatment File (Entries for up to 50 Treatment Days)

Daily Plan (i.e., Portals to be treated on a given day)
Treatment Action (Coded)
Meter Dose Given

Physician Message File

Up to 50 entries, each one associated with a treatment day, keyed to the Treatment File. Each entry consists of 201 characters of free form text.

Portal File (up to 24 Portals)

Type of Portal (Fixed, Offset or Arc)
Number of Times Administered
Specification for Treatment Setup:

Gantry Angle	Dose Desired
Collimator Angle	Mode (Clinac 12, 18 only)
Collimator, Upper	Energy (Clinac 12, 18 only)
Collimator, Lower	Wedge
Couch Angle	Shadow Tray
Couch Longitudinal	Electron Collimator (Clinac 12, 18 only)
Couch Lateral	Stop Angle (Arc Therapy only)
	Rads/Degrees (Arc Therapy only)

Portal Message—132 characters of free form text.
Meter and Given Dose factors for 8 anatomical sites-of-interest.

Sites-of-Interest File (8 entries)

Name of Site (6 characters)
Initial Value of Dose (Dose delivered before treatments using CART)
Cumulative Site-of-Interest Doses monitored by CART

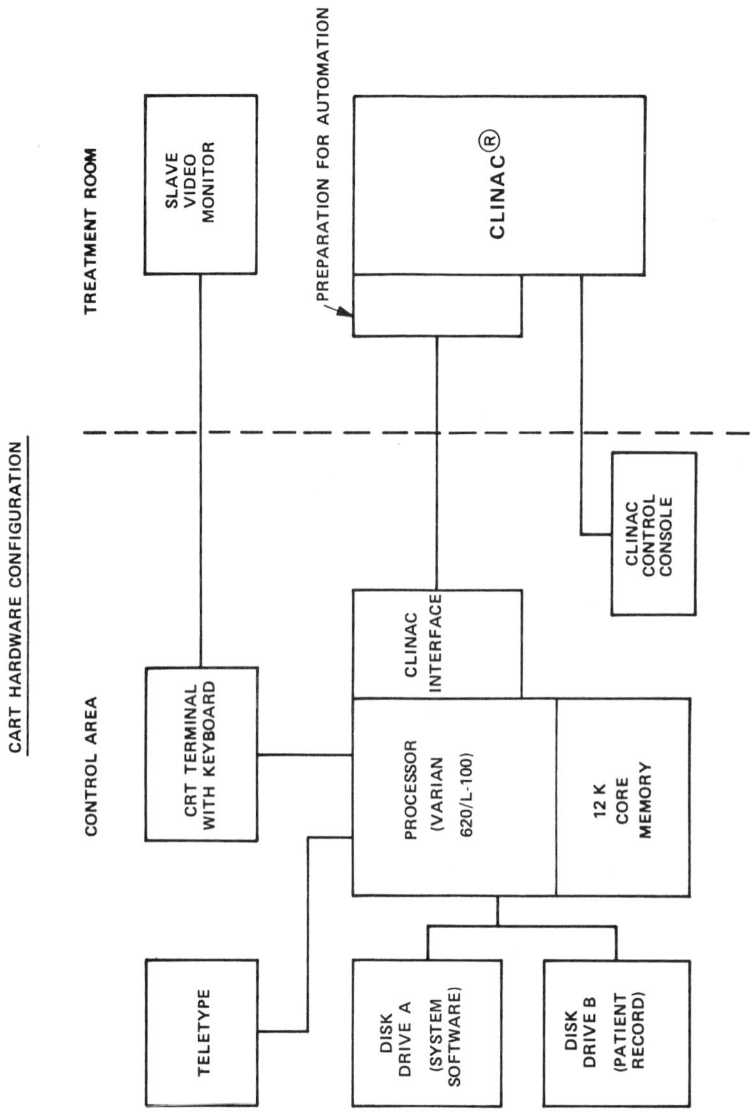

Figure 1. Cart Hardware Configuration

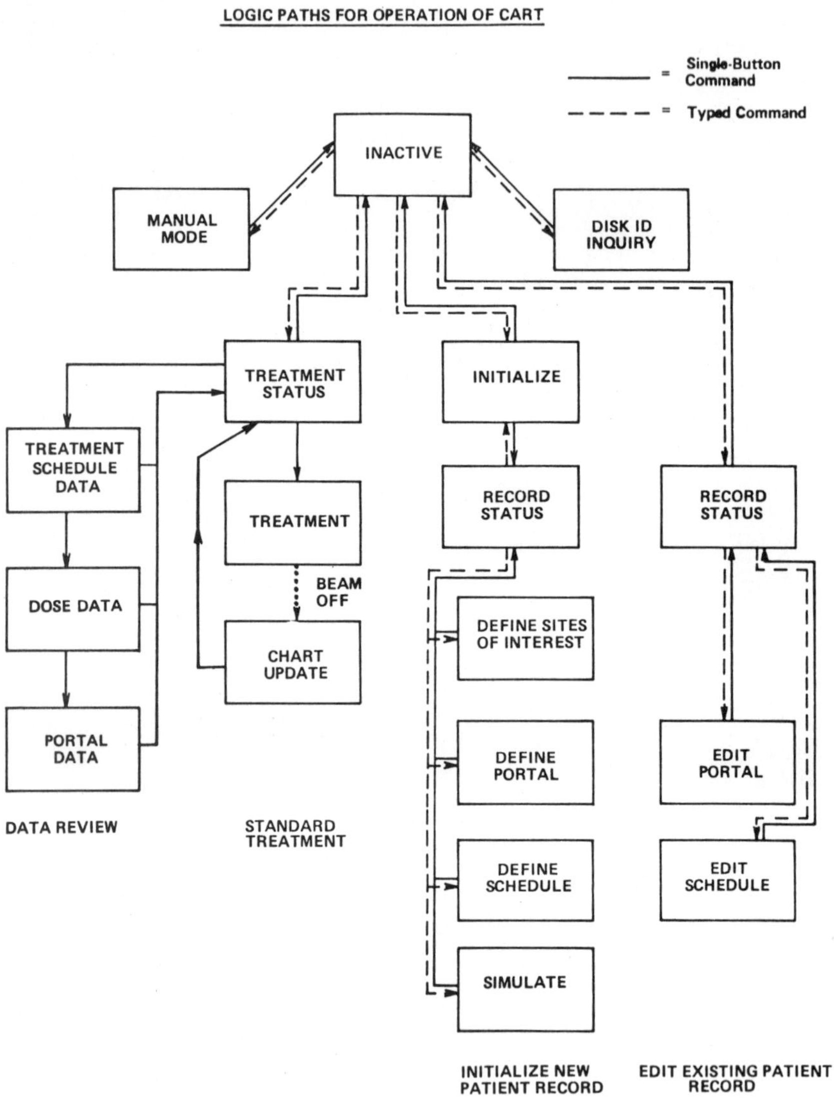

Figure 2. Logic Paths for Operation of Cart

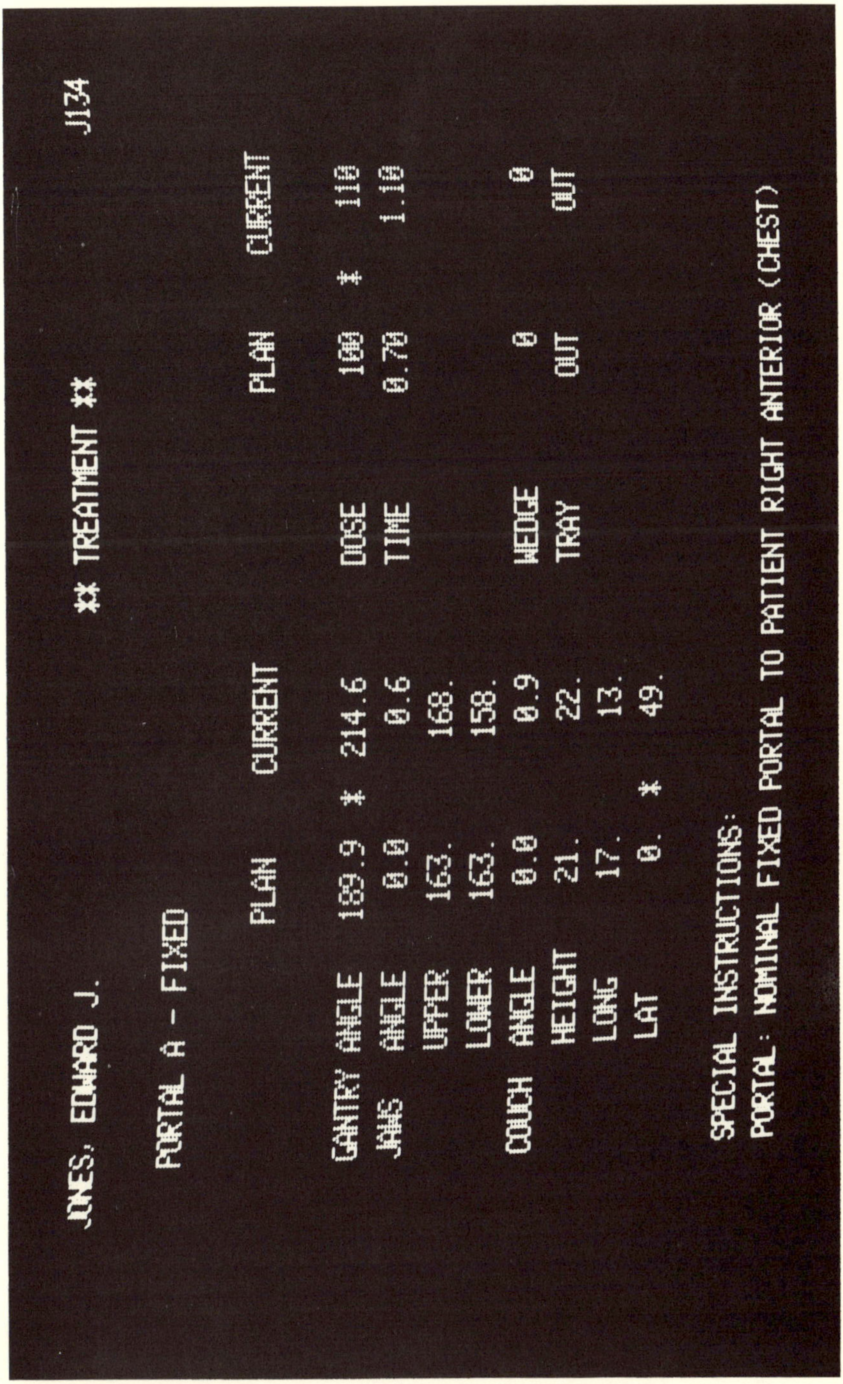

Figure 3. Cart CRT "Treatment" Frame

4. Computer-Assisted Entry, Verification, and Recording of Treatment Parameters for a 45 MeV Betatron

J. D. Steben
N. Suntharalingam

I. Introduction

Recently, the Thomas Jefferson University Radiation Therapy Center began treating patients with a versatile 45 MeV Brown Boveri Corp. (BBC) Betratron which is equipped with a BBC analog/digital readout device. In this machine, electron energies of 3, 5, 10, 15, 20, 25, 30, 35, 40, and 45 MeV are clinically available, as well as two photon beams at energies of 32 and 45 MeV. Despite helpful interlocks which guarantee prevention of many conceivable errors in setup, various other mistakes can still be made by the operator. It is desirable to strive further for high levels of accuracy and reliability with computer-assisted treatment verification. This will be implemented via an interactive operator-computer dialog. The approach to the problem at Thomas Jefferson University Hospital is herein discussed, and it is intended to commence computerization of the system within the next several months.

There is an existing Betatron automation package known as a "card system" available from the vendor, BBC (4), but several developments have led to a new approach. These developments will be discussed in the following section.

II. Description of the Proposed System

The computerized treatment system described in this paper is most correctly called a computer-assisted treatment system, rather than a computer automation system. The therapy technician must manually perform the patient set-up, and is assisted by the computer in recalling desired parameters and in guaranteeing the correctness of machine set-ups and dose parameters, etc. Correct patient position on the treatment couch is still an operator responsibility. The only control function by the computer is a passive one: interlocking the beam and/or possibly preventing machine motions if treatment conditions are not met. By contrast, the BBC-supplied card system for treatment automation actually drives the Betatron, automatically setting the great majority of Betatron parameters.

Automatic set-up is not desired in our clinical environment, however. Also, it was considered that the combination of video-terminal and mass storage input was more versatile than card-reader input. The proposed system is more analagous to the Varian CART/D system (2, 3) ("record and verify" but not "control," available for Clinacs) than the BBC card system. A further advantage of the proposed system, true also for Rush-Presbyterian Clinac and Theratron verification systems (1), is that the Betatron will be linked to a central data base for patient records, with the potential of greatly simplified paperwork and patient scheduling, and automation of record-keeping functions. The computerized patient data file is then available for other purposes, including research.

III. Operation of the System

It is planned to use the departmental PDP-11/45 central computer for the mass storage of patient records. The Betatron operator's keyboard/display terminal device will be operated as an intelligent rim node terminal to the central computer for a variety of purposes, as shown in Table 1. Figure 1 illustrates usage of a mini as an *intelligent terminal* (terminal mode). For convenience of program development, it is planned to use a PDP-11/10 mini-computer (possibly with a GT 40 as the terminal), and recent lower core prices indicate an optimum core module of 16K 16-bit words.

Figure 2 represents the verification mode used for automatic entry and subsequent verification of the treatment parameters. The method is that during the initial treatment set-up, a "snapshot" of treatment set-up variables and other parameters will be made by the computer, on a keyboard command from the operator. The computer reads the analog and digital signals, displays them, and, if acceptable, stores them (auto entry). These treatment data can later be edited manually if necessary. The computer subsequently monitors the set-ups, assuring that the same conditions have been met. The beam can be interlocked until verification is complete.

IV. Specifications

The parameters to be monitored during set-up are shown in Table 2. Most positional parameters are presented as analog signals to the computer, and most other parameters are read in digital form. Thus 5 rotational and 7 general coordinates and 10 additional treatment parameters will be monitored. As shown in Figure 3, a purchased BBC readout device will be interfaced to the PDP-11 mini (probably an 11/10).

Table 3 specifies some of the interactive keyboard functions, illustrating the dual mode of the terminal. Table 4 indicates the mode information available in frames of the video display and other output. Table 5 lists security specifications.

It is planned to pool patient data on local storage (floppy disk or DECtape) if such is available, prior to the treatment period, and then to update the main disk at the end of the day's treatments. These operations would be done in terminal mode, and have a slight edge in reliability compared to keeping all information active on the central system disk. Advantages include (1) duplicate copy of the active record, and (2) insensitivity to a conceivable system-crash.

V. Programming Aspects

It appears desirable to write the program in a higher-level language, probably Fortran but possibly Basic, both of which are available on PDP-11 family mini-computers. Accordingly, assembly level subroutines to handle data acquisition, using any system macros required, will be kept as brief as possible. It is estimated that the overall core requirement will be roughly 8K without collision-avoidance software and less than 16K with it. The assembly-coded verification routines developed by Wachtor et al. (5, 6) require more like 4K of core, in a form containing somewhat less dialog than is here specified. A considerable programming effort is involved.

VI. Further Discussion

The costs of developing this system have been estimated at $45,000 to $50,000. Hardware (such as a PDP-11/10, 16K core, videoterminal, videomonitor, DECtapes or diskettes, A/D conversion and Digital I/0) would cost around $20,000 at current prices. It is estimated that there will be about $25,000–$30,000 of developmental effort required, 40 percent for engineering and 60 percent for software.

One clinical concern is to attract technicians who are fairly intelligent and to allow nothing to distract them from active patient-care during the setup and treatment. The proposed system should speak to this need as well as minimizing errors in set-up.

Recognizing that technician-acceptance is essential to successful verification, the effort will be made to develop the system so that with the aid of the automatic retrieval and display of set-up parameters verified setups are at least as fast as manual setups.

Verification can be thought of as insurance, using a moderately demanding day-to-day setup procedure to avoid an occasional more major error in treatment delivery.

REFERENCES

1. Chung-Bin, A., Kartha, P., Wachtor, T., and Hendrickson, F., Proceedings of Fifth International Conference on the Use of Computers in Radiation Therapy, Dartmouth College, August 18–23, 1974.
2. Varian Associates, 1973. Private Communications Regarding the Varian CART™ System.
3. Kipping, D., and Potenza, R., in *Proceedings of the Fifth International Conference on the Use of Computers in Radiation Therapy*, Dartmouth College, August 18–23, 1974.
4. Von Arx, A., and Kuphal, K., Proceedings of International Meeting on Computers in Radiology (Brussels, 1969), pp. 183–189. Basel, München, Paris, and New York, 1970.
5. Wachtor, T., 1974. Private Communication.
6. Wachtor, T., Chung Bin, A., and Hendrickson, F., *Proceedings of the 26th Annual Conference on Engineering in Medicine and Biology* (Alliance for Engineering in Medicine and Biology, Arlington, Virginia, 1973), p. 383.

QUESTIONS

SILER: Do you have any results as yet on the accuracy of your manual setups, and secondly why has the automatic setup been ruled out?

STEBEN: We've been in contact with the Chicago group who have made a study of manual setups and we're aware that errors can be made. Of course, our technicians are better than anyone else's technicians, but then everyone feels that way. The reason why automatic setups have been ruled out is basically that it involves quite a bit more challenge. You do not want to collide with the patient. You would be at a major disadvantage if anything went wrong with an automatic setup. That expresses the philosophy: we want to avoid any major error. Our physicians show a strong concern for patient safety. As for record and verify applications, however, we felt this is one way we could do it now and move right ahead.

Table 1. Some Capabilities of Betatron Therapy Control Station

Function	GT40 Mode
1. Enter a new treatment	Processor
2. Verify and start treatments	Processor
3. Display (at GT40) or list (Line Printer)	Terminal
Treatment parameters	Simultaneous
Treatment history	with Betatron
Patient data	Operation
4. Pool patient data for treatment (Disk → Dectape)	Terminal
5. Schedule treatments	Terminal
6. Update treatment records (Dectape → Disk)	Terminal
7. System management and other functions	Both

Table 2. Betatron Parameter Readout

A. DIGITAL

1. Type of radiation X, E				1 bit
2. Equalization filter $X_0 - X_4$, $E_5 - E_9$				10 bits
3. Energy step	01	-	12	5 bits BCD
4. Nominal dose	0000	-	9999	16 bits BCD
5. Maximum time	00.0	-	99.9 min.	12 bits BCD
6. ECC. E = 0				1 bit
7. Radius $R = R_1 = 110$ cm (can be changed)				1 bit
8. Radius $R = R_2 = 120$ cm (can be changed)				1 bit
9. Long-field (LF) selected				1 bit
10. Pendulum (P) selected				1 bit
11. Localizer inserted				1 bit

B. ANALOG

General:

1. Shutter Y 030 - 200 mm
2. Shutter Z 030 - 200 mm
3. Shutter angle ±60°
4. Isocentric height H 00 - 60 cm (actually 100 to 160 cm)
5. Table longitudinal Q 000 - 185 cm
6. Table lateral S ±00 - 99 cm
7. Table height V 00 - 36 cm

Rotational:

8. Rotation angle actual ±120°
9. Rotation angle left ±120°
10. Rotation angle right ±120°
11. Rotation angle speed 000 - 199°/ min.
12. Rotation radius R 100–135 cm

Table 3.
Interactive Keyboard Functions; Specification

General:	Typed characters are displayed on video screen
Verification Mode:	Enter mode by a CONTROL/characters signal (such as perhaps CTRL/V or several characters) typed on keyboard. Enter simple and short commands to access various frames, etc.
Terminal Mode:	Enter mode by typing a CONTROL/character signal (such as perhaps CTRL/T) typed on keyboard. A variety of terminal functions, such as 1. Machine schedule for day 2. Schedule of patients 3. Patient pooling and file updating are to be available to the operator, since the machine will behave as a general purpose terminal to the PDP-11/45.

Table 4.
Some Specifications for Verification Displays

Readout display mode:

A. via Ascii video-display terminal with 2nd TV monitor in treatment room, hard-copy available

B. keyboard input is echoed on screen (lowest line)

Display frames:

A. patient data:
name, diagnosis, etc.

B. treatment schedule:
treatment schedules today; fields, etc.
overall treatment schedule

C. machine setup parameters (for each field) simulate (provide) live display by fast auto-display (to rewrite the screen; <1 sec writing, <2 sec total), when any significant parameter change has occurred in A/D inputs which are monitored. Desired and actual values will be displayed. (The timing requires a 4800 Baud or 9600 Baud Ascii terminal.)

D. other treatment parameters (for each field): dose, time, particle, field shaping foil/absorber, and energy, and field (or letter).

E. patient dose information (current and cumulative)

F. Many terminal functions (in Ascii terminal mode, whether or not monitored by mini-computer) such as: scheduling patients, viewing the day's schedule, etc.

Table 5.
Some Specifications for Security

Auto-manual switch:	a hardware (key-operated) switch to disable the interlocks on treatment (in case it is ever necessary to disable the verification, or to run without the computer)
File Entry Authorization:	a key switch can be implemented to read a status bit or a password. Any changes to a treatment schedule are to require appropriate clinical authorization.

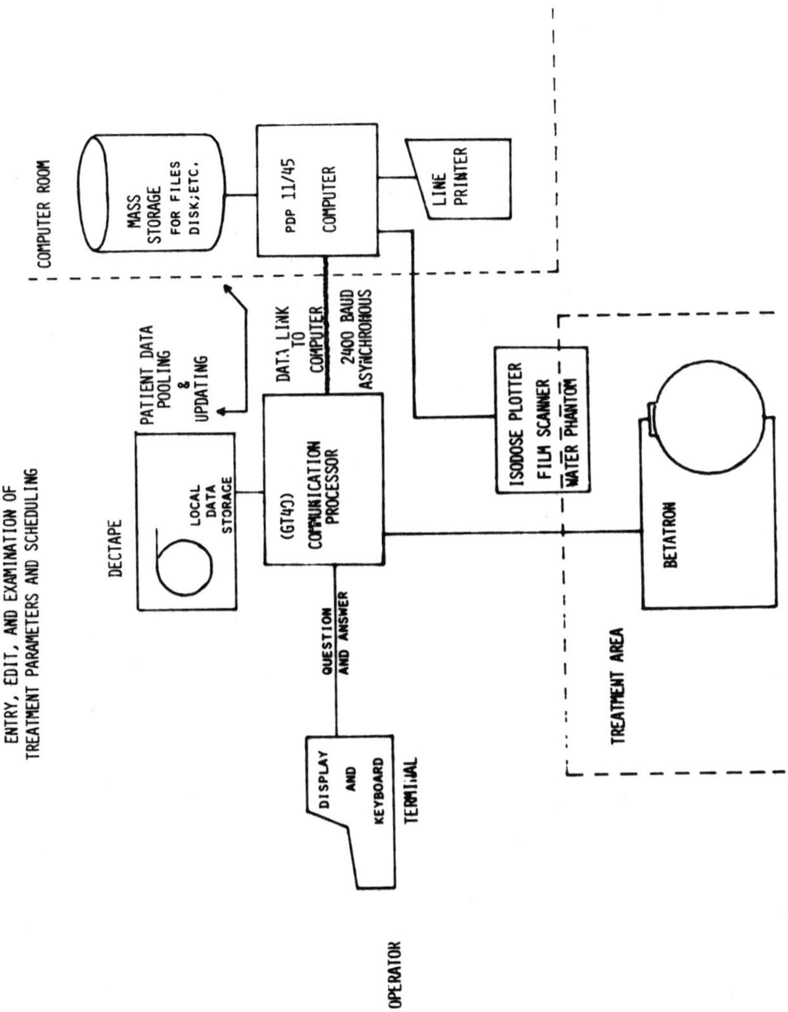

Figure 1. Entry, Edit, and Examination of Treatment Parameters and Scheduling

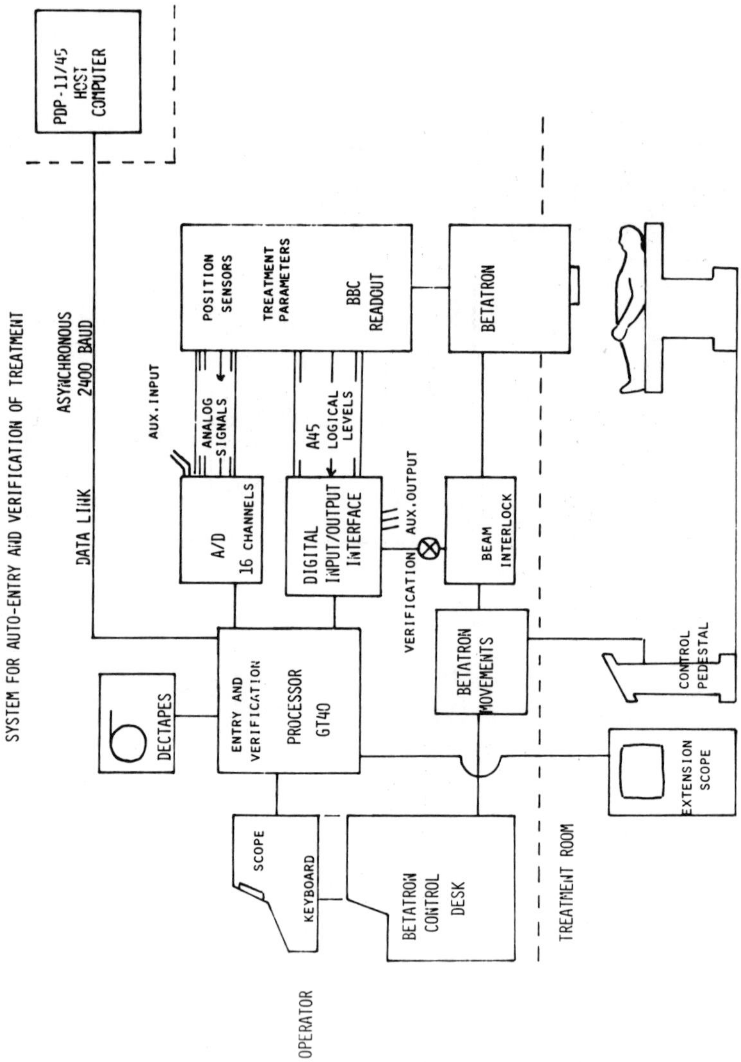

Figure 2. System for Auto-Entry and Verification of Treatment

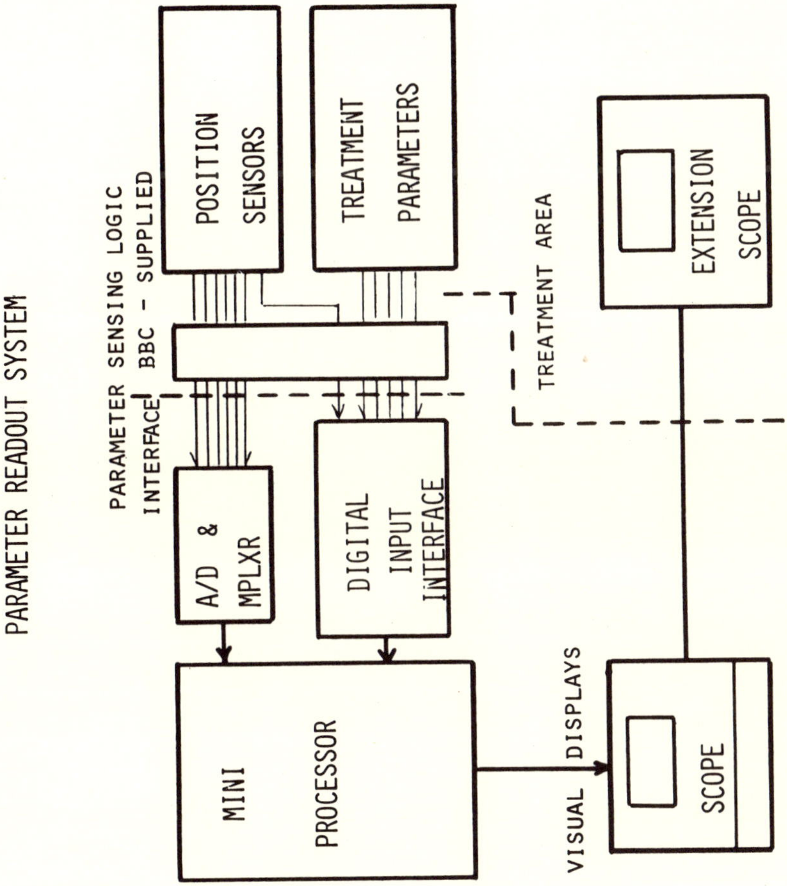

Figure 3. Parameter Readout System

5. A Dedicated Computer for the Checking of Field Settings and the Maintenance of Records for Treatments Given on a Linear Accelerator

M. E. Rosenbloom
R. E. Bentley

Abstract

A PDP-8 computer has been interfaced directly to an SL-75 medical linear accelerator for the checking and recording of treatments. The system compares set-up parameters (field size, wedge angle and sense, orientation of treatment head, gantry, and patient couch) against data entered on a punched tape. An error message is typed when any quantity set differs from its expected value by more than a preset tolerance, and treatment is inhibited. Records are automatically maintained of the dose given to each patient, and can be reproduced on demand.

The system has been run for a trial period with a limited number of patients under clinical conditions.

A brief description is given of the hardware and the programs used.

The overall objectives of the system and its integration into a clinical environment are discussed.

Introduction and Objectives

A PDP-8E computer has been interfaced to an MEL SL 75 medical linear accelerator. We already have a computer for treatment planning.

Table 1 summarizes our objectives, which fall under two major headings: the reduction of human error in, and the documentation of, radiotherapy treatment.

Set-up data will pass from the planning computer to the computer interfaced to the accelerator. A number of set-up parameters will be verified by the computer against these data and the given dose recorded. The computer will perform the arithmetic operations associated with giving and maintaining a record of dose to the patient. These we feel are the major areas where human error can jeopardize treatment.

The computer will facilitate the recall and documentation of treatment. Initially information will be stored locally, but we would like to consider using this computer as a terminal to a remote and autonomous computer data base handling rather more than radiotherapy treatment data.

Description

From the outset we recognized a severe financial restraint, which we interpreted as a challenge to see what we could do with very limited hardware.

We chose the PDP-8E on the grounds of low capital cost and familiarity. It is equipped with 8K of core store. There are two terminals, a visual display unit and paper tape reader in the radiographer's control area, and a teletype just out of earshot. We hope to add magnetic tape storage shortly.

Table 2 lists the parameters checked by the verification program, i.e. field size, collimator and gantry angles, and wedge number. The same table also shows the error messages. The wedge sense is derived from the gantry and collimator angles. Tolerances are program constants.

The program will allow all variations of set-up which are clinically acceptable; for example, a field may be rotated by multiples of 90° if square, by 180° if rectangular, and not at all if wedged. Allowance can also be made for the patient being reversed head to toe.

Field data is fed in as a short length of paper tape each time a patient appears for treatment.

Dose is not checked in advance, since this is frequently varied by the therapist at very short notice.

The link between our planning computer and the "record and verify" computer duplicates the existing link between treatment and planning. In this way each set-up is compared with the original prescription This is significantly different from the approach where the computer uses the first set-up as a pattern for the subsequent course of treatment.

The link between the computers is the paper tape, which bears the patient's name and hospital number as well as the set-up data in coded form. It is produced on the planning computer, which is quite separate from the "record and verify" system. A program is used to punch the tape from clinical data typed in by the planning technician. Table 3 illustrates the difference between the data input by the planning technician and that punched on the tape. We hope to link the preparation of tapes more closely to the planning program.

The second point to stress is that no indication of the correctness of treatment is given while the patient is being set up. The only indication of an error occurs on attempting to start the treatment. An audible warning is given, which persists until treatment is stopped by the radiographer. At the same time a simple diagnostic message is given. The radiographer has a choice of three actions: she can re-enter the treatment room and change the set-up, she can give the treatment despite the warning, or she can override the verification by a single command.

We have resisted the temptation to "close the loop," on the grounds that we want radiographers to retain as much as possible of the responsibility of setting up. Because the system gives no indication at all until the last possible moment, we can argue that we have maintained the maximum incentive for her to get the settings correct. Furthermore, by leaving the override at her discretion, we feel that we have left her as much responsibility as she had in the absence of the computer.

The third point to stress is that the interaction with radiographers is conversational. There is no instruction manual.

Progress to date

So far the system is very much at the development stage. We are still extending both the hardware and software. The verification program is very nearly in final form, but as yet the record program is limited to a statement of cumulative dose in monitor units and the number of treatments for up to four fields. An important contribution to design and evaluation, however, is assessment under clinical conditions, i.e. operation by radiographers during their treatment of patients. Because the system has not evolved to the stage where it can give its full benefit in return for the effort of operating it, we have made our trials so far on a strictly limited basis. The first, with minimal hardware, was made last year, when the treatment of seven patients was followed from beginning to end. The second, with improvements in hard and soft ware, had been in operation since the beginning of May 1974. Only some six patients at a time are followed, but these are replaced as they finish their treatments.

A second function of these trials is to make the introduction of the system as gradual as possible—so that we can incorporate radiographer's suggestions into the system, thus allowing them to feel that they have played some part in its evolution.

Discussion

A surprising result of the two runs, in which completely different teams of radiographers were involved, is that considerably different error rates were encountered. In the first run, out of 193 fields treated, seven significant alterations were made to field settings as a result of warnings by the computer. Some of these were serious, usually a parameter being quite different from its intended value. In the second run (of some 600 fields so far) there have been two minor adjustments to the gantry angle and two isolated incidents when the field dimensions were completely wrong. Errors of addition are frequently made but invariably spotted by the radiographers themselves at a later date without the assistance of the computer.

It has never been easy to convince the radiographers that use of the computer was not to be interpreted as a lack of confidence or as a first step toward making them redundant. We have always been aware, as they were not slow to point out to us, that the first impact of the project on them was an increase in work load before the benefits promised were obtained. They have cooperated with us on our limited trials and have become more tolerant as their worst fears were not realized. On the occasions when errors were prevented, they appeared more pleased that they had been avoided than upset that they had been spotted. We feel fairly optimistic that when the computer takes a fuller part in the record-keeping and reduces the considerable burdens of arithmetic involved, they will agree it is worth the effort of identifying the patient and fields to be treated.

With a project of this nature it is difficult to define our end goal. We feel that ideally this system should serve as the terminal or interface to a remote computer acting as a data base for the department on a broader basis.

QUESTIONS

RAGAN: I was impressed with the minimal hardware for all you've accomplished. Could you give us some estimate of hardware cost?

ROSENBLOOM: Something like $20,000. But I think we should be fair here. The system doesn't accomplish, as it stands, what we hope it will, because we haven't got the mass storage, and we must have it. So we must add this cost, to do what we want to do—i.e. a full treatment record of dose given. We must add something like a dual-deck tape or some form of disc.

Table 1. Objectives

1. Reduction of Human Error in:
    - (a) Communication from planning to treatment
    - (b) Setting up of individual treatment fields
    - (c) Recording of dose given
    - (d) Arithmetic operation prior to and after treatment
2. Documentation of Treatment:
    - (a) Local storage of data for subsequent display or printout on demand
    - (b) Transfer of data to remote and autonomous computer data-base

Table 2. Verification Program

Parameters Checked	*Error Messages*
-length	-wrong length
-width	-wrong width
-wedge number	-wrong wedge
-head (collimator) orientation	-wrong wedge direction
-gantry angle	-wrong head angle
-turntable/couch angle	-wrong gantry angle or combinations of above

Table 3. Tape Producing Program

Input Data and Questions	*Parameters Derived and then Punched on Tape*
-length	-length
-width	-width
-wedge number and sense	-head (collimator) orientation
-gantry angle (±) angle	-gantry angle
-headtwist	-turntable/couch orientation
-patient along or perpendicular to isocentric axis?	
-wedge in plane of treatment or at right angles to compensate for obliquity along tumor axis?	

Session IIIa: General Discussion. "How can record and verify computer systems add reliability to and decrease the cost of the radiation therapy? What needs to be done in the next five years?"

Moderator
B. Bjarngard

BJARNGARD: I've asked Dr. George of the National Cancer Institute to make a short introductory statement to focus on the problems that we want to discuss.

GEORGE: I'm not a big enough man to resist pointing out to today's discussants what's been pointed out to me again and again relative to our record, verify, and control systems. In many languages, people have said: "But Doctor, until you lock the coordinates of the patient into the coordinates of the treatment system, everything you've said is completely meaningless." And I don't think that any of the people who have made presentations today have explained to me how they've ensured that the coordinates of the patient are really related to the coordinates of the treatment system they have been describing.

In answering the question how we can improve reliability and cost-effectiveness, it would appear that we're going to have to refrain from this enormous reluctance on the part of radiotherapists, technologists, computerniks, and so on, to avoid at all costs the control part of the loop. Until we can close the loop with the control of the setup and until we develop systems for repositioning the patient accurately, you don't know that the patient's coordinates are locked into the treatment system.

One can't help noticing the cost of record and verify systems which possibly have no relevance to the patient's coordinates. I think it brings the message home very hard that we sooner or later must go all the way. To go all the way and incorporate the full loop of proper patient repositioning, immobilization and security, integrated into control and then record and verify, would make this work meaningful and perhaps cost effective.

If you tell an attorney that you have a system which you *hope* indicates that the patient is where you want him to be, I'm afraid that's not going to hold up very well in court. It's not defensible. To reiterate, I feel that much of this work is certainly very important, but primarily in context of eventual development of the closed-loop system with control and repositioning.

TING: Another point here is very important. If I'm a technician, and setting up patients, and if the light field indicates I'm one centimeter off on the couch, I am supposed to adjust the couch to have the light field correspond to the ink mark on the patient. However, in the back of my mind I remember that the computer is recording what I'm doing, so I'd better not make that adjustment, otherwise somebody is going to know that I made a one percent error in my records. Therefore, I might tell the machine to go ahead and treat. I'm not going to make the change because the computer is recording. But when the light field doesn't correspond to the ink mark, the patient is not properly positioned on the couch—so until that problem is resolved, I think verification is not well justified from a technician's point of view.

GOITEIN: I also wanted to address the same problem, because I take great issue with the statement that the patient has to be fixed to the couch in order to make this sort of thing work. I would not argue with anybody who says that patient immobilization and support is very necessary, but I believe that we're taking a ten-year step backward if we require that the patient be nailed to the couch before we can treat him.

One of the great advances has been the provision of tables that can be inched in position, can be raised, lowered, moved left, right, up, down. And this ability to inch the patient in instead of lugging him or her around on a sheet on a stretcher has greatly improved and simplified patient setup. What is necessary is to be able to tell the computer that my patient has now been moved accurately and precisely into a coordinate system; he's centered midline; he's straight up-down; he's lying ready. And then the computer can establish this as the origin and after that point one may say, "Now I'm going to do a right anterior oblique" and move three inches up and two inches over. This is the sort of thing that computers can then check on. But demanding that the patient-coordinate system be a fixed thing within the room is in my mind a tremendous error.

GEORGE: I said a repositioning system. I never demanded the patient to be nailed to the couch. But I would be very intrigued to hear you describe the way you're going to do it without locking him on the couch . . . Such a system would be ideal, of course.

FREY: I'm really astonished by the second run, which Dr. Rosenbloom mentioned, of two errors out of 600. When you think that if you say to the patient, "Here is the table, now please get up on it," I would be surprised if the patient would be within two or three centimeters longitudinally, laterally, anywhere, in getting on that table. Either you have a tremendous range that you consider acceptable, or else perhaps the other alternative is the one that Joe Ting said; maybe the technicians are unwilling to go on record as contradicting the computer.

ROSENBLOOM: We don't say that there were no errors in any treatments bar two out of 600. What I said was that there were 600 treatments in which the errors in the parameters which we were monitoring were not out significantly to the extent that they were by any definition wrong. The whole thesis of my argument is that we *have* to rely on radiographers. We can only take some of the responsibility away from them.

STEBEN: I just wanted to answer the points that have been raised by preceding speakers as to the positioning of the patient on the couch. I certainly agree that this is a problem. First of all there is the question of immobilizing the patient. I think this is somewhat an independent question in the sense that the great majority of our betatron patients have not been immobilized. In fact, I don't believe more than one or two out of the hundred or so that we've treated have been immobilized. So that is a separate legitimate concern in itself. In particular if you're treating a head or pituitary or some other case where a very precise positioning is required, I think you do require immobilization. Now the other thing that changes from day to day is the patient contour. Particularly the middle part of a large patient can shift a centimeter or more if the patient is just lying flat. I know that's a separate problem which we haven't quite solved, but it is relevant and it should be studied.

Basically, the coordinates that can be freed, I think, are the two lateral couch motions and the couch rotation. I think that if one relaxes the tolerance on these, it will be helpful. On the other hand, one should prevent the patient from being set up half off the couch. Basically, however, the lack of rigidity of the patient I see as a separate problem. You can't add verification and patient rigidity at the same time. You've got to get the patient in position first, or the technician will never buy it.

NEURATH: I think one can look at verification of patient setups in steps. One doesn't have to do all things at once. A Theratron-80 has ten axes. Most of our patients lie basically parallel to the stretcher. Therefore, the longitudinal and lateral positions of the stretcher are the only variables that depend greatly on where the patient lies. If you verify 8 out of 10 axes, I suggest that you are being an 80 percent help to the technician.

I have one question on the very interesting data of Chung-Bin and his group (which we haven't been able to verify, although we didn't do it for as many patients), regarding the rather large number of what he calls "accidental errors." Do you mark your patient with the total outline of the field? That points up the difference between different institutions. If you mark it up completely, we find that the number of errors are very small when we let the technicians set up the patient to correspond to the marked field.

CHUNG-BIN: The techniques we used are mainly isocentric. We definitely mark the center. But the edges of the field are at the depth of the tumor. So it's really not practical to mark on the skin. Especially, you cannot mark an oblique field on the skin—so, actually, we don't mark; we only mark the isocenter from the front port.

SUNTHARALINGAM: I believe, Mr. Chairman, what we are trying to discuss here is whether record and verify computer systems add reliability to radiation therapy. And I was wondering whether we can go step by step. What are we doing today? Today we are relying—and I believe this is true across the world, not necessarily only in the United States—on radiographers or technicians setting up reproducibly from day to day and delivering the treatment. Occasionally the clinician may go into the treatment room to verify that the patient is being treated as prescribed. The next step is to have the computer record the data, rather than to rely on what the radiographer enters on a form. This is subsequently the patient's next treatment. By doing this, we have taken one step.

Immobilization and patient-treatment gadgets are essential items in radiation therapy. They are going to vary from department to department. It's going to take time. I think if it goes step-by-step, I certainly feel that record and verification is going to lead to good quality radiation therapy.

PRASAD: The question I would like to ask the Rush-Presbyterian group is in regard to the report of various errors. What do they mean in terms of dose delivered to the point of interest?

WACHTOR: This is a very interesting question which another coauthor of our paper, Mr. Kartha, has addressed himself to. He is in the process of publishing an analysis of what happens when these types of errors are made. I don't want to go into a complete rehash of what he has done. But if any of you has in your institution some dosimetry computing capability, try some interesting cases like reversing the wedges 10 percent of the time. Calculate that out and see what happens to your isodose contour. You'll be surprised that nothing happens. I mean, so little happens that you won't really be able to see it.

The same thing applies if 10 percent of the time you treat with a field that's twice as big as it should be. The same thing applies if you miss that entry port by maybe 15 to 30 degrees. You're not going to affect your isodose contour very much.

However, if you do set up the *time* wrong several times and you treat for perhaps three minutes more than you were supposed to over a period of the treatment course, you could affect the dose to the tumor by perhaps 200 rads, which could be highly significant. I think perhaps there should be some more analysis done on what actually should be verified. The thrust of Mr. Kartha's paper is that although many things really do not matter, some things do matter.

GRIEM: I think the group at Rush-Presbyterian and the group at Marsden have made some very important contributions. I think the other important contribution has come from St. Louis, and that is that tumors don't grow in squares and rectangles. And we're seeing more and more shaped fields. As we start to look at the accuracy of a mantle treatment, and the possible errors analyzed node for node in the field, it's important that we think about the problems which Dr. George brought up, and that's how we do set up the patient accurately each day. We've used a system the group at Michael Reese have developed, and that is some reflecting tape and a sensor that looks at this reflecting tape to see if the patient moves during treatment. That seems to work quite well. We don't bolt the patient to the cot.

RAGAN: Both the group at Tufts and the group at Rush have a multiuser or time-shared system on which their verification is done. I'd like each of them to address the problem of how much the degradation of other functions is. What is the response time of their other functions? What is the implication of doing machine verification on the same machine?

NEURATH: I think it's fair to say that for the verification there is no degradation on our system that has ten users. It uses one port for a fraction of a second, so you know you could treat quite a few patients. What takes time isn't the automatic setup but the collision-avoidance calculations.

WACHTOR: We are not doing anything with the automation right now, but on the matter of doing verification and monitoring on time-sharing computers, even the way that we crudely do time-sharing, the program is doing several swaps in a fraction of a second in the CPU. Monitoring two different machines on our unit doesn't make any difference. You do not even know that there is a monitoring verification going on.

CLIFTON: We were asked in this session to consider the questions of both cost and reliability, and of radiation treatment planning. Having listened to some of the discussion, I wonder whether in terms of cost and hence of reliability, we could get some comparative measure of the amount of funds that are actually spent on proper training of technicians or radiographers. It seems to me that we might get a lot more payoff from that than from vast expenditures on automation in order to try and use less skilled technicians.

FREY: I can suggest a far more cost-effective way. Judging from the change in the error rate when technicians know they are being checked, I think all we need to say is "You are now being checked," and we'll decrease the error rate by a considerable factor.

CHUNG-BIN: What is the training of technicians in this country? It turns out that there are several training schools—good training schools—in the United States. We ourselves have a training school. And most of our technicians are supposed to be certified, genuine, good-trained technologists. So usually people say, "I have a better technician than you have," but you really cannot say that because it doesn't matter how careful you are, you always have that chance to dial wrong; it is just a matter of being human, not a matter of how well you're trained.

BJARNGARD: If I remember right, the spread was from half a percent error rate to 5 percent between individuals in your table.

CHUNG-BIN: The error rate is about 2 percent per parameter. That is very much what psychologists have published about repetitive tasks and how frequently mistakes are made.

BJARNGARD: But there was a range of 10 between individuals, to the extent that you looked at it.

CHUNG-BIN: Yes. But you average this out.

KIPPING: In response to the question of the load that control setup places on a computer—I can't talk about the time-share computer, but I can give some fairly accurate numbers on a dedicated system. On the CART I system, which is a 620-L computer—which is roughly like a PDP-11/20 in terms of power (1.8 microseconds cycle time)—for control setup we normally run through the algorithm every 50 milliseconds. For a Clinac-4 without a beam stopper, it takes approximately 30 percent of the CPU time to run through the algorithm. For a Clinac-4 it takes about 40 percent. So that gives you an idea of the load. Our rough perception of the load that it takes for verification is significantly less than one percent of the CPU time.

SMITH: I was rather concerned to hear what Mr. Wachtor said about hardware reliability problems and I'd like to ask him to explain that further.

WACHTOR: The largest problem that we've had is that we got into this game very early, and we wrote our own time-sharing operating system. In a multi-user operating system, operating in an unprotected environment, this provides for a lot of crashes. Someone does something wrong on a FORTRAN program and the whole thing goes down. When this occurs, the technicians who are interfered with in their use of the computer for verification get quite angry at us and to retaliate will not use the verify system for the next hour. Things of that nature. The hardware problems have been ordinary types of hardware problems—a disc goes down or the CPU has gone down, or the problem is that the terminal has gone down. We had a tremendous problem in June—we were down from June 6 virtually through July 1 with innumerable problems—but outside of that one major disaster, hardware reliability has been fairly good.

ELLIS: I understood Mr. Wachtor to say that if he reversed the wedge, it didn't make any difference to the isodose distribution. There's something wrong somewhere—I can't believe it.

WACHTOR: If you have the ability to calculate this on a computer or do the hand calculations, try it. Reverse the wedges 10 percent of the time and you will be amazed how little the result changes.

HOLT: One comment on reversing treatment parameters is that you might very well run the risk of changing your time-dose relationships, which could be very important because you're changing gradients. But what I really wanted to comment on was the fact that while I'm a strong believer in the monitoring of therapy setups, I would also suggest that part of this could be included in the equipment itself. Now that the new generation of therapy equipment already has a computer built in that will monitor those devices for verification, there are a lot more important features than field size or distance. There are machine parameters, as the bending magnet current, which are perhaps as important as, if not more important than, some of the parameters we've been discussing.

And if one looks toward the future, I think we should insist that the manufacturer build stability into the dosimetry equipment, i.e. the equipment in the machine that displays the dose in a monitored way, to be compatible with the standards that we demand as far as precision is concerned.

Session IV: Contributed Short Papers on Automated Treatments

1. Computer Operations for Support of Pion Radiotherapy at Los Alamos

A. Lundy
M. Minor
S. Shlaer

A facility for testing the value of negative pions for radiation therapy of cancer is starting operation as part of the Clinton P. Anderson Meson Physics Facility (LAMPF) at the Los Alamos Scientific Laboratory in Los Alamos, New Mexico. LAMPF is a linear accelerator approximately one kilometer long which is designed to accelerate one milliampere (average current) of protons to an energy of 800 MeV and provide beam to several targets simultaneously on a non-interfering basis. The radiobiology and radiation therapy facility is a self-contained facility for studying the biological effects of negative pions and for evaluating their usefulness for cancer therapy by conducting clinical trials with patients. The facility includes laboratories for dosimetry, treatment planning, cellular radiobiology, animal preparation, plus patient waiting room, examining rooms, consulting rooms, a simulator room, mask and mold room, patient staging areas, and the pion treatment room.

The negative pions are produced when the high energy proton beam from the accelerator impinges on a carbon target. Since large quantities of other radiations are also produced by the target, a system of large focusing and bending magnets penetrating through a dense shield is used to filter out unwanted radiations and to transmit pions of appropriate energy to the treatment room. The resultant pion beam has a fixed vertical downward orientation. The beam cross section at stopping depth in tissue is rectangular and very narrow on one axis ($\sim 1\ 1/2$ cm) so a horizontal scanning technique will have to be used to treat nearly all tumors. The well defined penetration range of pions coupled with their large dose deposition near the stopping point will require that scanning techniques also be used to scan the tumor vertically.

The following computer uses are planned in the facility (status as of August 1974 as indicated):

1. Control and monitoring of the pion beam line (operational).
2. Experimental data acquisition: data-taking on experiments for beam-line tuning, beam characterization, and dosimetry studies (semi-operational).
3. Beam-line modeling: ray-tracing programs to predict channel performance and aid in beam-line tuning (operational) (1).
4. Treatment couch and beam energy degrader control: dynamic control of scanning functions during treatment to achieve semi-optimized dose distributions tailored for each patient (scheduled mid-1975).
5. Pion beam treatment-planning: an interactive code designed for easy operator utilization. The code corrects for inhomogeneities and will calculate the three-dimensional dose distribution given sufficient time. (Basic computational code with graphic film output (2) is operational in batch mode on a CDC 7600 at present. Conversion to run on the biomed facility computer is in progress.)
6. Simulator data-logging: automated data-logging of couch and collimator settings to minimize time required for initial treatment-room setup of patients. Semi-automated patient contour measurement. (Scheduled late 1975).
7. Patient record-keeping (probably late 1975).
8. Treatment parameter data-logging and monitoring: checking of all pertinent treatment parameters during treatment and print out of parameters at the end of each treatment to go in patients chart file (in progress, scheduled September 1974).
9. Communications link to UNM Cancer Center for transmitting treatment plans, patient data, etc.: Two-thousand baud auto-dial link planned. This is to allow easy exchange of clinical data, including treatment-plan plots between people at the Cancer Center at Albuquerque who will be directing the clinical work and the staff at Los Alamos. (Scheduled mid-1975.)

The development of the computer system was influenced strongly by the experience of the LAMPF staff in developing a real time multi-tasking operating system for the accelerator control computer (3) and by experience in developing a multi-computer experimental data-acquisition system for nuclear physics experiments (4). The particular computer used is a Digital Equipment Corp. (DEC) PDP-11/45 with floating point hardware multiply and divide, 96K of memory (8K MOS), and using DEC's RSX-11D real time, multi-tasking operating system. Peripherals are listed in Figure 1.

The 20 × 20 inch graphic digitizing tablet, the 20-inch electrostatic printer-plotter, and one of the storage display terminals are located in the treatment-planning room. Some computer-interfaced knobs will also be located in the treatment-planning room to allow changing beam parameters quickly in the treatment planning code.

Another storage display terminal is located in the physics counting area to allow beam-line and experimental data-acquisition program control from that location.

Nearly all special hardware interfacing is done using commercial hardware built to the international CAMAC standard (5, 6, 7). The CAMAC System is diagrammed in Figure 2. This system has proven to be extremely flexible, allowing rapid connection of new apparatus and reconfiguration of existing apparatus when needed. All interlocking which bears on personnel safety or machine hardware protection is hardwired but monitored by the computer through the CAMAC interface. A software-controlled interlock is also provided on the beam. The channel-control system involves 96 binary (on/off) command channels, 264 binary data channels, 43 pulse motor drives, and 128 analog data channels. CAMAC interfaced programmable buttons and knobs with alphanumeric displays based on hardware developed for accelerator control (8) have been installed on the console to permit very easy operator interaction. Software has not been completed for these as yet. A color character display scope with a light pen on the console is used to display channel operating parameters, and the light pen will ultimately be used to make control program selection. This also is CAMAC interfaced as are two IBM 729IV magnetic tape drives. The CAMAC branch highway is interfaced to the computer through a locally designed microprogrammed branch driver (MDB) (9). This is a small computer with 1536 words of 16-bit memory. The code to handle all routine CAMAC branch highway operations resides in the MBD. (MBD units are commercially available). A datascan program is used to scan all the data from the process control equipment at a rate of at least once per second and updates a core buffer in the PDP-11. Separate display programs use data from this buffer to generate displays scaled with proper engineering units.

The codes to monitor proper channel performance during radiation exposure provide for two levels of action. An unexpected binary indication may be programmed either to shut off the beam or to present a warning message to the operator. Similarly, analog data may have two tolerance ranges specified, one in which only a warning message will be presented and another in which automatic beam shutoff will occur.

A treatment-parameter logging program will provide a hard copy printout (which can be placed with the patient's chart) of all pertinent control settings and the date and time of treatment.

The details of just how patient set-up verifications will be done have not been perfected, but it is planned to enter data into the system at the time treatment planning is done and to require operator entry of the data again at the time of treatment to check for verification. It must be possible to change the treatment plan readily at the time of treatment while making accidental change nearly impossible.

Control of the beam-scanning functions during treatment is a complex task which must be done with very low probability of undetected error. Special hardware to handle this task is being planned, and a microprocessor may be utilized. The problem is complicated by the varying RBE over the pion-stopping region and the desire to treat tumors which vary in vertical thickness as a function of horizontal position. This implies nonlinear vertical-scanning functions which vary during the treatment as a function of horizontal beam position and tumor thickness in order to deliver a treatment of uniform biological effect throughout the treatment volume. The scanning velocity must also be scaled to the instantaneous pion beam intensity from the channel.

While medical record-keeping is planned on the system, this is keyed to work to be done at the UNM Cancer Center in Albuquerque. They have installed a PDP-11/40 and have a 20-million-word disc on order for it. That both the Albuquerque and the Los Alamos facilities are new and have not previously handled patients should make the development of an acceptable medical-records system somewhat easier.

Beam-line tuning studies at the facility began in February of this year, dosimetry in April, and radiobiology work in June, and the first work with humans (treatment of skin nodules on terminal patients) is scheduled for September. This rapid schedule has been dictated by the desire to do radiobiology experiments which require several months of follow-up, before a scheduled accelerator shut-down of several months in the first part of 1975. This schedule has interfered somewhat with an orderly development of the computer system, but enough experience has been gained to prove the feasibility of real-time, multitasking operation of the system.

We believe a computer system such as that described (of which there are now probably several commercial vendors) offers many advantages for a conventional radiation therapy department. One can start with a true mini-computer of modest cost doing a single task. As demand increases, a multitasking operating system can be added, and memory expanded as needed. Experience and programs developed with the smaller system remain usable. Machine verification and automated set-up, treatment-planning, patient record-keeping and billing, and special research studies are all possible on a single system without time-scheduling problems. The use of a standard hardware interfacing system like CAMAC offers easy interfacing of a wide variety of special equipment and makes the interfacing problems independent of the brand of computer used.

REFERENCES

1. Crandall, K. R., *TRACE: An Interactive Beam-Transport Program.* LA-5332, Report, Los Alamos Scientific Laboratory, Los Alamos, N.M. (1973).
2. Shlaer, W. J., PIPLAN, A Treatment Planning Code for Pion Radiation Therapy. LA-5433-MS, Report, Los Alamos Scientific Laboratory, Los Alamos, N.M. (1973).
3. Butler, H. S., *Proceedings of the Instrument Society of America*, 1970 Conference. Philadelphia, October 26–29, (1970).
4. Anderson, H. L., Bevington, P. R., Buchanan, J. A., Butler, H. S., Chrien, R. E., Kirsten, F. A., Synder, J. N., and Thomas, R. F., LAMPF Data-Acquisition System. LA-4504-MS. Los Alamos Scientific Laboratory, Los Alamos, N. M. (1970).
5. Costrell, L., ed. "CAMAC tutorial issue," *IEEE Transactions on Nuclear Science*, NS-20:2 (1973).
6. Shea, R. F., ed., "CAMAC tutorial issue," *IEEE Transactions on Nuclear Science*, NS-18:2 (1971).
7. U.S. AEC Reports, TID-25875, TID-25876, and TID-26488. Available from Louis Costrell, National Bureau of Standards, Washington, D.C.
8. Hartway, B. L., *IEEE Transactions on Nuclear Science*, NS-20:3, 531-535 (1973).
9. Biswell, L. R., and Rajala, R. E., *Design and Operation of a Microprogrammed Branch Driver for a PDP-11 Computer*, LA-5144 Report, Los Alamos Scientific Laboratory of the University of California, Los Alamos, N. M. (1973).

QUESTIONS

DAHLIN: Are you working in the field of narrow-beam surgery or narrow-beam therapy, too, with the pions?

LUNDY: No, the interest is primarily in larger tumors, and in fact, a pion beam probably is not particularly well suited for narrow-beam work.

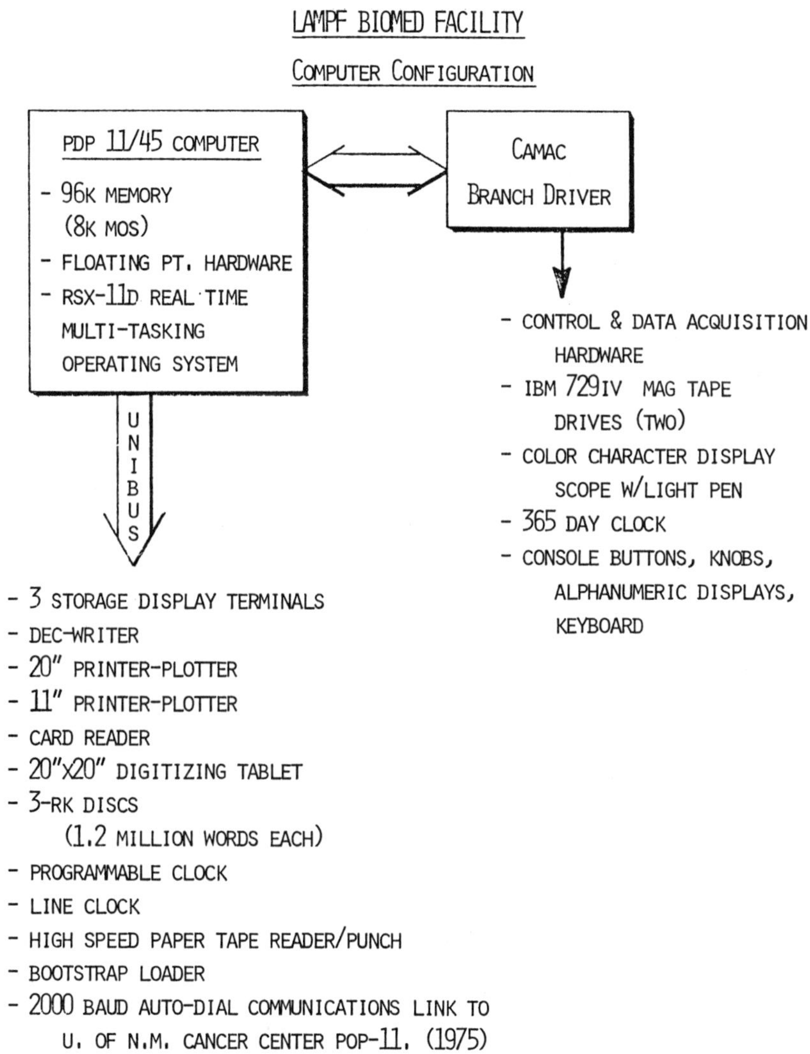

Figure 1. Lampf Biomed Facility Computer Configuration

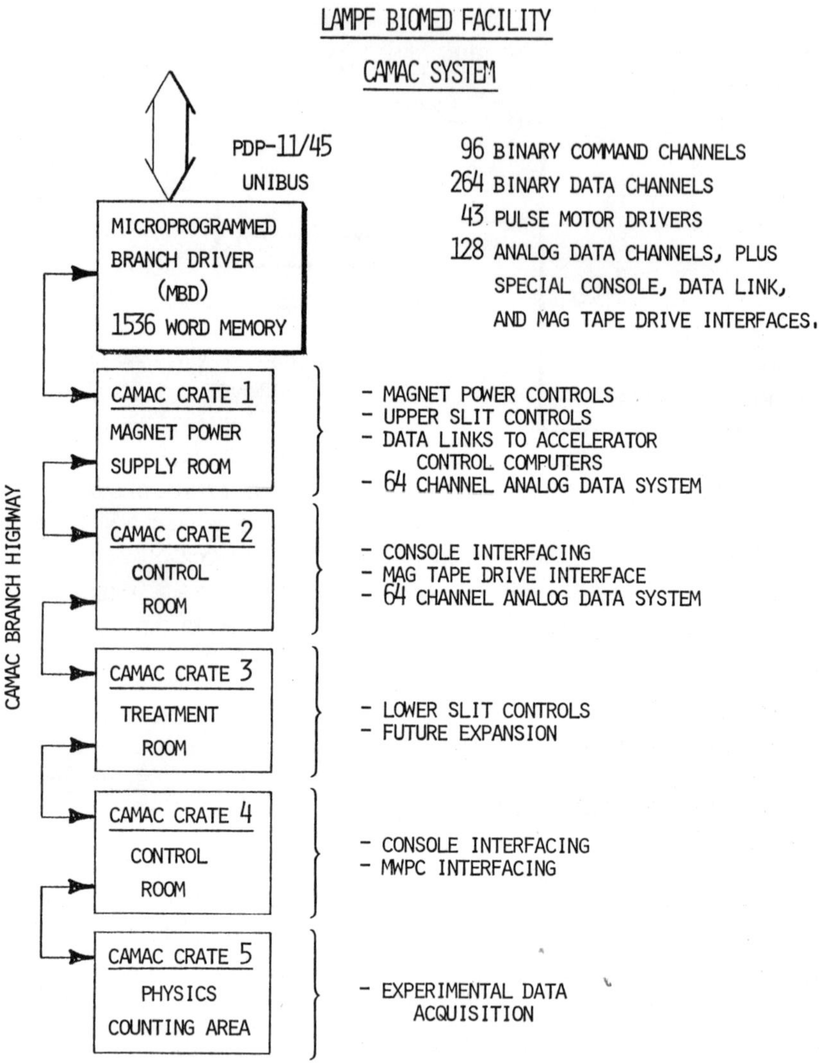

Figure 2. Lampf Biomed Facility CAMAC System

2. An Integrated Approach to Simulator and Treatment Unit Automation

C. J. Karzmark
D. C. Rust

The automation of radiotherapy treatment units using digital mini-computers has proceeded via treatment-prescription verification, since this is most easily implemented. Prescription verification can reduce treatment-delivery error but in itself is likely to increase costs. In justifying automation of the treatment unit from economic considerations, therefore, one usually cites higher utilization factors along with a higher dose delivery rate. The chances for error increase under these high treatment rate conditions, taxing contemporary treatment surveillance practice. This burden can logically be assumed by the mini-computer. It is our contention, however, that treatment-unit automation with interactive simulation as an integrated part of the system is more readily justified on economic grounds than treatment prescription verification only (1).

For improved space utilization an orthovoltage treatment unit can be efficiently combined with a megavoltage simulator. To this end we have constructed and installed a simulator closely duplicating the Varian Clinac 4 treatment unit. The simulator will provide the initial input for an automated Clinac 4 treatment unit. The simulator has been installed in a room together with an overhead mounted orthovoltage treatment unit so as to conserve space and accommodate two functions: simulation of patients for megavoltage therapy, and orthovoltage treatment. The Clinac 4 treatment couch incorporated in the system is shared for these two functions. The orthovoltage treatment unit is positioned overhead in a remote corner of the room when not in use.

Our studies have indicated that improved patient care can be achieved and savings achieved by using megavoltage treatment facilities exclusively for treatment while employing separate treatment simulators to provide tumor localization and treatment plan verification (1). Additionally, they suggest that automation of certain aspects of simulation and treatment would likely affect further economies in some environments. Moreover, since the simulator would, in many çenters, require less than full-time use, it was thought economically beneficial to incorporate a suitable orthovoltage treatment unit in the simulator room, using the treatment couch for both megavoltage simulation and orthovoltage treatment. We believe that this facility, only recently activated, will be efficient in the use of space, equipment, and personnel.

In order to test our hypotheses, we have constructed and installed a simulator closely duplicating our Clinac 4 treatment unit together with an overhead-mounted orthovoltage treatment unit (Philips RT 255). The 250 KVP constant potential orthovoltage treatment unit (2) is ceiling-mounted and positioned out of the way when using the simulator. The Clinac 4 treatment unit and simulator have identical couches, and computer-readable transducers are being installed on gantry, treatment head, and couch motions of both units. A Digital Equipment Corporation PDP-11 computer system incorporating two central processors has been installed for the automation role described below as well as for additional radiotherapy department tasks. A block diagram of this system is illustrated in Figure 1.

Each Clinac 4 patient will be given a file number badge upon registry. The simulator room will be equipped with a computer terminal which is used to initiate the patient's daily therapy record, including treatment prescription. Positional parameters will be sampled directly from simulator transducer positions corresponding to the treatment prescription. Once agreed, this treatment information will be stored on disk file for daily access and updating during the course of therapy. It will be accessed and treatment parameters set for each treatment. A record and confirm operation will be incorporated, although the technologist will provide vernier positioning and have final override authority.

Figure 2 shows the Clinac 4 simulator positioned over the Clinac 4 treatment couch. The associated diagnostic unit is capable of 125 KV and 300 mA exposures. The retractable film cassette holder, which is mounted opposite the treatment head and rotates with the gantry, provides source-film distances (SFDs) over the range of 95 to 150 cm with the isocenter located at 80 cm source-axis-distance (SAD) from the target. Although our Clinac 4 simulator has been constructed using a simple structural framework, its external dimensions coincide with those of the treatment unit by the use of Clinac 4 fiberglass covers. Many of the components of the Clinac 4 have been incorporated in the treatment head with the 125 KVP diagnostic tube.

REFERENCES

1. Karzmark, C. J. and Rust, D. C., *Radiology*, *105*, 157-161, 1972.
2. Wichmann, H., *Medicamundi* (Rome), *11*, 61-62, 1965.
3. Wichmann, H., *Fortschritte auf dem Gebiete der Rontgenstrahlen*, *106*, 614-617, 1967.

QUESTIONS

GOITEIN: Why did you choose to read out the CLINAC-4 and not the orthovoltage unit in that room?

KARZMARK: I believe your question refers to the positional parameters of the orthovoltage unit. I guess we don't regard it as so important. The orthovoltage unit is for palliative therapy. It's not used frequently, but we feel we should have the facility both for training and for the few cases where it is appropriate. I don't think the treatment procedures are quite the same or quite as precise for most of the orthovoltage treatments.

FREY: Do you feel that you can trust adequately the setup parameter values from the simulator to be put into the computer and then use these same numbers to set up the Clinac in the other room? If not, what techniques are going to be used to make sure that you have appropriate calibration between them?

KARZMARK: As I understand your question, Harvey, I think that eventually the electromechanical transfer of the coordinate positions from the simulator to the record on the disc back into the treatment unit will be done faithfully. If you're talking about this question that we've tossed around earlier about the precise patient position, then I don't think they will be. As I envision this, the purpose of the prepositioning is to give you the approximate positional locations. And it is the technician's responsibility to provide the final orientation. I think that precise setting of the gantry angle is possible and useful. The x-y positioning of the patient will clearly have to be zeroed in by observation, in my opinion.

ACKNOWLEDGMENTS

This work has been supported by Research Grant CA 05838 from the National Cancer Institute, N.I.H.

We are indebted to Varian Associates for donating many of the components for construction of the Clinac 4 simulator.

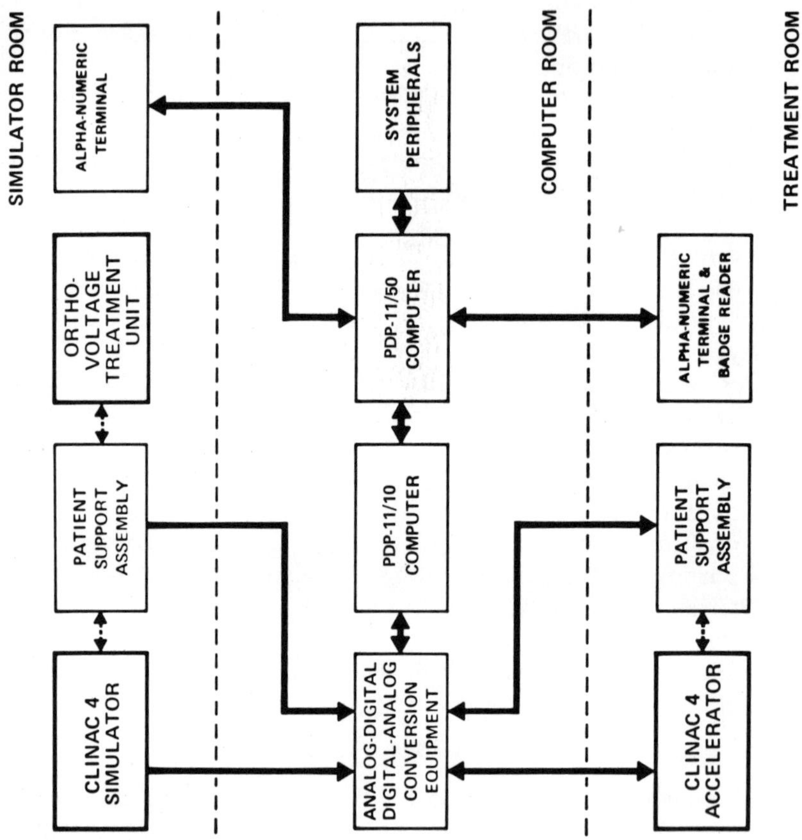

Figure 1. Functional block diagram of Clinac 4 radiotherapy automation system illustrating equipment located in simulator, computer and treatment rooms.

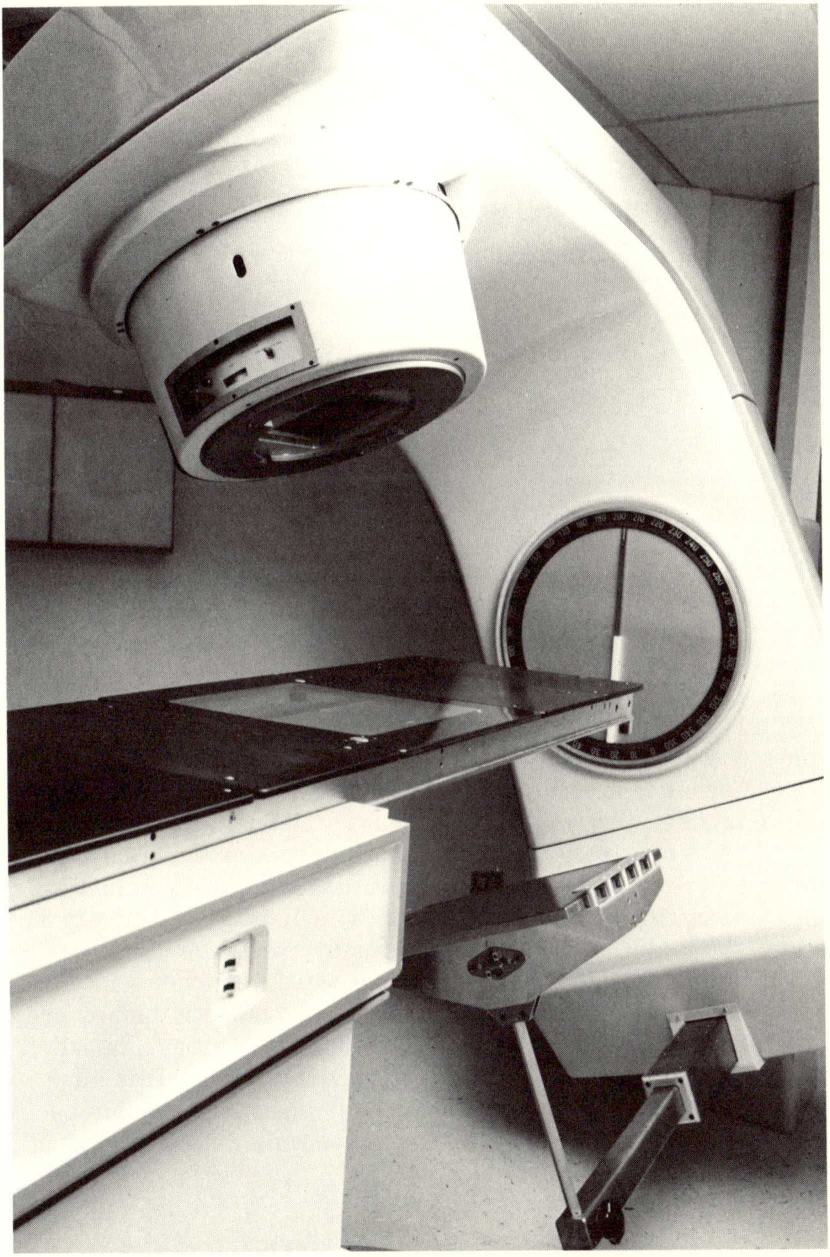

Figure 2. Clinac 4 simulator including treatment couch and retractable, demountable, variable SFD film/cassette holder.

3. The Potential of Computer Control to Improve Dose Distributions in Radiation Therapy

B. Bjarngard
P. Kijewski

Introduction

From the very beginning of radiotherapy a great deal of ingenuity has been applied toward delivering a maximum dose to a tumor volume while sparing adjacent healthy tissue. A solution to this problem was especially urgent during the days when only orthovoltage machines, with their poor depth-dose characteristics, were available (1). Even with high energy photon radiation as provided by modern machines, however, the freedom to shape dose distributions is limited. While multiple field techniques are important advances from a single field or parallel, opposed fields, they have the limitation that in practice no more than a few fields can be set up for any one treatment. One way to overcome this limitation is to change field parameters continuously during treatment. This is done in rotational treatments. In fact, the gantry angle is the only machine parameter one can change on present-day therapy machines while treatment is in progress. There are nine adjustable parameters on a modern therapy machine: three couch translations, couch rotation, two field-size adjustments, field rotation, gantry rotation, and dose-rate adjustment. Moving the collimator jaws independently brings the total number of adjustable parameters to eleven. One can speculate as to how much better dose distributions could be shaped if machine parameters other than gantry angle could be changed as well. It is the purpose of this paper to explore this possibility.

Many essential features of the technique of changing machine parameters during treatment, hereafter referred to as dynamic treatment (2), can be discussed without elaborate calculations. Simplified geometrical considerations give a good insight into some of the things one can do with this technique.

In the past, dynamic treatment techniques have been based on machine control by means of mechanical devices or electronic hardwire schemes (3). These methods are inflexible and cumbersome. Recent developments in computer technology have drastically expanded the possibilities to translate dynamic treatment into practice.

1. Motion of Collimator Jaws

1.A. General. One of the simpler forms of dynamic treatment is a displacement of the collimator jaws while the radiation beam in on (2). Quite a variety of dose distributions can be generated in this way, and this simple technique will become part of many more complex schemes. Assume that a field size a*b is set up, and just as the beam is turned on, one of the collimator jaws starts to move toward the center with a velocity v(x) and continues until it comes in contact with the other jaw. This is illustrated by Figure 1. It is apparent that a high dose will be deposited in the right portion of the field and very little dose in the left portion of the field. This dose distribution is not unlike that of a wedged field.

The dose at any point in tissue can be calculated as follows. The point x_0 (Fig. 1) is exposed to radiation for the time it takes for the edge of the beam to move from $x = 0$ to $x = x_0$:

$$t = \int_0^{x_0} \frac{dx}{v(x)}$$

If we assume that the dose rate $\dot{D}(d)$ at the depth d with open collimators is independent of the lateral position (x_0) and is caused by primary photons only, the total dose is

$$(1) \qquad D(x_0,d) = \dot{D}(d) * t = \dot{D}(d) \int_0^{x_0} \frac{dx}{v(x)}$$

1.B. Constant jaw velocity. With a jaw moving at constant speed across a radiation field, i.e. v(x) constant, one can show that the angle θ an isodose contour makes with the central axis is given by

$$(2) \qquad \tan\theta = \frac{\partial D}{\partial x_0} \frac{\partial D}{\partial d} = \frac{1}{x_0 \left(\frac{1}{D}\frac{\partial D}{\partial d}\right)}$$

The term in parentheses is the percentage decrease in dose with depth and can be taken from depth dose tables. For the special case that the dose changes with depth as $e^{-\mu d}$ the wedge angle θ on the central axis ($x_0 = \frac{b}{2}$) is

(3) $$\theta = \tan^{-1} \frac{2}{\mu b}$$

This result is interesting in that it indicates that the wedge angle is independent of jaw velocity. However, the wedge angle does depend on field size. Taking a typical field size of 20 cm and $\mu = 0.06\text{cm}^{-1}$, the wedge angle is $\theta = 59°$. This angle represents the maximum angle that can be obtained with a moving jaw technique for this field size.

A lesser angle can always be attained by adding a flat field. The relationship between the new wedge angle θ' and the fraction f of the total dose on the central axis contributed by the unwedged field is:

(4) $$\tan \theta' = (1-f) \tan \theta$$

1.C. Variable jaw velocity. Using equation (1), it is possible to deduce the dose distributions one gets when the jaw velocity v(x) changes during irradiation. Since the integrand is always positive, the dose must increase monotonically from one end of the field to the other. There can be no dips in the distribution, and the maximum is always at one edge of the field. If both jaws are permitted to move, however, the maximum dose can be anywhere in the field. To calculate the resulting dose, equation (1) is applied to both jaws independently. Figure 2 illustrates the motion of the jaws.

Fields with two or more dose maxima can be achieved by combining two or more exposures. In conclusion, fields with a single maximum are easy to generate, and they are the ones most often encountered. More complex distributions are possible, but are more difficult to execute.

1.D. Extension to two dimensions. Above it was assumed that only one pair of collimator jaws was moving, with the orthogonal pair remaining stationary. It is possible to move all four jaws simultaneously. For instance, if the four jaws move from an original position of a rectangular field to being completely closed, the isodose lines in a cross-sectional plane will look as shown in Figure 3. The dose along the dotted lines in Figure 3 can again be calculated from equation (1), by considering each jaw separately.

Limitations of this technique are that the isodose contours are approximated by squares, and that the intensity increases monotonically toward the maximum. Additional intensity peaks can be added by repeating the procedure for each peak.

When the dose distribution in a patient has been perturbed by an irregular surface or the presence of inhomogeneities, this technique can be used to compensate for the perturbation. This is the dynamic treatment equivalent of the compensator.

2. Linear Motion of Treatment Couch

The lateral or longitudinal displacement of the couch during treatment is a basic form of dynamic treatment. If the couch is moved without changing any other machine parameters, a longer field than is normally available can be treated. However, the dose at the beginning and end of the motion only gradually increases toward the maximum.

The slope at the edges of the dose distribution is determined by the field size. The larger the field, the more gradually will the dose increase toward the maximum. The reason is that the edges of the treated region are exposed to the radiation field for a shorter period of time than is the central region. Adding jaw motion to the motion of the table will produce a flat field. The technique is illustrated in Figure 4.

So far it has been assumed that the width of the field was fixed during motion. If these jaws are moved as well, irregular field outlines can be generated.

3. Rotations

3.A. Rotation with simultaneous motion of the collimator jaws. The advantage of conventional 360° rotational treatment is that the tumor dose is high compared to the dose to surrounding tissue. Good uniformity across the tumor volume can be achieved, especially if the volume is centrally located in relation to the surface. In clinical situations where it is not possible to execute a complete rotation, one can retain the advantage of distributing the surface dose by executing a partial rotation. However, compared to a complete rotation the region of uniform dose becomes smaller and the maximum dose moves away from the axis of rotation toward the surface. One technique to overcome these disadvantages of arc therapy is the use of wedges to improve the dose distribution (4, 5).

Note (Fig. 5) that in the absence of wedges, beams of equal intensity directed at points A and B will result in a lesser dose to B, since there is more overlying tissue at this point. The wedges are arranged in such a way that a higher-intensity beam is directed toward the deeper-lying part of the tumor volume. In this manner the dose at A and B in Figure 5 can be equalized, resulting in a much more uniform tumor dose and a maximum near the axis of rotation.

It is possible to replace the arced-wedge technique with a dynamic treatment procedure by manipulating the position of the collimator jaws during rotation. The sequence of events is shown in Figure 6. At the beginning of the rotation the field is small and aimed at point B. As the gantry rotates, jaw number 2 is moved to increase field size, and points closer and closer to A are exposed to the beam. The angle at which the field size becomes maximum is adjusted so that points A and B receive equal amounts of dose. The gantry then moves with constant field size to the complementary angle on the other side of the vertical, at which point jaw number 1 is moved so that the field size decreases again. At the end of the motion the field size is the same as at the beginning of the gantry motion. The complete exposure results in uniform dose distribution in the form of a cylinder with an elliptical cross-section and a maximum near the axis of rotation.

Nothing of what has been said above requires that the axis of rotation fall within the irradiated volume. The proper use of rotation and moving collimators is equivalent to a rotation around another axis. The technique is to move the jaws during rotation in such a manner that the radiation field conforms to the tumor volume.

3.B. Motion of the collimator jaws through the isocenter. By moving the collimator jaws through the isocenter, dose distributions in the form of a hollow cylinder can be produced. Consider the simple case of a complete rotation with one of the jaws always in such a position that the region in the vicinity of the axis of rotation is shielded by this jaw for all gantry angles (Figure 7). Only scattered radiation can reach the core of the volume, resulting in a low dose near the center and an isodose contour in the form of a hollow cylinder. The cylinder does not need to have a circular cross section if the jaws are moving during rotation. A cylindrical shell can be irradiated by doing only a partial rotation.

3.C. The multi-section collimator. So far we have looked only at the shape of the dose distribution in a two dimensional plane. Because of the outline of the radiation field, the three-dimensional extension of the isodose contour will be in the form of hollow cylinder. In case the tumor volume cannot be readily fitted to such a simple shape, one has the option of generating several such cylindrical contours, and joining them. The result is schematically illustrated by Figure 8.

The same result can be achieved with a multi-section collimator, as described by Ueda and coworkers (6), who control the sections by mechanical devices. This makes the system somewhat inflexible, and computer control is ideally suited to adjust such a multiplicity of machine parameters.

The action of a single pair of sections of a multisection collimator is the same as for the standard set of jaws already discussed. Only now one has the option of simultaneously generating a number of adjacent cylindrical dose volumes (Figure 8), which may have different diameters. Also the axes of the individual cylinders can be in different position. Only in the case of very long tumor volumes will it be necessary to adjoin two or more separately exposed dose distributions. The alternative of a simultaneous couch translation and rotation is considerably more complex, but might prove to be viable.

Partial rotations pose a special problem for a multisection collimator. The difficulty arises when some of the cylindrical dose volumes lie at a substantially greater depth than others. Those parts of the tumor volume lying closer to the surface receive a larger dose than those lying deeper inside the tissue. The most obvious way to overcome this problem is to make the treatment arc smaller for sections that irradiate tumor volume closer to the surface. The gantry still moves through the full arc, but the sections corresponding to more superficial volumes are kept closed until the appropriate angle, at which time they move through a sequence of positions corresponding to the shorter arc. As a consequence, the exposure time is reduced and hot spots are avoided.

Summary and Conclusion

We have discussed various techniques to optimize dose distributions by changing machine parameters when the radiation beam is on, a method commonly referred to as dynamic treatment.

The dose distributions that can be achieved by moving collimator jaws or the treatment couch or the gantry show that these simple techniques by themselves can be of value. Treatment schemes that require the simultaneous motion of several machine parameters are more difficult to visualize but ultimately more useful. The procedure we find most promising is a combination of collimator jaw motion and gantry rotation. It permits the deposition of a dose distribution in the form of a solid or hollow cylinder at an arbitrary depth. Several methods, including the use of a multisection collimator, can serve to extend this technique to get dose distributions in the form of several adjoining cylinders, each of which can have a different diameter and axis position.

We have not discussed all possible combinations of machine motions and have limited the discussion to photon beams. Furthermore, our treatment of the subject has been conceptual rather than based on a complete analysis of the dose distributions. However, even with these limitations we conclude that dynamic treatment offers interesting opportunities to optimize dose distributions in radiation therapy and deserves further study.

REFERENCES

1. Wachsmann, F., Barth, G., Lanzl, L., Carpender, J., *Moving Field Radiation Therapy*, University of Chicago Press, Chicago (1962).
2. Neblett, D. L., Schaeflein, J. W., Haymond, H. R., George III, F. W., Ahten, E. R., Mackinney, J. G., in *Proceedings, Fifth International Conference on the Use of Computers in Radiation Therapy*, Dartmouth College, August (1974).
3. Ilfeld, D. N., Wright, K. A., Salzman, F. A., *Am. J. Roentgenol., Rad. Ther. and Nucl. Med., 112:* 792 (1971).
4. Welker, K., *Strahlentherapie, 128,* 514 (1965).
5. Welker, K., *Strahlentherapie, 132,* 497 (1967).
6. Morita, K., Kimura, C., Takahashi, K., and Ueda, T., *Strahlentherapie, 147,* 487 (1974).

QUESTIONS

CUNNINGHAM: Your suggestion of this dynamic collimator is not at all far out. In fact, it's about twenty years old. It was done about the late 1940's, I think, by Wilson in England, and much more recently but still a fair time back, by Takahashi in Japan. They called it "Conformation Therapy" in the latter case.

KIJEWSKI: We are all very well aware of that. The shortcoming of their technique is that it's done in a mechanical fashion. The collimator jaws are controlled by cams, which makes the system very inflexible. And we think if you use a computer and control the individual sections in that manner, you have much greater flexibility and control when you move the jaws.

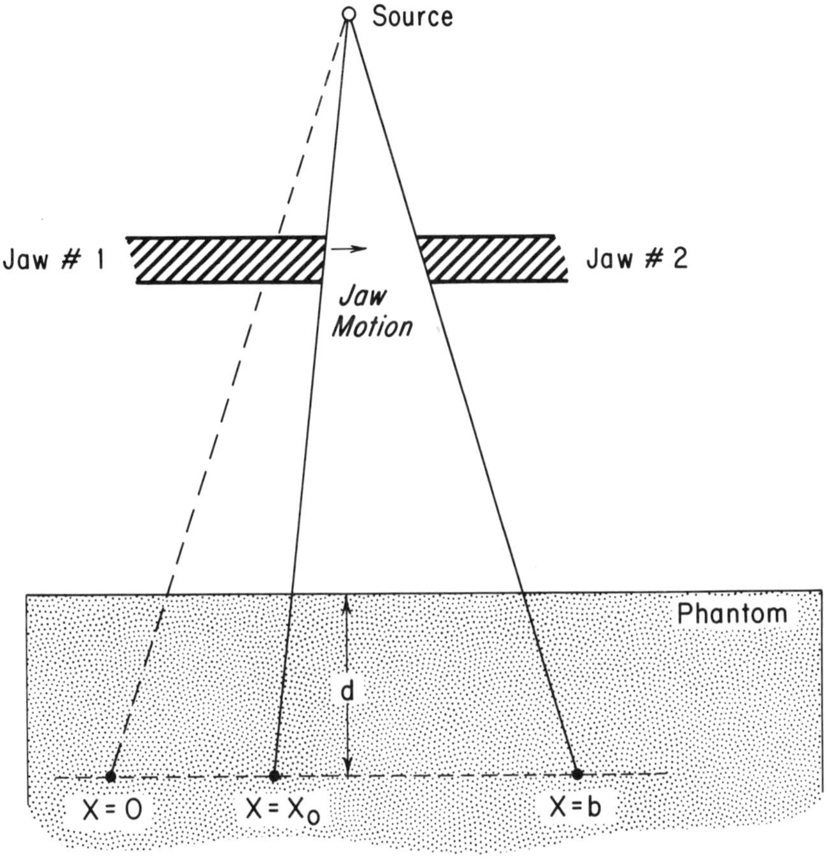

Figure 1. Motion of a single collimator jaw to produce a wedge shaped dose distribution

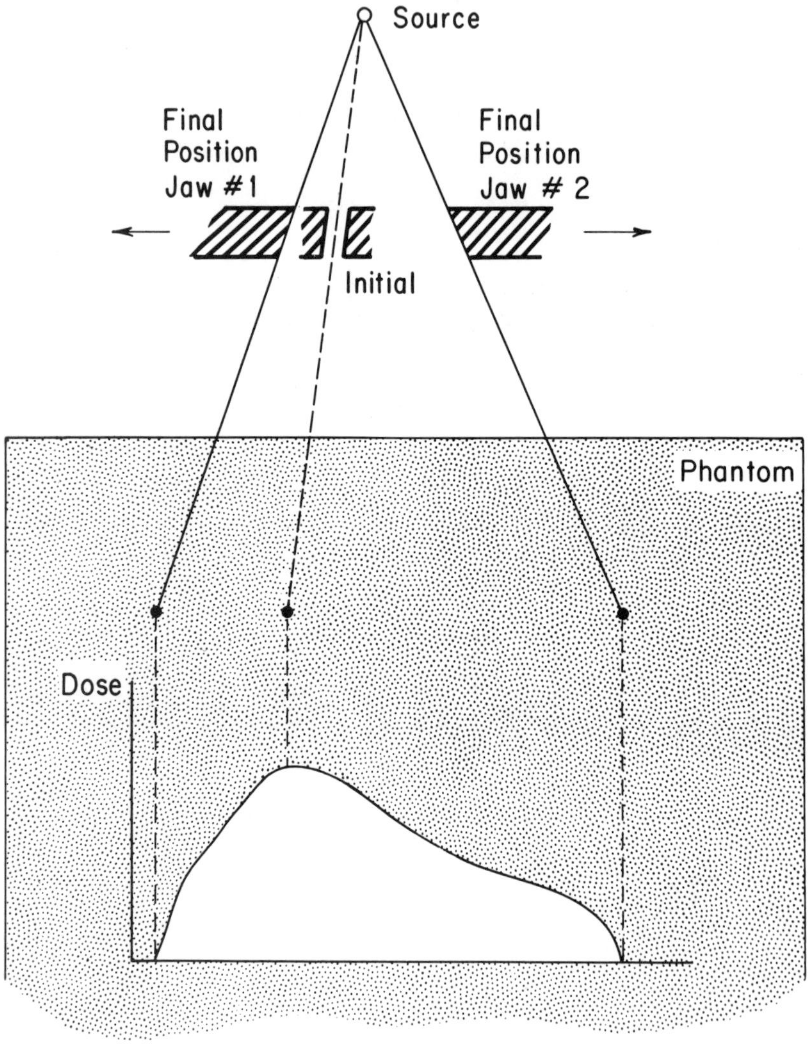

Figure 2. Dynamic treatment equivalent of a one dimensional compensator with simultaneous motion of two independent collimator jaws

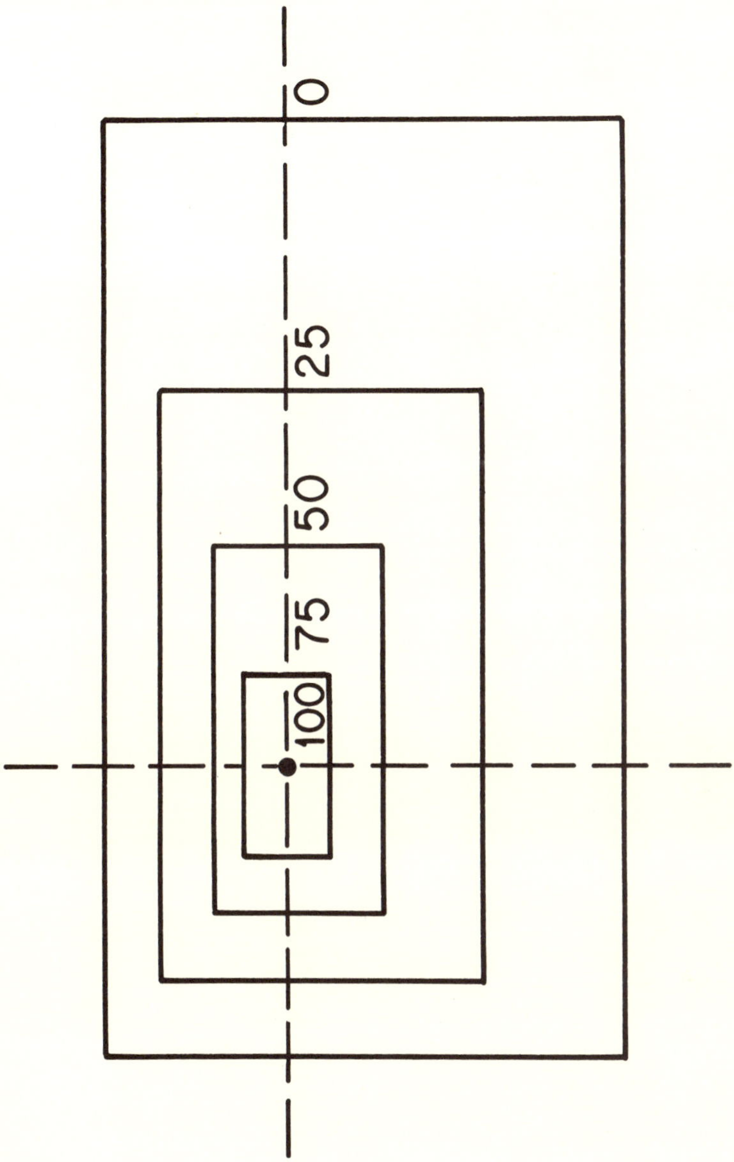

Figure 3. Isodose contours in a plane perpendicular to the central axis obtained with the motion of four independent collimator jaws

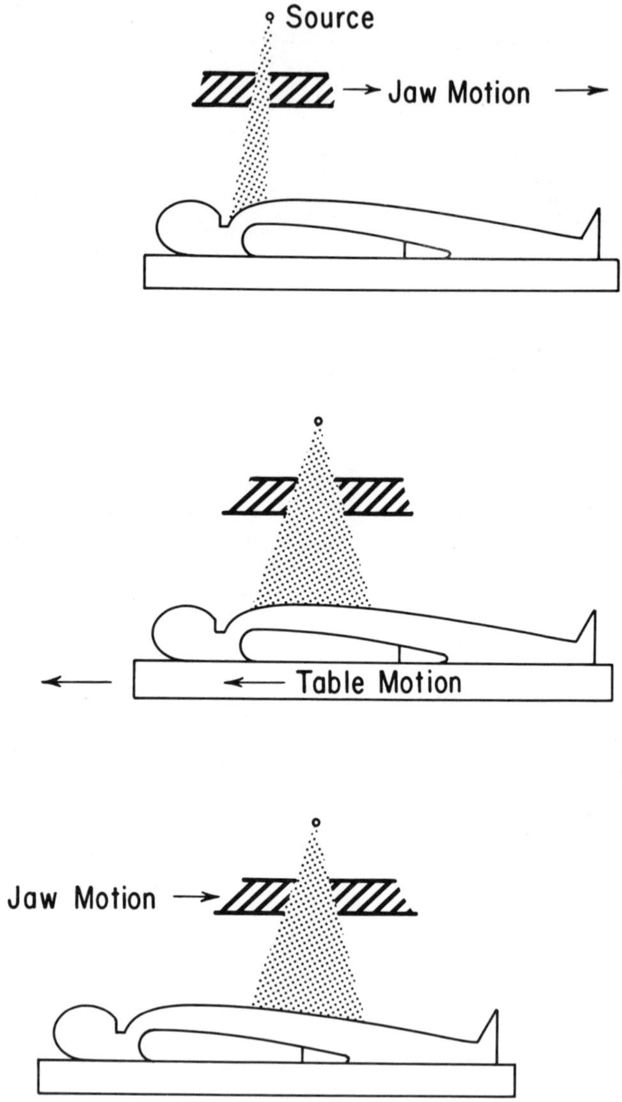

Figure 4. Large area flat field generated with jaw motion and table motion

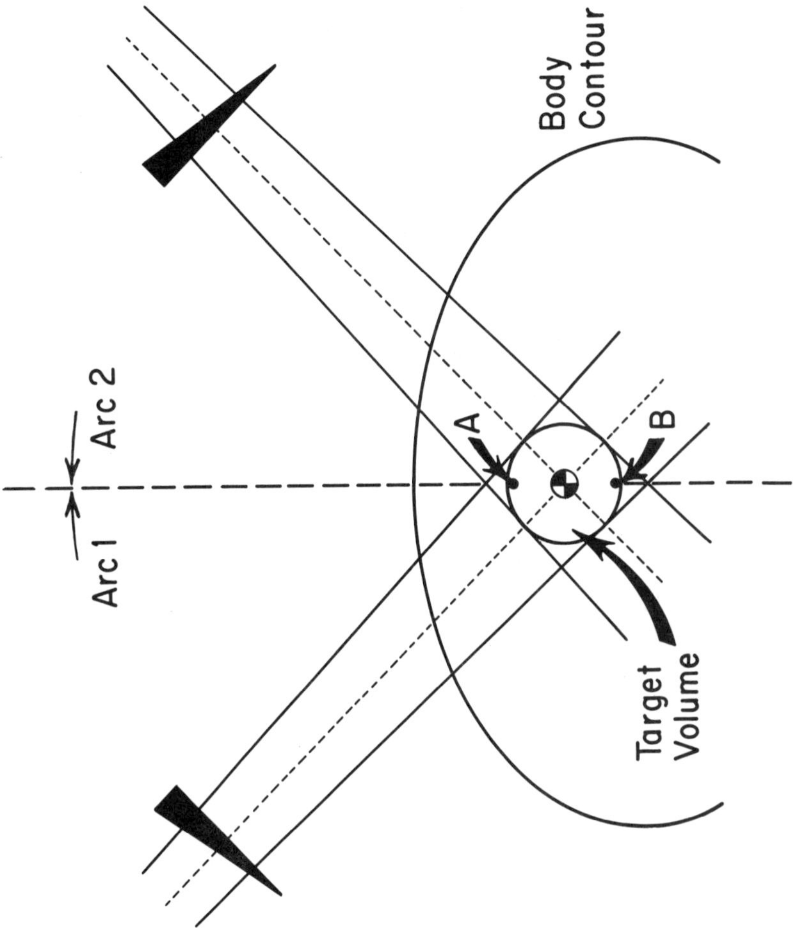

Figure 5. Partial rotation with wedge shaped fields

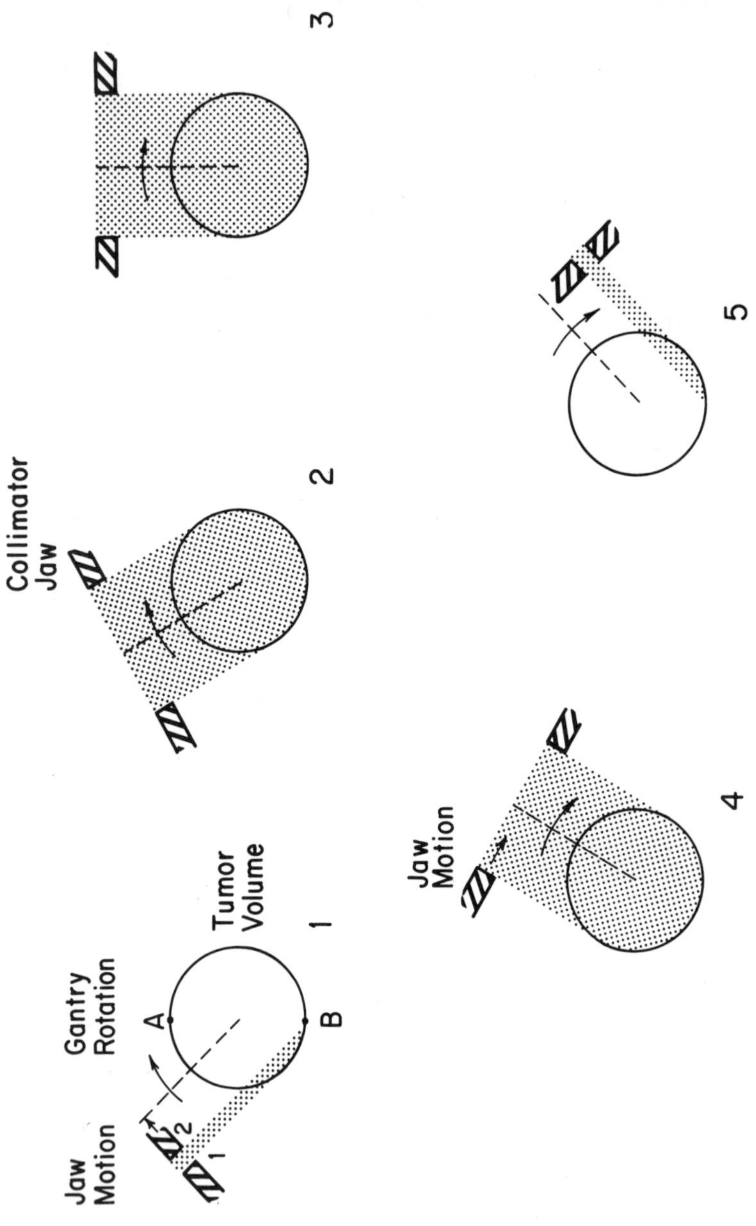

Figure 6. Partial rotation combined with simultaneous collimator jaw motion to generate a dose distribution in the form of a cylinder with elliptical cross-section

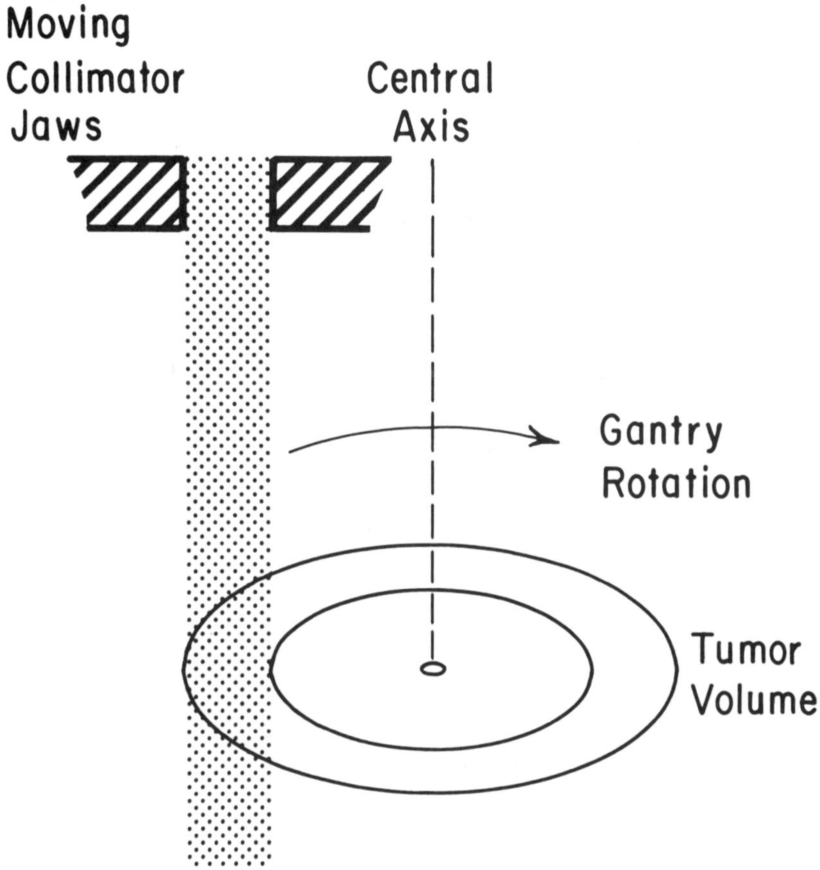

Figure 7. Simultaneous motion of collimator jaws and gantry with one jaw covering the central axis to generate a dose distribution shaped like a hollow cylinder

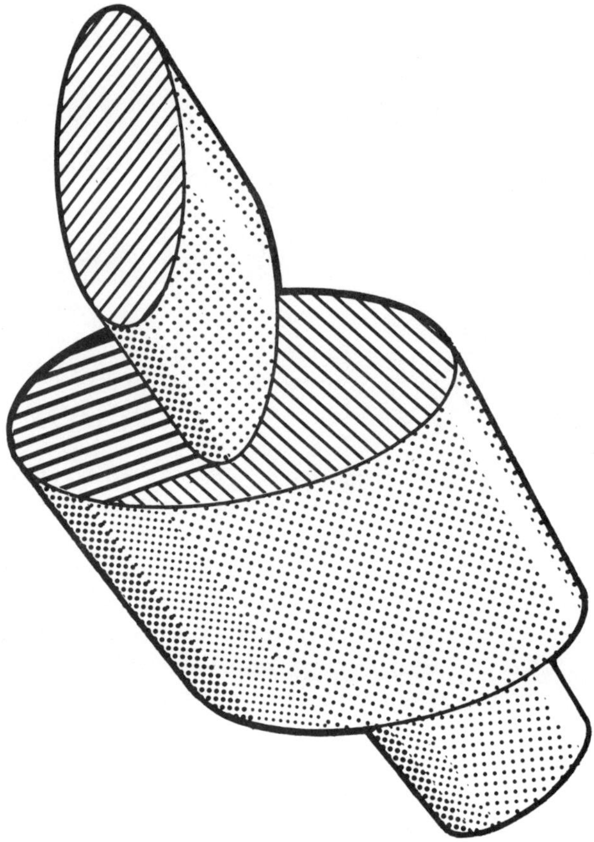

Figure 8. Dose distribution in the form of several adjoining cylinders obtained with a multi-section collimator

4. The Hardware and Software Used in the Automation of a Theratron-80 Cobalt Machine

P. W. Neurath
R. M. Seymour

INTRODUCTION

This paper is a detailed design record of the installation of an automated Cobalt-60 teletherapy machine at the Tufts–New England Medical Center.

The hardware consists of interrelated subsystems which are discussed under six headings; the cobalt machine, the computer, the machine-position sensing, the interfacing hardware, the operator controls, and the safety systems designed to protect the patient.

Five sets of programs support the system: (1) one which senses and directs the cobalt machine, (2) one which detects and avoids intramachine collisions, (3) MUMPS, (4) the patient record-handling system, and (5) the operator-interaction programs.

System operation is described, focusing on an initial period in which twenty-seven patients were treated in an automatic setup mode.

HARDWARE

Theratron 80 Subsystem

Function. A cobalt 60 treatment machine with multi-axis, control of motion, and sensing.

Selection criteria. A machine equipped for motion of both source and patient, capable of performing all current therapy techniques. The axes to be speed-controllable to allow full proportional control of motions, and gentle acceleration of the patient. For safety, several normal manual controls should be able to stop or override the automatic system. An Atomic Energy of Canada, Ltd. (AECL) Theratron 80 was purchased (Fig. 1). It featured (1) position readout and control for ten axes of motion, and (2) digitally controlled solid-state control circuitry with potentiometer feedback. Additional indicators were brought out, including door status, beam status, hand/console indicator, computer/manual indicator, and power on/off indicator.

The cobalt source is contained in the head, which also includes the X and Y beam shaping collimators, and a system for rotating the collimators. The head can swivel, and is swung around the patient by the gantry (arm). The entire arm assembly, including a counterweight, weighs about 8000 pounds. The couch has five movable axes: (1) stretcher lateral and (2) longitudinal, parallel to the floor; (3) stretcher vertical; (4) couch rotation about the source axis; and (5) stretcher rotation.

Before the cobalt source is exposed (beam on), a set of six conditions must be met; (1) hand control set to "console," (2) treatment room door closed, (3) treatment "mode" selected, (4) clock set, (5) "reset" button pushed, and (6) clock started. Any change in status causes the beam to go off.

A collision detection device exists in the form of a strain gauge attached to the stretcher. If the gauge detects a change in a stretcher load while the arm is moving, power to the axes is disabled.

A switch can exclude the computer from affecting manual operations. In computer mode *any* manual operation stops the Theratron and overrides the computer.

Equipment performance. Specifications were that any axis could be commanded by presenting a six-bit speed command and strobing one of the ten lines for selection of the axis. However, starting current surges require all axes to be brought to full speed by steps covering up to 2 1/2 seconds. The manual controls simulated this but are overridden for computer control.

The strain-gauge collision detector triggers during any motion involving both the couch and the arm, and must therefore be ignored during multi-axis motions. This is AECL's solution in their 780 model.

Circuitry for computer control of the beam was installed by us. Strain reliefs, cables, and switches proved inadequate in our clinical environment, and a make-to-signal emergency switch on the hand control contributed to unsafe operation. AECL has recently modified this.

Except for the starting-current problem, circuitry failure rate is about two boards per year, with 90 percent of the circuit boards covered with two spares.

The buried cable connecting the console to the couch had to be replaced because of insufficient wire gauge.

Interlocks prevented some motions, such as restricting arm rotations when the head was swiveled beyond 3° to prevent the head from hitting the stretcher base during rotation. However the safe limit is

7°. No indication is given when the interlock has been activated, so that a treatment may have its rotation stopped without warning.

Suggestions. For installation of an automated treatment system, the hardware and interfacing problem requires competent engineering support.

It is probably cheaper to buy an all-electric-drive manual machine and adapt it with custom computer interfacing, but faster to purchase a complete system. However, the local service organization is unlikely to be familiar with such sophisticated equipment.

PDP-11/20 Subsystem

Function. Machine control and patient record handling.

Selection criteria. Cost and data base sharing with a departmental information system using MUMPS.

Equipment selected. Digital Equipment, PDP-11/20, 28 k (now 44K) core, Extended Arithmetic Element (EAE) integer multiply/divide device, multiple disc drives, two Dectapes, easily interfaced bus and addressing structure, line clock, 56 million character Diva disc system (Fig. 2).

Normally runs under control of MUMPS-11 (1, 2), a terminal oriented disc-based time-sharing system. Every $1/60^{th}$ of a second MUMPS yields control to our Theratron Operating System (TOS) for maintenance of ongoing functions and initialization of new ones.

Peripheral devices appear as addressable "memory" in the top 4k of core. Their interrupts are hardware vectored to addresses identified by the location which is jumped to. This eliminates the need for "polling" devices and saves interrupt processing time at the expense of address space.

The 28k core is the maximum supported by the 16-bit word length of the computer (28001–32000 reserved for devices). This was apportioned to:

12k MUMPS operating system
4k Theratron Operating System
12k Seven User partitions

Additional user demand required expansion of the partition space. A memory mapping box was installed to manipulate the upper two bits of the 18-bit addressing capability of the UNIBUS. MUMPS is an interpretive system with a user's program serving as data, instead of containing executable statements. The operating system resides in low (unmapped) core, and only data exists in mapped areas. The mapbox then points the system to the desired 8k page by activating the upper two bits to an address above 16k.

The KW-11-L real time clock causes an interrupt every power line cycle. MUMPS uses this 16.7 millisecond unit as a basis for switching between users in time-sharing, and TOS uses it as a real-time approach to control. A clock pulse may be delayed up to a millisecond by other interrupt processing, but is never skipped.

DR-11A general purpose interfaces present a word of data to external devices, and to read from external devices. They provide a "data ready" signal on the output side, to allow protection against picking up an incomplete word. The input and output sides are separate.

Equipment performance. The PDP-11 requires separate branch-on-condition statements after operations generating the conditions, compared to the Data General Nova line, where each instruction can carry a "skip-on-condition" suffix allowing faster coding.

As hardware, the 11 had a poor first year. We assumed most service functions ourselves to avoid long shutdowns requested by the manufacturer's service representatives. Providing interdepartmental computing services has forced "professional" attitude upon system operation, and every effort is expended in keeping the system on line between 8:00 A.M. and 5:00 P.M. System and mainframe maintenance must therefore go on after hours. Hardware failures are rare, and usually triggered by an outside factor—for example, a recent voltage spike on our power lines.

Suggestions. Our independence from service contracts, based on having competent technical people, has allowed us to continue to use and expand a cpu which is no longer made, and to explore safely the "used computer" market to ease cost.

Analog-to-Digital Subsystem

Function. Read position of the machine.

Selection criteria. Lineal accuracy of 1/4 cm in beam placement. For gantry angle, that translates to .08°, or 12-bit accuracy, as the most demanding case.

Equipment selected. DEC AD-02, a modification of their AD-01 12-channel 12-bit A/D 15 microsecond per channel speed (165 microseconds for 11 channels) ±5 vdc swing, derived analog ground. Potentiometers on the Theratron were 10k ohm Computer Instruments Corp., No. 135556, models 205 and 206. Connection to the moving axes was by precision chains (arm, lat., long, stretcher, and couch rotation), by gear drive (head swivel), and by direct connection of linear pots for collimator X and Y. The number of leads from sensors was limited by the number of slip rings installed on the Theratron.

Equipment performance. The electronics perform well, but no indication is given if a pot-wiper lead breaks, since the A/D will maintain the last reading, with only slight drift. The attachment of some of the pots to the Theratron was inadequate and was reworked.

Suggestions. Replace the entire system with digital encoders, if 12-bit units are available. The accuracy of the system is limited by the pots. The open connector problem is being corrected by trace leads installed in the cable to detect an open circuit.

Operator's Interface Subsystem

Selection criteria. Operator interaction was defined in five classes:

(1) Hard copy—A printer record of treatments

(2) Soft copy—Interactive dialog on a CRT

(3) Buttons, lights and buzzers—Binary input/output systems for showing Status and requesting responses

(4) Emergency and pause—Special button inputs, special circuits for safety, and software provision for overriding all other functions.

(5) Treatment clock—A simple, easily read clock system for beam timing to the computer.

In all cases an effort was made to "human factor" the hardware design or selection.

Equipment selected. An Ann Arbor video terminal was selected for the soft function, to obtain (1) 1200-baud speed, (2) multiple displays in various parts of the treatment area, (3) multiple keyboard stations for the single terminal, (4) silence, (5) reliability, (6) low cost. The video terminal has a 32 $\times$ 16 screen, sufficient for most messages ("ENTER PATIENT'S NAME," "VERIFY TREATMENT TIME," etc.), with characters large enough for easy reading. A fully controllable cursor allows increased visual impact by planned placement and isolation of messages. The ability to clear the screen aids our effort at patient data privacy.

Hard copy was initially based on the idea of printing self-addressing labels. This proved impractical. A redesign of the printed form allows use of Univac-type thirty-character-per-second terminals.

Two operator panels were constructed (Fig. 3). The smaller is located within the treatment room, and the other, with the digital clock, serves as the main control panel. Whenever possible, functions duplicated on the two boards share the same button position. The buttons are merely input signals to the computer; if a function is added or dropped, the only hardware change needed is replacement of the label on the button. Also, pushing any button (other than emergency/pause) has no effect unless the program is looking for that particular button to be pushed. Button options are illuminated, and pushing one is acknowledged by extinguishing the button.

Each panel contains a Sonalert, to allow either a quick "beep" or a prolonged scream to alert the operator. To bring all controls to the panels, the Theratron's "reset" button is hard-wired to one of the panel buttons.

The panels are tastefully executed in oiled walnut and anodized aluminum, adding to their acceptance.

At the top of the two panels are buttons labeled "EMERGENCY" and "PAUSE/CONTINUE." The emergency button causes (through software) the Theratron to be shut down (motions stopped, beam extinguished, power turned off).

The pause/continue button causes a software halt of the system. When pushed again, the system resumes whatever it was doing, unless something major was changed during the pause. These buttons are illuminated when activated.

The treatment clock is an input and display device for the computer. All timing is done via software. Digitran Mini lever switches permit fast and accurate setting of the treatment time. Feedback to the operator is provided by four Dialite light emitting diode digits.

Alternatively, the computer can "prompt" the operator with a previously stored time on the CRT and the operator can accept. In this method a day of normal treatments would not entail manual setting of the "clock."

Equipment performance. The Ann Arbor terminal broke down twice in two years, and is temperature sensitive. The flexibility of the button reassignment has proved itself many times. The lever switches unfortunately have 0 as the upper arm position and 9 as the lower.

Suggestions. We are changing the emergency circuit from a normally open system to a normally closed system. This will cause an automatic shutdown in the event of a cable failure.

Interface Subsystem

Function. To match signal levels between external devices and the computer, to provide protection from damage to computer or devices from out-of-range voltages, to provide amplification for driving long cables, and to perform data conversion and buffering as required.

Equipment selected. The interfaces share a mounting panel (DEC H911-J), a 64-slot connector assembly designed to hold standard DEC logic modules, with wire-wrap pins available for interconnections and power supplies for both 5 and 15 volts.

The logic is made up of DEC logic boards, eight serving as line-drivers. There is a time-delay and a one-of-ten switch for use in assembling the Theratron control signal. Thirteen slots serve as cable terminators.

A second section of the interface consists of five integrated circuits on a board within the card frame of the Theratron. These are line-drivers for transmission of status back to the computer and inverter circuits for enabling the beam and for shutting down the Theratron.

To prevent accidents due to computer failure, the Theratron power is turned off unless the computer toggles a specific line everycycle. If three consecutive toggles are missed, with either the line high or the line low, a timer closes the emergency circuit.

A similar toggle action is used for final beam control.

Equipment performance. The wire-wrapped construction of the interface has proven reliable, easy to document, and easy to change. Use of DEC logic modules allows diagnostic swapping with other parts of the PDP-11.

Suggestions. We are moving the one-in-ten function to the Theratron end of the circuit to allow error-checking and to free up some wires, and are providing a system that requires Theratron commands to be followed immediately by their complement. The signals will be exclusive OR'd, and any discrepancy will inhibit the command, start a timer, and notify the computer. A second error within a second will cause direct shut-down of the Theratron.

DEC logic cards could ideally be replaced by fewer, more complex boards with more gates, which would reduce costs.

Ancillary Equipment

Selection criteria. The selection of cables, connectors, and cabinets, etc. was all too often haphazard. The computer being located 150 feet from the Theratron, approximately 160 separate bits of information had to be routed that distance. To allow separation of the panels and the Theratron, we decided upon six separate cables, each with at least 32 lines with some extra capacity for power and ground feeds. Belden 8769 22-gauge, 38-conductor cable, with the wires mated as 19 pairs, each pair shielded by foil, was used, at a total cost of over $700.

Cinch DC-37 plugs and sockets terminate the cable, chosen for low cost. These are 37-pin versions of the RS-232 connector used on terminals and modems. Since 19 pairs plus shield equal 39 leads, one pair of each cable is not brought through the connectors.

The computer-end equipment is mounted within the PDP-11's H950 cabinet. The interface is behind a front panel, and its power supplies are mounted on an aluminum plate on a rear door. For connecting the outer cables to the interface, lengths of the 19-pair cable (stripped of their outer jacket) join the Cinch plugs to terminal boards plugged into the interface. Flat "ribbon" cables join the interface to the DR-11's within one of the computer's BALL-ES drawers.

At the Theratron, the machine control and potentiometer feedback cables are brought from Cinch plugs to a dozen terminal strips mounted on an inner door of the Theratron's control cabinet.

The two operator panels each have 6-foot Belden cables which plug into the cable from the computer. The wire for the beam "reset" function directly joins the outer panel and one of the Theratron terminal strips.

Suggestions. The connectors are wrong for this application. They lie on the floor and are kicked and stepped on. There is no provision for locking the connection other than taping the connectors together.

The unjacketed cable within the computer cabinet is unprotected, yet too stiff to move about during maintenance. We therefore conclude that for long cable runs with indefinite knowledge of final signal load, a system using multiplexors and two (send and receive) lengths of coaxial cable would be better. If a multiple wire cable must be used, the use of proper connectors is a must.

Safety Subsystems

From the project's inception, an overriding concern for all design features, both hardware and software, has been patient safety.

The initial feeling was to shut down the system at any malfunction. Thus the original operating system upon detection of an error sent speed zero commands to all axes, and then turned off the Theratron.

The Theratron was modified to have a normally closed relay in parallel with its emergency circuit (Fig. 4) driven by rectifying a signal from the computer. Thus the signal had to change at regular intervals or the relay would drop out, shutting down the Theratron. This circuit is called the "computer alive" line. The toggling of the bit is done by program TOSAXM, and circuit values were chosen to drop out in less than 50 milliseconds. By inhibiting the toggling, we can arrange for the computer to shut down the Theratron on purpose. A new version of this circuit is being installed, using IC timers.

To prevent the computer from trying to direct the Theratron when it is not available for control, the status indicators detailed below are routed back to the computer.

Indicating	*Options Yes/No*	*Action Inhibited if No*
Theratron power	on/off	any motion, beam
Beam status	on/off	
Control status	system/hand	any motion, beam
System status	Computer/manual	any motion, beam
Door status	closed/open	beam (turned off, if on)

The activation of any indicator (except beam) physically breaks the computer's control of the listed action. The indicators are also used to ascertain that commands are executed. If the beam does not go to a commanded state (either on or off) within one second, the

Theratron is shut down. The pause button is available as a convenient manually controlled safety system. If the operator detects a questionable activity, this switch allows suspension of operations, followed by trouble-free resumption if desired. The programs allow the beam to come back on if interrupted, unless the machine is moved manually during the pause. In that case the remaining and elapsed beam time is available for storage and interactive dialog with the operator.

An error during swapping in the collision-detection package, or its execution, shuts down the system.

The computer can operate the cobalt source. To ensure against accidents, especially those caused by a programmer working on developing the treatment programs, the Theratron has one switch which must be manually activated to allow a beam sequence. This is the reset button on the Theratron's control panel. For ease of operation this has been brought out to the computer's control panel, but is hardwired directly to the Theratron. For the beam to come on:

(1) The hand control must be in the "console" state (hardware interlock).

(2) The Theratron must be in "computer" mode (hardware interlock).

(3) The door must be closed.

(4) The beam-permit bit must come up (software/hardware interlock).

(5) *Then* the reset button must be pushed (hardware interlock).

(6) *Then* the beam will go on, if the beam toggle starts. The beam toggle is similar to the computer alive toggle, explained previously.

Additional safety features and systems being installed are devices which require the computer signal to be received, followed by its one's complement. If any two errors occur within a specified time period, currently one second, the Theratron is shut down and the computer is told why. The motion programs have been given more ability to decide whether an axis is not responding properly. The pause programs look for nonmanual motion. To deal with accidental cable disconnects, the must-be-complete emergency and power-on signals are routed through multiple cables to provide a high-priority shutdown command if a cable separates.

As a final precaution, a hold-while-moving dead man's switch is being provided for the technician, and will have to be depressed for any patient setup motion by the computer. This will provide an additional necessary safety feature.

SOFTWARE SYSTEMS

Theratron Operating System (TOS)

TOS functions are subroutines of two classes. The voluntary functions are those called upon by a program running under MUMPS. They are:

(1) Turn on lights on operator panels.
(2) Read buttons currently being pressed by operator.
(3) Read a/d to determine current position of Theratron.
(4) Move a block of ten words within the TOS table area.
(5) Read the clock switches.
(6) Present a number to the clock display.
(7) Move a single Theratron axis at a specified speed.
(8) Move the entire Theratron from its current position to a new position specified by a movement vector, in a specified time span.
(9) Count down the clock display (beam turn-on optional).
(10) Invoke collision detection (pulls in non-core resident program).
(11) Invoke collision avoidance (pulls in non-core resident program).

The involuntary class functions are:

(1) Sample and process requests for "pause" or "emergency" actions.
(2) Sample current position of moving Theratron, update speed commands as necessary to correct for deviation from planned path (following No. 8 above).
(3) Continually update Theratron with current speed commands (including zero), and tell it that the computer is still functioning.
(4) Check for new function requests by the MUMPS program, clean up local tables, and indicate completion of on-going functions.

Although seen by the MUMPS program as distinct functions, many of the functions call each other for services, to save program duplication.

MUMPS

The MUMPS-11 Data Management System is a single-language, real-time, multiprogrammed, time-sharing system for the PDP-11 series of computer (1).

The hardware environment of our MUMPS system is detailed in Figure 2.

Collision Detection (3) and Avoidance (4)

To allow the computer to move the Theratron required the development of programs that could detect and avoid possible collisions between parts of the machine and the patient. The mathematics of a

10-degree-of-freedom machine moving in space required the use of higher-level languages than either assembler or MUMPS. The size of the problem required computer space which could not be allowed to exist as overhead. To meet these problems, the MUMPS operating system was modified to permit the entire primary-user partition area (about 12k of core) to be swapped to the disc, and to be replaced by a precompiled Fortran program from the disc. After the spatial calculations are performed, the MUMPS partitions are brought back.

The collision problem was divided into two areas, detection and avoidance. Collision detection is performed by dividing the planned motion path into ten fixed positions evenly spaced along the planned path through which the machine travels. For each of the ten positions the entire machine is mathematically modeled by equations or table look-ups and analyzed to find points of intersection between the machine components. If none is found, the motion is allowed.

If collision is computed, collision avoidance will be invoked. During the test period, the collision-avoidance programs were too large to fit the operating system. The incidence of probable collision was, however, low enough to require, in that event, a simple manual setup. The collision-avoidance method currently involves swinging the patient to known "safe" zones, moving the arm, and then bringing the patient back to the final position. The collision-avoidance and collision detection programs are alternatively swapped as described above.

Patient's Treatment Record

There are four types of data concerning a patient's treatment on our system. They are the prescriptions for treatment, the machine-movement data, the daily record of delivered treatment, and a summary of the relative doses delivered to various sites, cumulated daily and weekly.

Prior to or during the first treatment, the patient's prescription is stored on the computer's disc file. Subsequent treatments are allowed until the prescription is satisfied.

Daily Treatment Operation

(1) Identify patient to computer. From the machine's schedule, which is currently implemented as a Departmental Information System package, the next expected patient's name is displayed on the CRT. The technician must respond with "Y" via the keyboard, otherwise the system will ask: "initials, name, or number? " If the next patient is listed on the machine schedule (which is displayed if the technician types a "? "), then only the first and last initials are required. The system will then display a name with those initials. If an "N" (no) is entered, it will display the next name with those initials. If it runs out of names, it will again request "initials, name or number." The technician may also respond with the patient's name, either in full or with just the first few letters of the last name. The system will access the entire patient file, and display names which match the selection criteria. If only one is found, it prompts with it and asks "OK? " A negative answer again brings back "initials, name, or number." If multiple names are displayed, the technician is requested to enter the particular patient's number (shown with the name lists). This will uniquely identify the patient to the system, and his record will be retrieved.

If the treatment day is over, a response of "QUIT" to the system will shut the system down for the night.

If the patient is as yet unknown to the system, the technician would ask one of the interviewers to "admit" the patient, a two-minute process.

(2) Verify field. Once identified, the options are: treatment in normal order of stored fields; skip any number of stored fields; rearrange treatment order; add fields (described in "New Field Entry" section); and treatment over, unload patient. The system will prompt with the number of the next expected field, or will ask "Field number? " Once a stored field is requested and its data retrieved, the "Start Set Up" button on the operator's panel will light. If the collision detection/avoidance programs cannot produce a safe path, the button does not light, but a sonalert beeps and the video terminal says "Please move Theratron, I can't do it."

(3) Setup. Once the field is identified, the technician has the option of automatic setup (initialed by pushing "start setup") or manual setup. If the machine is moved by hand after "start setup" lights, the button is extinguished. If "start setup" is pushed while the Theratron 80 is unready for motion, the video screen displays the controls which must be set before motion is allowed. Automatic setup must be followed by the technician's final adjustment of stretcher lateral and longitudinal to bring the beam to the prescribed position. This adjustment is required by the lack of a positive patient-positioning device for the couch.

(4) Record changes. The system will compare the position with stored data. Minor stretcher discrepancies are allowed, and stored for application to the next field to be given to this patient. Arm angle or field-size changes produce questions on the video terminal, which must be answered before treatment can proceed. The final question, assuming that the change is valid, is whether to modify the stored prescription ("is this a permanent change? ")

(5) Time entry. When the setup is completed, the clock displays the stored prescription, and the "enter time" button is lit. If the clock switches are set to zero, or to the value displayed, when the button is pushed, the prescribed value is used for the treatment. If another time is entered on the switches, the system requests verification via the video terminal, and asks if the change is permanent. There are three available responses: Yes, No (today only), and Port. The port option indicates that an X ray (port film) of the treatment is being taken. That indicates a short (set on switches) exposure with the X-ray film in place, followed by an exposure of the difference between the prescription and the port time. The difference is calculated and displayed (after the port exposure) and may be changed as above.

(6) **Deliver treatment.** Successful completion of time entry lights the "reset" button. Once this button is pushed, the computer turns on the beam and the clock display counts down the exposure. The machine will move as the treatment requires. The treatment will stop if (a) the clock reaches zero, (b) the treatment-room door is opened, or (c) the pause or emergency button is pushed. Either (b) or (c) allows an interrupted treatment to resume.

(7) **Record delivery.** The computer monitors the beam and stores the final time and any other pertinent data on the disk. During the trial period an adhesive label was printed for insertion into the patient's record. Control is then returned to the "verify field" section of the program.

(8) **Unload.** When no more fields are requested for the patient, the "unload" button lights, and if pushed, the machine swings the patient away from the arm and lowers the couch to make dismounting easier. The unload position thus serves as the starting position for the next patient.

New Treatments

A new field entry is made during the verify field process by requesting a field number not already assigned to that patient. This produces, e.g., a "New field 30 . . . OK? " message. If affirmed, the system waits while the technician manually sets up the field. When it is set up, the technician enters the treatment time. It is verified via the video terminal, which also asks: "Fixed, Rotation or Other?" If the technician types "F," the treatment can start (the "reset" button will light). If "R" or "O" is specified, dialog to describe the method is entered. A rotary treatment will swing the arm about the patient, at a speed to bring it to the starting position at the end of the exposure.

At the initial treatment, the Theratron's position is read and stored, and the technician is asked to describe the field and any equipment (bolus, blocks, etc.) used. This data is stored, and subsequent executions of the field produce reminders about the equipment on the video screen.

At the end of the field, control returns to the "verify field" program section.

Trial Period Operation

For two weeks in March 1974 all patients assigned to the automatic machine were treated under computer control. An engineer was in attendance at all times to assist the technician in data entry and to detect and prevent errors before the technician or patient were affected. By the end of the first week all errors which that patient base brought to light were programmed out. The second week approximated a fully operational system, with the technician performing all interaction and control functions.

As described earlier, the collision-avoidance program was unusable at this time. If collision detection indicated a "hit," automatic setup was bypassed and the computer told the technician to set up manually. This occurred with about 10 percent of the setups. In addition, the engineer would occasionally request the technician to proceed manually to avoid possible collisions involving unmodeled accessories on the Theratron.

Technician response to the system included concern for the patient, unwillingness to wait for slow responses by the computer and dislike of the terminal operations. Also expressed was the feeling that installation of the system is inevitable, regardless of their wishes. As the system became more reliable after the first week, their confidence in its technical ability to move the patients increased.

Response time came to be a problem. Between the acceptance of a field and illumination of the "start set up" button, there was a three-second delay while collision detection occurred. For the first week, if the technician walked from the video keyboard, outside the treatment room, to the button inside the room before it lit up, he would start a manual setup. Demonstration of the total time saving gained by waiting one more second eliminated this habit.

During patient motion, the technician would either adjust the patient's pillows and retrieve the lead blocks, or hold the manual control box, ready to take over when the machine appeared to be getting too close. The engineer was permanently stationed over an emergency switch for the same reason.

A problem with the collimators not achieving the last millimeter of travel cropped up, but was circumvented by the engineer advising the technician when the rest of the machine was in position. The computer was therefore programmed to "beep" at the end of a successful setup. For the majority of patients, only the first setup of the day required some lateral and stretcher longitudinal adjustment. Subsequent fields for that patient came close enough to elicit praise from the technician.

Default-beam timing by computer was readily accepted. The technicians always checked the displayed time with the chart, but familiarity may lower their attention to this in the future, so this option is questionable and may be eliminated.

The terminal dialog to identify the next field was timed to occur during the exposure to save time. The safety circuit would trigger, however, if collision-detection was performed during an exposure, so the visible three-second delay remained.

The Continuing Effort

Following installation of the new safety features and debugging of some changes to MUMPS, the Theratron Operating System, and the Collision Detection programs, we plan to resume automated setup treatment in late 1974. The new form of treatment record being tried has the computer print the entire planned treatment schedule at the first visit. As treatment follows the plan, the technician simply initials the printed form daily. A complete new form is printed if any changes are made. The new form shows all previous treatments, the revised planned treatments, and a detailed description of the changes. The collision detection and avoidance program are being rewritten to improve performance, storage, and speed. Collision detection calculation might be bypassed if it had been previously calculated and proven safe.

After a period of practice and adjustment, we intend to begin dynamic treatments, moving the patient and source to achieve tailored dose distribution. We will need to develop or adapt accurate three-dimensional treatment-planning programs or simulation films to implement this treatment ability.

ACKNOWLEDGMENT

This work has been supported by NIH grant Nos. CA12178-03 and 1 ROICA 14960-01.

REFERENCES

1. Digital Equipment Corporation, *"MUMPS" Programming Manual*, Maynard, Mass. (1972)
2. Digital Equipment Corporation, *MUMPS-11 Language*, Reference Manual, Maynard, Mass. (1972)
3. Kreifeldt, J. G., Neurath, P., Seymour, R., Hsieh, D. C., "Collision Detection Programs for a Computer Controlled Theratron 80 Radiotherapy Machine," American Association of Physicists in Medicine, Chicago, December 1972.
4. Hsieh, D. C., "Collision Detection and Avoidance Programs for a Theratron 80 Radiotherapy Machine," Thesis, Tufts University (1973).
5. Kiel, R. A., "Collision Detection and the Theratron-80," Thesis, Tufts University (1974).

QUESTIONS

KARZMARK: I wonder if you could estimate how much time—man hours, weeks, months—was consumed in converting your MUMPS system so as to accommodate the control function for the Theratron. Also, would you comment on the vulnerability of the MUMPS system to software crashing, originating from Theratron operations?

SEYMOUR: The time required for initial MUMPS to Theratron conversion was not that great. I would estimate—looking at the programs, not counting one last bug which chased us for a year—about two man months, with hands held by DEC and Medi-Tech, who developed our MUMPS. What was the second part of your question?

KARZMARK: The vulnerability of the MUMPS system to crashes.

SEYMOUR: Well, the assembly routines which are core resident theoretically don't crash. They've been debugged and tested and no numbers you give to them will cause them to crash, since they are in there all the time. Therefore, they will not crash as long as they're not fiddled with by somebody using a view command under MUMPS.

The external Fortran package is allowed to crash as long as it doesn't wipe out actual operating-system code. At the end of ten seconds, MUMPS takes back over and says, "Well, the Fortran program must have made a mistake." The stack pointers are probably all screwed up, and it resets the machine to the state that it was before we were swapped in, and resumes control. That's been working pretty well. And the one bug that took a year was only affecting the swapped Fortran program, so MUMPS never crashed.

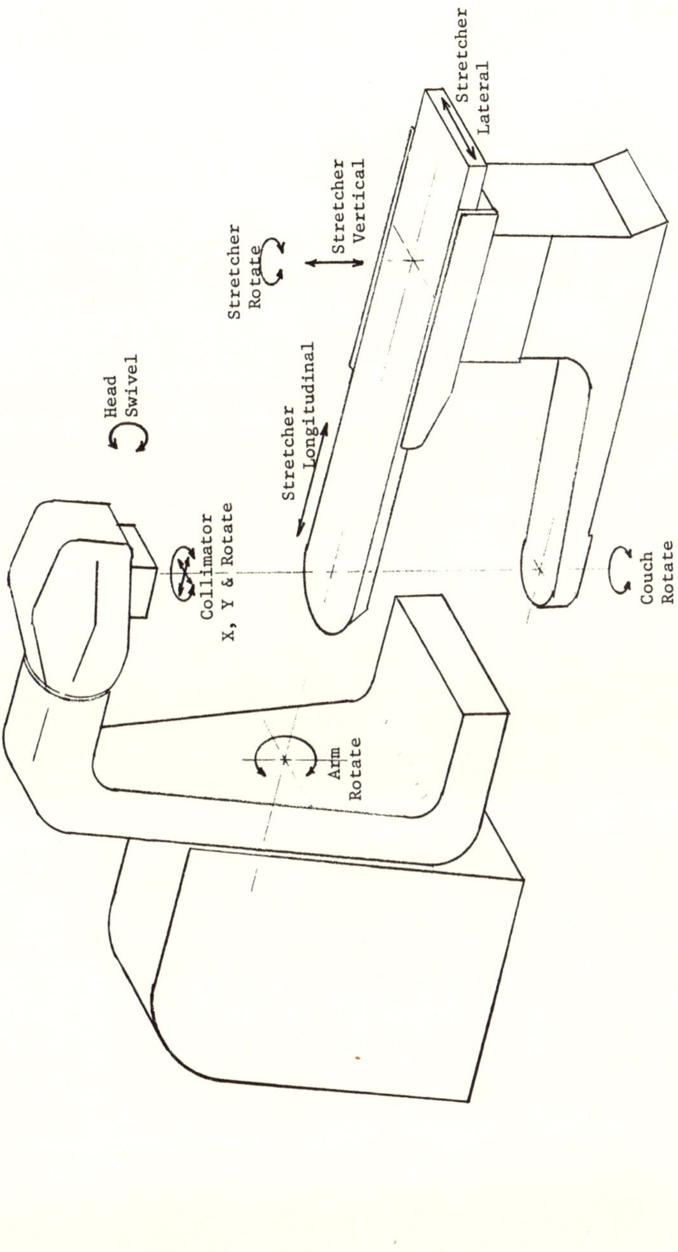

Figure 1. Theratron 80, Showing 10 Movable Axes

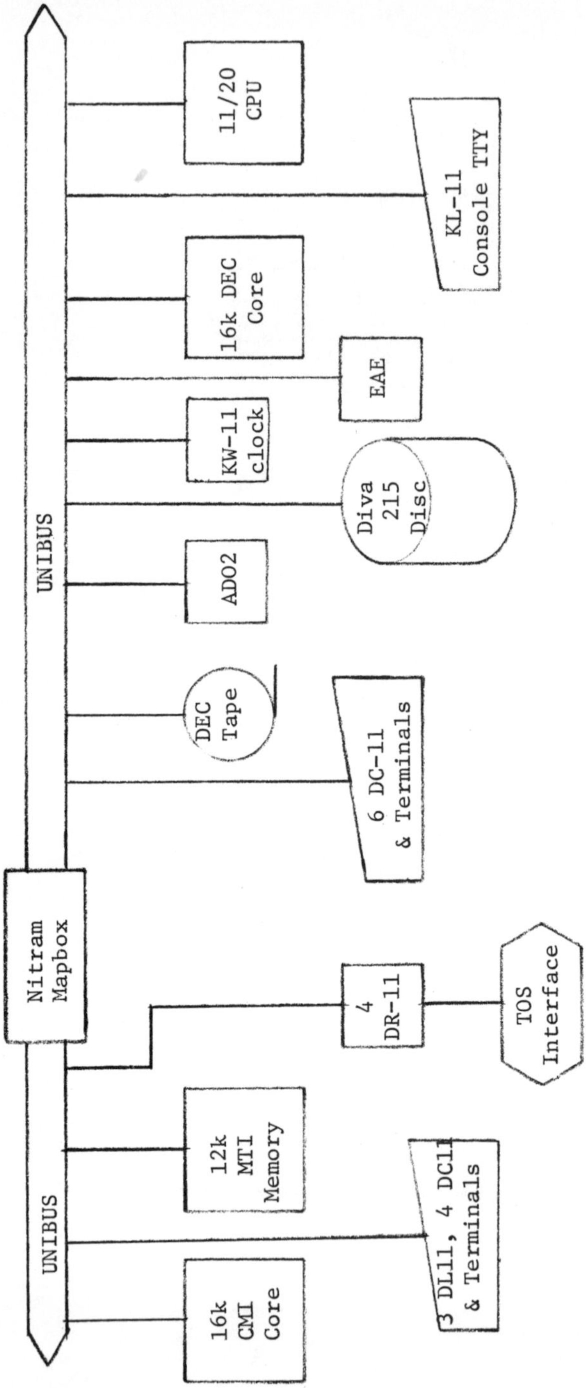

Figure 2. PDP-11/20 Hardware

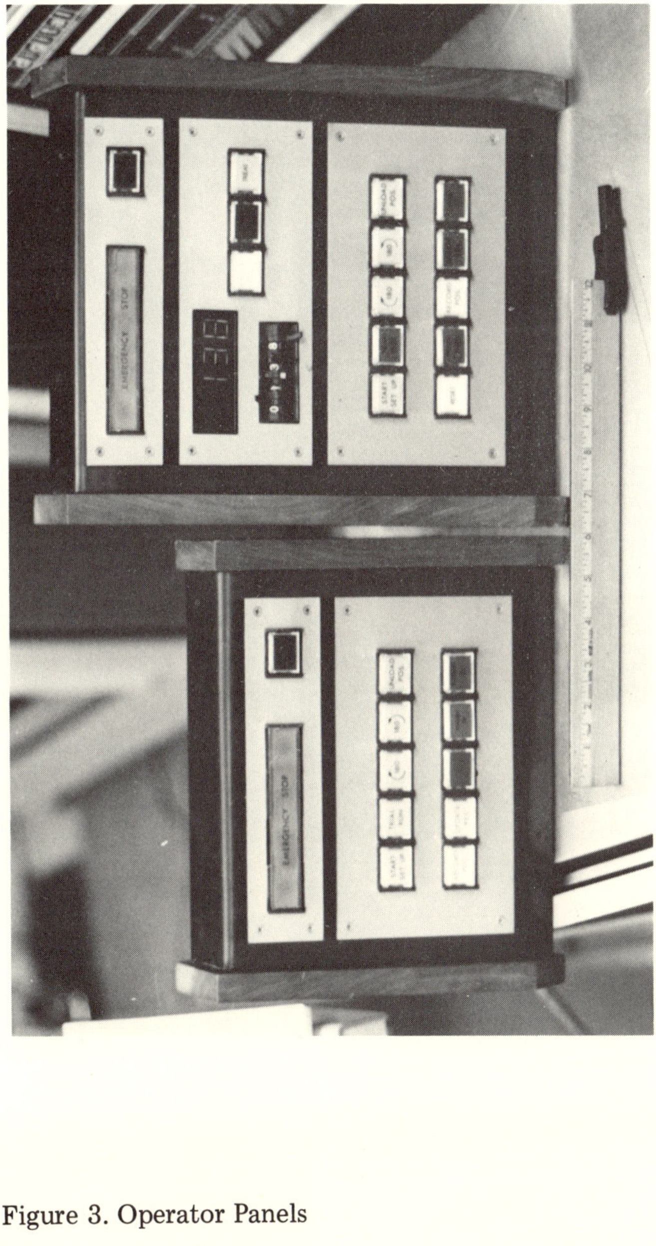

Figure 3. Operator Panels

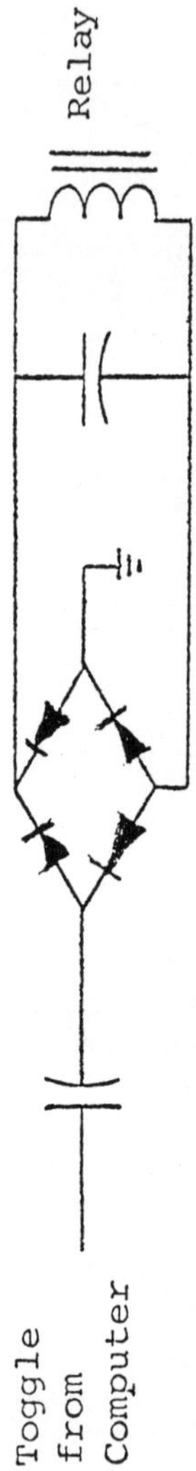

Figure 4. Computer-Alive Circuit

5. Dynamic Treatment

D. L. Neblett
J. W. Schaeflein
H. R. Haymond
F. W. George, III
E. R. Ahten
J. G. Mackinney

Introduction

Dynamic treatment is a phrase used to describe radiotherapy treatments administered during the coordinated movement of one or more axes of the therapy machine. Rotational therapy is an example of dynamic treatment where a single parameter, the gantry angle, is changed during the course of treatment.

Commercially available units are equipped with computers that can read the treatment unit's position and control simultaneously the movements of all the axes. All of the treatment unit's parameters can be coordinated by the computer, which positions the source by moving the gantry, determines the collimation by opening, closing, and rotating the jaws, and establishes the patient's relative position by moving the stretcher in the longitudinal, lateral, and vertical directions. With the computer able to control simultaneously all the axes of a treatment unit, innumerable nonlinear dose-distribution shaping techniques are possible.

The first implementation at our institution of dynamic treatment was a simulation of the dose distribution created by inserting a mechanical wedge filter—that is, a dynamic wedge. In the simplest case, the dynamic wedge is produced by the coordinated movement of two axes—for example, the closure of the collimator jaws and the lateral movement of the stretcher. The technique used to produce a dynamic wedge is to deliver uniform dose to the entire field with the jaws open, then produce a wedge-shaped addition by closing the jaws and simultaneously moving the stretcher so that the edge of the collimator is always coincident with one of the edges of the field. The following sequence of figures is presented to illustrate the idea. Figure 1 shows the collimators and a cross-section of a patient with a representation of the dose-distribution delivered to the volume from a single static field. Figure 2 shows the dose-distribution if the collimators are closed incrementally during the beam-on period; instead of being flat, the dose-distribution is pointed like an arrow or double-sided wedge. Figure 3 shows the effect of moving the patient at the same time that the collimators are being closed. In this sequence the stretcher and patient are moved in coordination with the jaw motion so that one side of the treatment field is always aligned or coincident with the edge of the original fully open port.

The relative motion makes it appear as if only one side of the collimator is moving, but actually both are closing simultaneously. In Figure 4, the smooth dose-distribution similar to that produced by a mechanical wedge filter is obtained by using extremely small increments instead of moving in large increments.

In the above example the simple geometry allowed a wedge-shaped dose-distribution to be produced by moving only two axes in a linear fashion. This would be the case if one were treating a patient vertically and moving the stretcher horizontally. In the general case, the coordination algorithm must take into account all the treatment unit's axes of movement, which are: (1) gantry rotation, (2) collimator rotation, (3) upper collimator (jaws) closure, (4) lower collimator (jaws) closure, (5) stretcher longitudinal, (6) stretcher lateral, (7) stretcher vertical, and (8) couch rotation.

To coordinate the patient movement with the closure of the collimator, the following relationships are used:

Formulas

For simplicity and ease of understanding, the movement relationships are broken down into a number of steps.

The Y axis represents movement perpendicular to the central ray and coincident with the axis of gantry rotation.

The X axis represents movement perpendicular to the central ray and to the Y axis.

These variables, X and Y, are used to translate the collimator rotation, upper and lower collimator opening, and actual treatment source-to-surface distance (SSD) into a more usable form:

$$\triangle Y = \frac{\triangle CLJ}{2} \frac{SSD}{80} \sin\theta + \frac{CUJ}{2} \frac{SSD}{80} \cos\theta$$

$$\triangle X = \frac{\triangle CLJ}{2} \frac{SSD}{80} \cos\theta + \frac{CUJ}{2} \frac{SSD}{80} \sin\theta$$

Where CLJ = collimator lower jaw
CUJ = collimator upper jaw

θ = collimator rotation angle

Since the collimators close symmetrically about the central ray of the treatment beam, each side of the collimator provides one half of the collimator movement. The $\frac{SSD}{80}$ in the expression corrects for the actual source-to-surface distance and is needed because collimator opening is defined at 80 cm SSD. The collimator rotation angle is the degree of rotation of the collimator about the central ray of the beam from some reference point. The sine and cosine functions of the collimator rotation angle allow one to translate changes in field size due to the upper and lower collimator motion into the X and Y coordinate system.

The distances moved by the individual axes of the couch are represented by the following equations:

$$\text{Stretcher lateral} = (X \cos\phi + Y \sin\phi)\cos\alpha$$
$$\text{Stretcher longitudinal} = Y \cos\phi + X \sin\phi$$
$$\text{Stretcher vertical} = (X \cos\phi + Y \sin\phi)\sin\alpha$$

where α = Gantry rotation angle
ϕ = Couch rotation angle

Gantry rotation angle is the angle of rotation of the gantry about its axis of rotation. Couch rotation is the angle of rotation of the couch around a point directly under the isocenter.

These formulas provide the relationship to translate X and Y, generated above, into the three stretcher movements (longitudinal, lateral, and vertical). The equations indicate that to deliver a wedge-shaped dose-distribution, one must be able to coordinate the movement of the three stretcher axes with the collimator closure.

The algorithm for the dynamic wedge is designed to modify a flat field at 10 cm depth to produce a wedge-shaped dose-distribution. First a uniform "foundation" dose is delivered to the entire field with jaws opened to the desired field size. Then a wedge-shaped addition is produced by closing the jaws and moving the stretcher simultaneously.

A linear empirical relationship was used to determine the foundation dose and the maximum meter-setting necessary to deliver a desired maximum dose on the central ray with the desired wedge angle at a depth of 10 cm. The motion to produce the wedge-shaped dose-distribution is started at the completion of the foundation dose and ends with the completion of the maximum meter dose. The desired wedge angle and the maximum central axis dose are entered into the computer by the operator. The computer then calculates the required meter setting to be entered on the linear accelerator control console.

Implementation of the Movement Algorithm

The electromechanical characteristics of the direct current (DC) motors and associated mechanical linkages in the linear accelerator were important considerations in developing the movement-control algorithm.

Since the speed range resulting from the use of DC control voltages produced a movement which was too fast, pulse techniques were used to control the various axes. A minimum pulse height and width was chosen for each axis that would give a consistent movement. For low speeds this pulse was used to control the motors in a fashion similar to that used for stepping motors. For higher speeds the duty cycle was increased to 100 percent by increasing the pulse width, and finally DC voltage-level control was excercised. In this manner continuous speed-control range was obtained.

Because of the geometry of the treatment unit and the change in load on the motors with different patients and different treatment-unit positions, the voltage versus velocity relationship of the axes are not linear over the course of movement, even when delivering a linear dose-distribution to a volume. In addition, the output or dose rate from the accelerator is neither steady nor constant.

For the above reasons, the algorithm is designed to ensure that when a certain dose has been delivered, a particular axis has moved to its appropriate position. For the linear wedge, the relationship between dose and position is linear only for closure of the collimator jaw.

The dose from the integrated dose meter is constantly being compared with a calculated dose. If the meter dose is greater than the calculated dose, movement in the form of a small step is initiated; if the meter dose is less than the calculated dose, no movement is taken.

The movements of the other axes are nonlinear, and their positions are calculated or predicted as functions of the collimator jaw positions. In this case the position of the axis is compared with the position predicted by the meter dose. If the predicted position is less than the actual position, corrective action is taken. Since movement is in terms of small steps, it is possible to be slightly beyond the predicted position, in which case no corrective action is taken.

The correction of position of each axis is handled independently of the others, and action is taken only when needed. That is to say, the movements of the axes are coordinated with each other but independently controlled. This means that the starting or stopping of a control pulse can be initiated at any time regardless of the action being taken for the other axes.

The control algorithm is a cycle in which the dose-position relationship and the condition of the motor controller are considered separately for each axis. Is it in the middle of the pulse? If so, should the pulse be stopped yet? If it is not in the process of pulsing, then the dose-position relationship is examined and the decision is made whether to start a pulse.

Rotational Treatment Parameters

Rotational treatment techniques in the past have been constrained by the mechanical geometry of the treatment unit. Dynamic treatment techniques will allow the therapist several new treatment options.

It is now possible to coordinate the movements of the other axes with the movement of the gantry and the dose rate. The following list is the first of these relationships under investigation for computer coordinated rotational therapy. These relationships can be established individually but executed simultaneously.

1. Variable arc definition: Multiple arcs of rotation can be specified, each having its own start and stop gantry angle and rads per degree of specification.
2. Field size: The collimator jaw openings, both upper and lower, can be specified independently as a function of the gantry angle. This capability will allow oval-shaped and elliptical-shaped high-dose volumes to be delivered. For example, in the pelvis, narrow lateral and wider AP and PA fields may be desirable.
3. Collimator rotation: The angle of collimators may be adjusted as a function of the gantry angle. This allows an apparent axis of rotation that is askew from the mechanical axis of rotation of the gantry. This would be used for the esophagus, for example, by creating an axis of rotation coincident with the center of the esophogus.
4. Variable source-to-rotation axis distance: By moving the patient support mechanism in coordination with the gantry angle, it is possible to create a range of source-to-axis distances.
5. Off-center rotation: Head rotation, the ability to change the angle of the central ray relative to a ray through the source and the isocenter, is possible on many treatment units, usually cobalt units. By coordinating the movement of the patient-support mechanism with the gantry angle, it is possible to simulate this capability on a treatment unit that does not have the mechanical head-rotation option.
6. General position-coordination mode: In this mode the position of any axis of motion can be set as a function of the position of any other axis. This general motion coordination is to provide the capability for any future modes of dynamic treatment.
7. General dose-coordination mode: In this mode the position of any axis of motion can be adjusted as a function of the dose delivered.

Hardware

The equipment used in this set of experiments was a Varian 4 MV linear accelerator and a Varian 620f computer. To allow movement of the linear accelerator under computer control during the beam-on period, it was necessary for us to add some hardware logic to the treatment unit-computer interface, and temporarily to modify the ready relay in the linear accelerator gantry stand. The modification to the interface created a new state or mode called "dynamic treatment" of computer control. The standard Varian interface recognizes two states, "Auto" and "Home," which are initiated or created by depressing one of two switches that are added to the hand pendant motor controller. This modification allows the computer to supply the motor control signal to the DC motor controllers.

The ready relay in the gantry stand was installed to inhibit DC power to the motor controllers during the "ready" and "beam-on" condition of the linear accelerator. During these experiments the normal relay was replaced with a specially modified one. For clinical implementation of dynamic treatment, modification of the control logic for this relay with the appropriate safety interlocks will be required. Closing the deadman switch is also a necessary condition to supply voltage to the DC motor controllers. A new deadman switch will be provided on the outside of the treatment room for the clinical version.

Software

The programs are written in FORTRAN with no special assembly language or low-level languages used. The programs are running under VORTEX (Varian's multitasking real-time executive system). Under this operating system two programs are actually scheduled and run simultaneously. One very small program running at the highest priority pulses the treatment unit-computer interface every 50 milliseconds, so that if the computer fails, this pulse will not be transmitted and all electrical connections between the linear accelerator and the computer are severed and the treatment unit returns automatically to the manual or noncomputer controlled mode of operation.

The second program is the one that actually exercises the control over the linear accelerator. Currently, there is available a linear compensating filter program and the beginning of a rotation therapy program.

Results

Presently the linear compensating filter program is being used to produce dosimetry films in anticipation of clinical use. The rotation program is in the process of being coded. The films produced by the dynamic wedge are comparable to the dose-distributions produced by a mechanical wedge filter. Detailed analysis of the differences in the beam characteristics will be forthcoming; the primary concern up to now has been to generate accurately a dose distribution with the desired wedge angle.

Two significant results of the investigation are: (1) the motor control techniques, and (2) the development of position versus dose and position versus position-coordination techniques.

The dynamic wedge was initiated as a feasibility study for the general technique of using a computer to coordinate the various treatment-unit axes of movement.

These experiences can be generalized into a single dynamic treatment package which will be able to handle all possible combinations of axial movements.

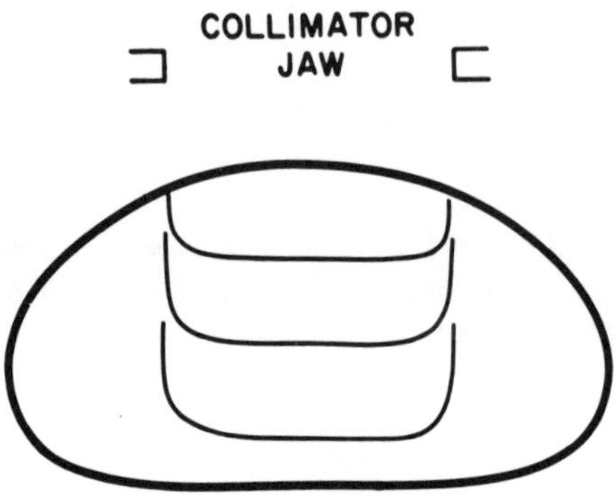

FIGURE I.

Figure 1. Isoeffect (Isodose) Lines from an Exposure from a Single Static Treatment Field with the Collimator Opened as Shown Superimposed on a Patient Contour

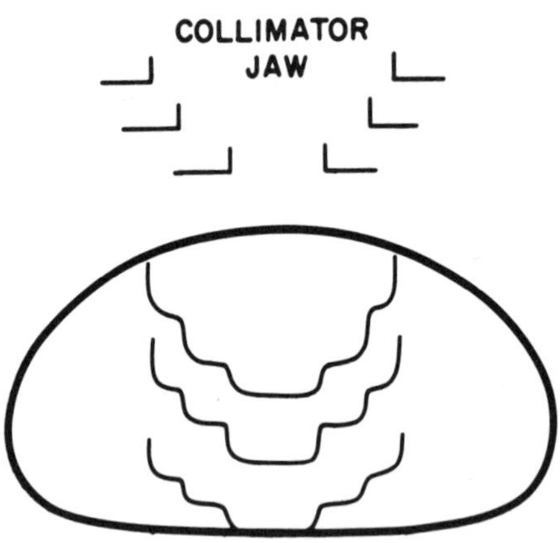

FIGURE 2.

Figure 2. Isodose Lines Superimposed on a Patient Cross-section from the Cumulative Effect of an Irradiation by a Static Treatment Field which has had the Collimators Closed 3 Times During Treatment

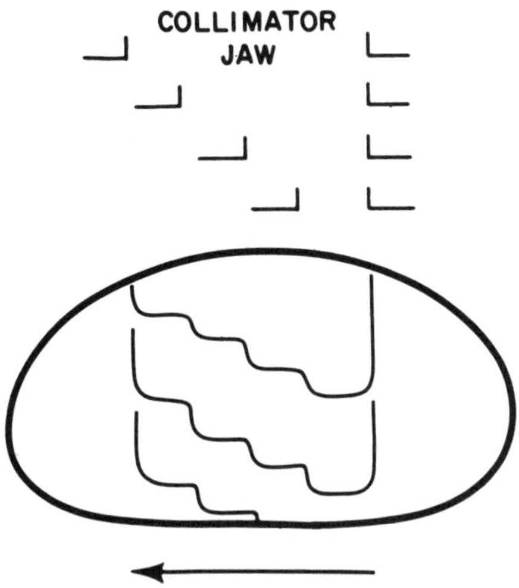

FIGURE 3.

Figure 3. Isodose Lines Superimposed on a Patient Cross-section from the Cumulative Effect of Closing the Jaws 4 Times and Simultaneously Moving the Patient During Irradiation.

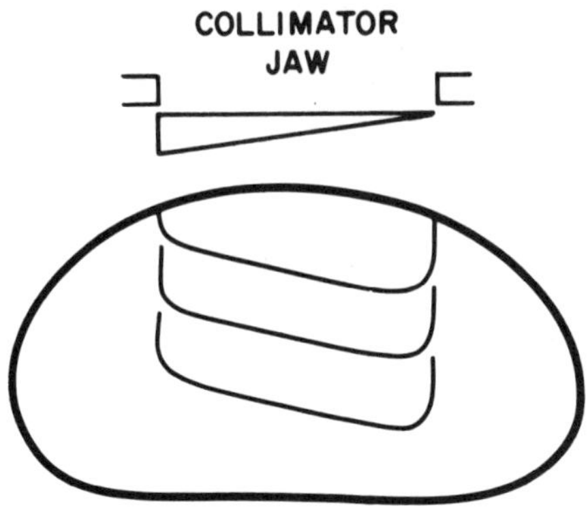

FIGURE 4.

Figure 4. Isodose Line Produced either by Continuously Closing the Collimators with the Coordinated Movement of the Patient, or Inserting a Mechanical Linear Compensating Filter

Session IVa: General Discussion. "How can we best make computer-controlled radiation therapy advance from a technically feasible project (if it is) to a clinically significant modality?"

Moderator
M. E. Rosenbloom

ROSENBLOOM: I feel there are a number of questions which are essential to answering this single question. The first one is the definition of our goals. Another is the importance of safety. And one very important question is really how much do we want computer-controlled radiation therapy? Do we think it will be cost effective when the development is complete? This is philosophical. We're in a better position now to answer the question of how far we have come. At the present state of the art, can we identify the major stumbling blocks? If we can see these, can we see our way to overcoming them? Dr. Glicksman has agreed to open the discussion.

GLICKSMAN: At the 4th International Conference, we were presented a problem of three-dimensional treatment-planning of the esophagus—of an esophageal lesion—and a number of institutions submitted plans for that. And as you remember, they were of all various types. But basically, the approach was how does one handle a three-dimensional volume that is moving posteriorly as it's moving inferiorly and with the kinds of critical organs around it that have to be protected? Today's session moved from the static approach to show that dynamic treatment—that is, moving the patient, moving the treatment source—can be feasible. Now we have to address ourselves to what is practical in this regard. Can we consider areas where there will be some payoff for this?

Since the esophagus was used before, let me ask: "How does one do 3-D treatment planning for pelvic nodes?" and "Would a dynamic approach give a significant improvement in our ability to deliver significant radiotherapy to pelvic nodes which are again in different planes of the patient?" And this is an area that we now handle very simply—we do parallel opposed fields and hope for the best.

There's yet another dimension to the challenge, and that would be to extend radiotherapy to organs that we do not even approach to treat well now. We're inundated with treatment techniques and discussion for Hodgkin's disease. There are 4,500 new patients with Hodgkin's disease each year in the United States. There are 21,000 patients with pancreatic cancer in the United States, and the mortality from this disease approaches 98 percent. We have a real challenge to extend the use of radiotherapy to such an organ. If we could define the volume that we have to irradiate without irradiating both kidneys, without irradiating the spinal cord, could we with the techniques that Bjarngard showed get our isodoses around that kind of target volume?

I think this will be the kind of challenge that would change this from a technically feasible, interesting experiment for a small number of institutions into a very practical and important contribution in the management of patients with cancer.

FREY: The article by Bengt Bjarngard and his group did one thing which I think harked back to an earlier time, which was thinking of hardware solutions to problems which perhaps now can be managed by software. The idea of uncoupling the jaws is something one has to do hardwarewise, but I think it was shown by Neblett that it can be done with the machine as it is set up by simply coupling two motions together. And I think the same thing can be said for the variable collimator. This can also be simulated by scanning the table longitudinally or in some other way as the collimator jaws are varied. Software is easy to write, whereas to get these kinds of hardware changes we have to have more acquiescence of the manufacturers, which I think may be more difficult. The other thing I would like to point out is that we have been attempting to simulate the mechanical wedges that we have available now—which just don't have straight surfaces. There's no reason why we need a uniform velocity, why we couldn't construct straight isodose lines with a nonuniform velocity, or do correction for irregular surfaces and construct surface contours as well in both directions. So I think there are a large number of possibilities.

KIJEWSKI: To answer your first point: To make hardware changes will be much, much simpler than trying to write the software with coupled jaws, especially when we go more to complicated techniques like combining collimator motion and rotation, for example.

In a simple case, like that of the wedge, that's not true. A combination of couch motion and collimator motion is quite simple. But if you couple that with rotation, we feel the independent collimators would be a much, much simpler solution.

To answer your second point: we've looked at a great deal more possible applications of dynamic treatment, but there's only so much one can present in eight minutes. Certainly a variable velocity of the collimator jaws is a very interesting topic, which we have studied.

NEBLETT: The wedge, of course, is merely a starting point. We are also playing with the use of Moiré patterns in the treatment position to produce contours with which we can begin to experiment with 3-D compensating filters.

CUNNINGHAM: I would like to make a very brief comment. It's with regard to dynamic treatment, which is really a rather exciting and interesting thing, and the computation of the dose distribution which you get under these circumstances. I have looked at this a little bit, and it's not as simple as one might expect. Sometimes you get surprises. You change your parameters in a particular way, and it doesn't necessarily give you the dose distribution that you expect unless you look at it from that point of view very, very carefully. The manipulation of the jaws or the treatment parameters, the couch and so on, that's fairly straightforward, but you have to close the loop through the dose distribution that you're going to get, and that's not an easy one.

MILAN: Would any of the speakers have any idea of the proportion of the total number of radiotherapy cases in which dynamic treatments would make any significant differences?

FREY: If this can give us merely a simple approach to compensate for surface irregularities, that in itself would probably be useful in 20 or 25 percent of the cases. And certainly the problem we have with the esophagus—this is something we really can't do appropriately and this is the sort of thing where we can follow an irregular cylinder through space. I would estimate about 30 to 40 percent of cases would benefit from this sort of thing.

PERRY: In answer to the question of dynamics, we've done a simple thing. With rotational treatments, we have used changing field size, changing output, and changing rad per degree, and in this way as a first step one can achieve a clinically useful end. We do this predominantly with patients who come to us with curative carcinoma of the prostate. In this manner we think we achieve a reasonably good dose distribution. We've checked *in vivo* with very small chambers as well as with lithium fluoride.

In regard to the question of the esophagus, one must use some 3-D approach, in the cervical esophagus and as one moves from the middle third to the upper third. In this setting, one must take into account where you're using fixed fields, a change in the gantry angle and the head angle in order to compensate for the change in the slope of the esophagus as well as its position; and again, as one weights the fields and adds or subtracts a wedge, one can achieve the proper kind of dose distribution.

Another thing that we have done in the static setting is to use the multiple leaf collimator to give irregular fields. But what we're trying to do now, and we need the funding, is to change the field dynamically as we move it through space. But this, of course, will take some doing, because in using a big linear accelerator the blocks are quite large, and of course there's a tremendous expense in getting the proper motion of these in space.

ELLIS: I think one of the biggest problems we've got is knowing exactly where the tumor is, the volume that we want to treat. With the esophagus I think it's probably easier but not absolutely settled. With the lymph nodes in the pelvis or para-aortic regions it's possibly easier than it used to be because of lymphangiography; but it's difficult to think of any other area where it might be very useful. Actually, the Royal Northern Hospital was concerned for a long time with trying to track the nodes along the para-aortic region and through the pelvis, and I understand that is working very well. In the esophagus it is very important, of course, to take account of the air in the lung, and I wonder how these dynamic methods would take account of air in the lung which varies with the patient's breathing. Some years ago, we published an article on fixed fields, taking account of air in the lung, estimated in the individual patients by Sievert dose meters put in the esophagus. Then with the four-field method we used compensators and found that it made an error of something like 30 or 35 percent to the dose if it was calculated as if the patient were water. So I feel that *that* is very important.

SUNTHARALINGAM: I believe the question we are posing to ourselves is: "If dynamic treatment is technically feasible, is it going to be clinically significant? " I'm still not convinced that it has been demonstrated that dynamic treatment is clinically usable. One of the assumptions I think is made in these hypothetical situations is that the dose rate remains constant. I am sure that we are fully aware that if you keep changing your collimator position, you are going to get a change in the dose rate. Film techniques have been used to show a single wedged beam produced using dynamic function. But I'm still not too sure whether this is adequate to tell us whether combining two wedged beams is feasible. You have to start with your target volume, you have to prescribe your isodose value that you want to administer to this target volume, and then you have to come up with the correct wedge angle that you want to use, combining wedged fields. And I'm still not too sure whether we have reached a new stage where this is a clinically usable technique.

FREY: First, let me answer Dr. Ellis, who said he couldn't think of any other place it might be useful. One that immediately comes to mind is this. I would be very happy if I could use rotation therapy for uterine cancer in such a way that I could change the collimator opening so that it would be wider in the AP direction and smaller in the lateral direction, and thereby conform the dose to a disease that tends to spread laterally. I think that's another thing that would be very useful and perhaps might increase the utility of external therapy in a place where we ordinarily have to use internal treatment.

In response to the last speaker, I think that this is a fairly simple problem, if we had the mechanisms to do these things. Right now people haven't addressed themselves to it because it's not required clinically just yet.

GRIEM: It seems that surgical staging of various diseases is becoming more fashionable, and what we've learned from Hodgkin's disease is now being applied to cancer of the prostate at USC and Stanford, and in cancer of the bladder at Northwestern. A number of cancer centers are now having the surgeons actually mark and identify where disease is, based on biopsy. Tumor localization using isotopes is certainly becoming more and more fashionable; ultrasound is being used, and now with the EMI scanner we're getting a better idea of where a tumor may be in the brain. I think as we develop some of the newer techniques for tumor localization, the radiotherapist is going to come to the computer expert and to the physicist and say, "I want to treat this and I don't want to treat the kidney or the spinal cord or the liver."

DAHLIN: Before this session is ended I would like to raise a question concerning the computer hardware. Many of us sitting here are very well familiar with computer techniques, and I am very surprised that no one has raised the question of introducing a microprocessor or computers on chips with this special type of computer-process controlling. If there is anyone here who is familiar with this special technique, it would be very good to have a hint about the future developments, because we know other similar applications in the medical field are going this way with the process control of specific devices.

HAHN: I think that microprocessors are certainly coming. The major advantage of them in the very near future, however, will be for things where you duplicate jobs very, very frequently. For intelligent terminals, for example, the trade-off at present is more expensive and more extensive programming. Our programming costs are in almost all cases greater than our hardware cost. I don't think that microprocessors are the answer now—but maybe three, four, or five years from now they will be. But they're basically, I think, valuable for repetitive processing.

LUNDY: We've looked a little bit at using a microprocessor controlling some of our scanning motions. I think Hahn's comments we would probably agree with. It may be harder to do, but we may do it anyway because of the interest. It seems to be a coming sort of thing. If you're going to build thirty systems, in that case it might be much more attractive.

I'm struck by some of the discussion here about dynamic treatment—that many of the factors that determine whether this is good or not are the same factors of whether pion therapy may be good or not. Now pions may have additional advantages of some higher LET, but I think that physicists working in this area—or at least, people that are somewhat removed from direct clinical work—would like more input from therapists on what we really do know about the dose distributions needed. How important is it to get a better dose distribution? Is it only going to be important if we can get better diagnostic information?

GEORGE: I'd like to respond to Dr. Lundy. I'd like to reinforce what was said by Mel Griem, and point out that in my view, progress in radiotherapy is toward more and more complexly shaped portals and, perhaps, combinations of modalities. And these combinations might include electrons, photons, mesons, neutrons, and various energies of these several modalities in combination with hyperthermia, systemic chemotherapy, and various types of sensitizers. We already see in the pi meson approach, the type of dynamic treatment that is needed. As dynamic treatment-planning becomes more sophisticated, we can present to the computer certain constraints. For instance, we're becoming aware that subclinical radiation injury is becoming more and more important. We're finding this out through the so-called recall phenomena of systemic chemotherapy: injury not clinically demonstrated previously but showing up when we give the patient Actinomycin-D or other chemotherapeutic agents—pericarditis, pneumonities, etc. So it is becoming increasingly important to apply constraints, particularly as we include "sanctuary therapy"—where we're treating brain, lung, kidney, gonads, etc.—to certain levels in combination with large-shaped fields, etc.

The complexity is already really beyond what is humanly possible to deal with, and when we mix radiation modalities and chemical modalities and try to practice a more responsible kind of therapy in terms of minimizing dose to normal structures, we'll have to use a sort of Monte Carlo approach, I believe, where the computer looks at all the possibilities and defines the arrangement which when implemented through computer control will maximize the dose to those regions we want to treat on the basis of EMI scanning, ultrasonic scanning, and increasingly sophisticated diagnostic and detection techniques. With ultrasonic scanning we're able to define the areas to be treated and define the anatomical location of normal structures with increasing accuracy. We are able to do it in digital form that can be computer-massaged, so to speak. We're digitizing contours, we're digitizing the position of the liver, the lung, etc. through scanning techniques; with EMI scanning, with transverse axial scanning, with radionuclides, with X rays, with ultrasound. There's even some possibility of using microwaves. I think we're almost beyond the position where the radiotherapist can use the conventional approaches.

ROSENBLOOM: I wonder if anybody now could say what he regards as the last word on the subject tonight. Who would like to take this on himself?

CLIFTON: I don't know whether I can say the last word. I sincerely hope not. I think this discussion will go on for some time. What I would like to do, however, is to follow up just a little of what Dr. Ellis said concerning the tracking cobalt unit that exists at the Royal Northern, or rather the Royal Free Hospital, as it is now. This unit has no computer, yet it is a dynamic treatment system. It is dependent on a cam-following system. It's used primarily for treating lymph-node systems, and one produces from the radiographs a contoured beam that is followed by a series of cams; the jaws of the machine and the treatment table are moved by another set of cams, the prescription of which is defined by the radiotherapist. This appears from a number of cases to be very successful. But now here comes the story—which may be the moral if you like. We've been discussing with them how they compute their dose distributions in three dimensions. This takes us not minutes but hours, of 360-65 computation time. What's more, having got the dose distribution in three dimensions, we've yet to figure out a suitable way of displaying it so anyone can understand what the devil it means. I think that we have to consider very seriously the other problems that go with making an all-singing, all-dancing, automated treatment machine.

Furthermore, listening to the discussion this afternoon, I would like to reiterate what Jack Cunningham said rather briefly, and that is, moving the jaws of collimators and things of this sort are fine, but we must watch that we don't throw out the baby with the water in the bathtub, because we are starting to compromise seriously a lot of basic dosimetry that we do not fully understand, when we start moving jaws and things in this matter.

III. Treatment Planning Systems

Chairperson: F. Dobrowolski

Session V: Contributed Short Papers

1. Classification of Systems for Computerized Treatment Planning

B. Olsen

Introduction

The purpose of this paper is to give a brief review of existing computer configurations for computerized treatment planning in radiotherapy. It includes a figure that shows the cost per year versus the number of calculated isodose curves per year.

In principle there are at least seven main configurations employed in radiotherapy, allowing seven different kinds of operation:

(1) Manual
(2) Batch computers
(3) Time-sharing terminals
(4) Small dedicated computers
(5) Medium-sized, multipurpose computers
(6) Remote-batch terminals
(7) Intelligent, remote-batch terminals

To avoid confusion, variants with chip computers are not discussed here, and neither are solutions with multiple local computers.

1. **Manual operations.** These are the basic methods of dose calculation. In case of computer failure they must always be practiced. They are, however, slow, restricted, occasionally inaccurate, and expensive.

2. **Batch computers.** These have a relatively long turn-around time. They are unsuited for on-line operation, but they have a cost advantage over other systems. In using batch computers there is no investment in hardware except for access to a card punch. As can be seen in Figure 1, they are highly recommended for use if the number of dose plans per year is small. They are thus generally the best solution for a developing radiotherapy center if specific local conditions do not suggest another solution.

3. **Time-sharing (TS) terminals.** The time-sharing (TS) terminals

used to be restricted with regard to such input and output peripherals as graphic I/O devices, but the situation has changed, and nowadays almost any function that can be undertaken by a dedicated system, perhaps with the exception of the direct monitoring of treatment machines, can be performed via a TS terminal. The hardware cost could be kept relatively low, whereas the running costs on the TS computer are deemed to be considerable. A typical hardware configuration would be typewriter, modem, and analog I/O. The response time for a single interaction may be in the order of a few seconds, which could be very frustrating.

The cost for the calculations on the large computer is roughly five times that of running the same problem on the same computer but in batch mode. The most important need for interactivity is in checking the input data. The ideal solution would be to use a system that allows interactive input in the time-sharing mode and then submission into the batch queue. Even a remote-batch terminal solution should be preferable, especially if it is also used for submitting other jobs.

4. Small dedicated computers (SDC). Here we talk about an 8 to 16 X-bit words stand-alone computer, where X in most cases is 16. Minimally it must be equipped with typewriter input and analog I/O. These computers are able to perform many of the tasks demanded by the radiotherapy center. Recent price reductions on memories and peripherals allow for a variety of configurations. Most of today's commercial solutions are of this type, but they severely limit the possibilities of advanced applications and further development.

In Figure 1 the costs of two different dedicated systems are shown, one of them home built, with a hardware cost of $40,000, and one commercial, costing about $120,000. Since the latter includes software, etc., it is not self-evident that the less expensive solution must necessarily be the preferred one. Other factors than those described above may contribute to the decision. Note that the costs are almost independent of the number of plans. It is estimated that the running expenses are around $1000 at 1000 plans/year.

5. Medium-sized, multipurpose computers (MS). These configurations are so well equipped (and thus expensive) that they normally require an operator. In addition to the minimum hardware of a dedicated system, they also have, for example, a card-reader and line-printer. Because they are more expensive than the dedicated computers, they should be capable of running different jobs more or less simultaneously. Higher-level operating systems and compilers are available without penalties in time. In order to justify the capital outlay, jobs might have to be run for other departments. Today the difference between the small and medium-sized installations is vague. These MS computers are not included in Figure 1 because the number of applications by which their cost can be shared varies considerably.

They may be advantageous, however—allowing analog I/O, complicated calculations, and splitting of costs between many users.

6. Remote-batch terminals (RBT). These are basically card-reader/line-printer terminals which make it possible to submit a job into the job stream of a distant large computer. The capital investment starts at approximately $20,000. They are competitive with time-sharing terminals after only several hundred plans/year and are to be preferred to dedicated systems if fewer than 1000–1500 plans are produced per year. Telephone costs are, of course, dependent on the distance to the computer.

7. Intelligent, remote-batch terminals (IRBT). For use in radiotherapy, these include a small dedicated computer (SDC). The different tasks may be distributed between the local minicomputer and a large computer via transmission lines. These terminals have all the advantages of a small computer on site as well as of the large computer. In the same way as for the TS and RBT systems, a suitable large computer must be available. As can be seen from Figure 1, this solution starts with an initial cost and has a slope which can be expressed as

$$\alpha(\text{batch slope}) + \beta$$

where α is the percentage of the plans computed on the large computer and β includes telephone and running costs.

Especially when comprehensive calculations (such as 3-D) and optimization and administrative programs (such as follow-up) are run, this solution is superior because it allows operations and has a flexibility in further development—not possible with a minicomputer.

Discussion of Figure 1

The figure is based on the following assumptions:

(1) The capital investments are distributed over a period of 5 years. Maintenance costs are included: approximately 7 percent of capital investments per year.

(2) Only external dose-planning is discussed. Other applications will, of course, help to reduce capital costs per dose plan.

(3) In the case of teletransmission (timesharing, remote-batch, and intelligent terminal), the telephone cost is included for a distance of 100 km in Sweden.

(4) Advantages and disadvantages of the different systems with regard to interactivity, quality of calculation and display, etc., are not taken into account.

(5) Differences in use and their implications for the manual work are not included.

(6) The cost is estimated for a 2-D case including tissue heterogeneities. A three-field technique is used. The spread of the cost

within a category depends on such factors as the efficiency of the program, the price level of the computer used, and whether the program allows and uses, for example, heterogeneity corrections.

Costs for manual planning are not included because they depend so heavily on salary and capacity and on the work load. The medium-sized computer and a remote batch terminal (RBT) are excluded because these configurations should not be used solely for dose-planning. The curves for RBT can be obtained by adding the appropriate part of the capital cost ($20–40,000) to the corresponding batch values.

The figure is greatly simplified. It does not take into account such important questions as other applications, the amount of manpower required to use the different configurations, or the cost of software and software maintenance and development.

Conclusion

In my opinion, the intelligent, remote job-entry terminal is the most general and attractive solution to the problem of introducing computers into radiotherapy. With the use of this terminal the local computer installations at various radiotherapy centers may become part of a medical computer network. Such a solution would simplify the program maintenance and development. The actual size of the local installation may be varied within broad limits ($30,000 to approximately $100,000 in hardware cost), depending on the current situation: the number of patients per year, the number of computer applications, and the accessibility of a large (regional) computer and its cost and service characteristics. The most natural way of introducing computers to radiotherapy is, however, to start with a batch, remote-batch, or time-sharing solution, especially if the number of plans is small.

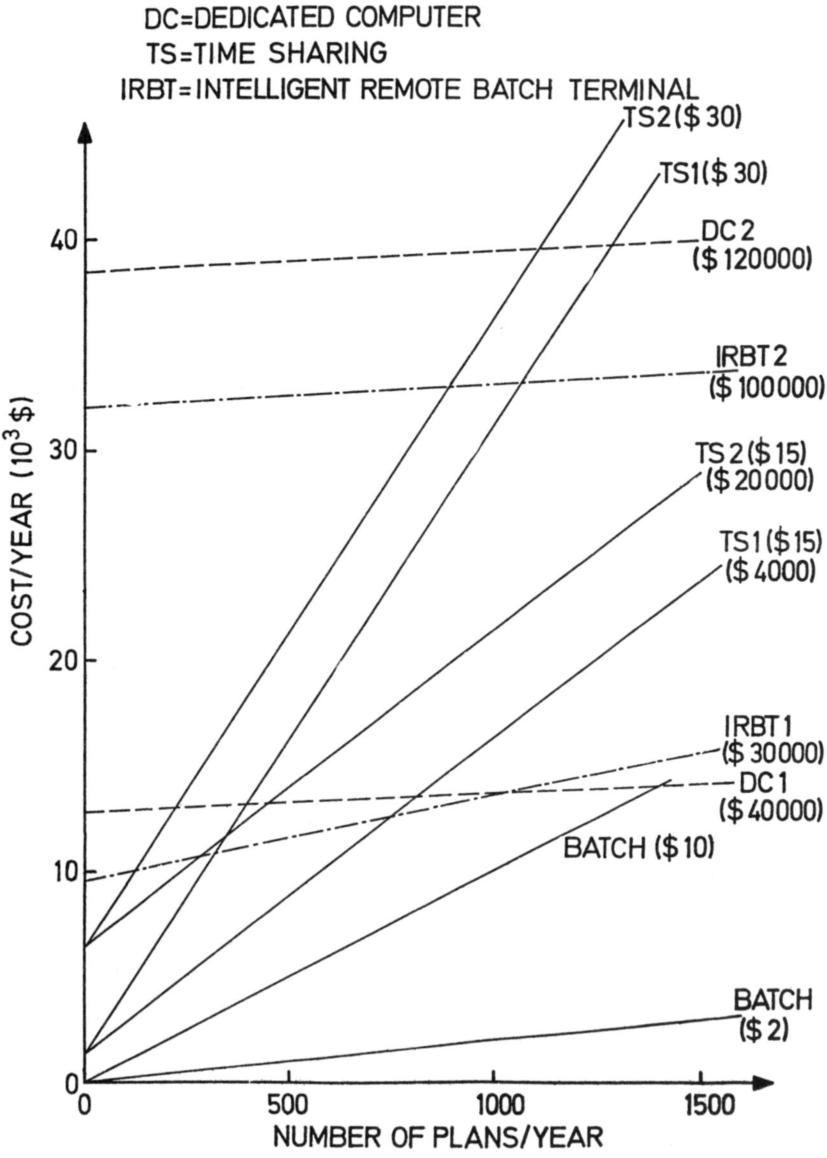

Figure 1. The Cost per Year vs. the Number of Calculated Isodose Curves per Year for Different Systems for Computerized Treatment Planning. The Capital Investment is Given for the Two Time-sharing Hardware Alternatives (TS1: $4,000 and TS2: $20,000), the Two Dedicated Computer Systems (DC1: $40,000 and DC2: $120,000) and the Two Intelligent Terminals (IRBT1: $30,000 and IRBT2: $100,000). In Addition the Assumed Cost per Plan is Given for the Time Sharing and Batch Alternative.

2. Treatment Planning in the British National Health Service

M. Cohen

Introduction

In this paper I shall try to draw a profile of treatment-planning in the United Kingdom, with particular reference to the use of computers. The work was initiated late in 1971 when the British Institute of Radiology, jointly with the Faculty of Radiologists and the Hospital Physicists' Association, set up a Working Party to enquire into the relationship between modern technology and radiotherapy. The Working Party was organized in three Task Groups, one of which, under my chairmanship, was asked to study the application of computers to treatment-planning.

The Task Group got off to a rather slow start, with a long questionnaire that promised a great deal but actually produced very little information. Then, toward the end of 1972, the Department of Health offered to fund a detailed survey, and my colleague Barry Barber, formerly a medical physicist and now Director of Operational Research at The London Hospital, was asked to travel the country gathering facts and opinions. Dr. Barber presented his report early this year, jointly to the Task Group and to the Department of Health. It is a massive document of some 150 pages plus 12 appendices. The report has not yet been officially accepted either by the BIR or by the Department of Health, and in any case the Task Group has still to produce its own report, which will incorporate or reject Dr. Barber's facts and conclusions as the Group thinks fit. My paper therefore draws upon three sources of information: Barry Barber's report, which I freely and gratefully acknowledge; some facts and inferences gathered independently by the Task Group; and other information that I have obtained specially for this paper. The opinions and conclusions will be my own and will not necessarily agree with those of the BIR Working Party when it produces its report.

Organization of Radiotherapy in the United Kingdom

In Britain, as you all know, we have a National Health Service, and this fact pervades all discussion of treatment-planning, medical-computing, or indeed any other aspect of health care. The Health Service is organized into twenty-one regions, each serving 2 to 3 million people, although the Scottish and Irish regions serve fewer people in larger geographical areas.

In the U.K. there is virtually no radiotherapy outside the Health Service. Radiotherapy is organized in centers, most of them in large general hospitals, a few in special cancer hospitals. There are sixty-five independent centers, plus or minus three or four. The uncertainty arises from the difficulty of defining an "independent" radiotherapy center. The term does not necessarily imply an institute or department located in a single building or even a single town. Many of these centers, especially outside London, have several satellite diagnostic and follow-up clinics with orthovoltage and/or low voltage X-ray sets. In terms of overall organization, treatment policy, and dosimetry, however, the main center and satellites function as a single unit, which provides a full range of radiation treatment.

Let us see how the patient load is distributed among the sixty-five centers, or rather among the fifty-nine centers in England and Wales for which statistics are collected by the Department of Health (Table 1). The source of this information is the so-called SH3 form, completed by every hospital, not simply for radiotherapy but for all specialties, and for both in-patients and out-patients. Unfortunately, the figures are suspect. A given patient may or may not be registered twice, once as an out-patient and again as an in-patient. Again, the out-patient figures reflect the numbers registering at a radiotherapy department, whether for radiation treatment or for some other purpose, such as diagnostic radioisotope tests, which are still given by some radiotherapy centers.

My own estimate—this has still to be verified—is that about 45 percent of the centers are small (<1000 patients/yr.), 40 percent medium size (1000-2500 patients/yr.), and only 15 percent large (>2500 patients yr.).

Cancer, Radiotherapy and Treatment-Planning Statistics

Turning to the evidence from cancer statistics, we may see that here again the data are not as helpful as we would wish. The last year for which published figures are available is 1967. One can make a reasonably good estimate on the basis of the constancy of the incidence rate and then add 10 percent to allow for the estimated proportion of cancer cases that are not notified to the National Cancer Registry. This gives about 160,000 new cases annually in England and Wales. It is usually considered that about 50 percent of all cancer patients in the U.K. have radiotherapy of some kind, and this confirms my previous statement that the number of new radiotherapy patients lies somewhere between the two extreme figures derived from the SH3 data. Ninety-thousand new radiotherapy patients per annum in England and Wales seems a reasonable figure, equivalent to about 1500 for an average center.

If we now consider our typical medium-sized center, after allowing for palliative and other cases not requiring detailed dosimetric planning, about 37 percent of the initial intake will be candidates for individual planning by computer if the facilities for such planning exist. Thus over 500 patients of the initial 1500 will benefit from such planning if available, and this number is important because it links up with the break-even point I shall mention later for in-house real-time computing.

The BIR Task Group

We now return to the BIR Task Group. Its task was to assess the present situation in the U.K. and to make recommendations useful to the radiotherapy centers themselves, to hospital authorities and regional health authorities, and to the Department of Health. The options open to us were five: (1) batch-processing, (2) time-sharing with alphanumeric I/O, (3) interactive/dedicated computer, (4) time-sharing with graphical I/O, and (5) manual planning. It must be stressed that the survey was conceived and carried out as a purely parochial exercise. There was no question of combing the world for new developments, nor of producing recommendations of world-wide significance. The object of the exercise was to elaborate a realistic policy for the implementation in the next two or three years, of a computer system or systems of radiotherapy throughout the U.K., in small centers as well as in large, in remote towns as well as the metropolis. Such a policy had to be based on systems actually available and in use in the U.K., or at least in an advanced stage of development. In the end the options came down to two—a batch-processing system based mainly on the ICL 1903T and 1904S computers belonging to Regional Health Authorities, or the dedicated real-time system based largely on the Royal Marsden Hospital system and available commercially in the U.K. as the RAD-8 system.

Department of Health Policy

My use of the terms "developed" and "implementation" leads me to mention the official policy of the Department of Health with regard to computing in the Health Service. This policy was laid down in a document published in 1972. The policy is based on three stages: *experimentation* within a single center so as to produce a prototype system, *development* of that system in at least two or three other centers, and finally *implementation* of the model system throughout the Health Service. Between the development and implementation stages *evaluation* is supposed to take place according to detailed criteria set out in the document. The whole process looks neat and tidy on paper but is open to certain objections. To begin with, only the first two stages are eligible for funding by the Department of Health. When the Department recommends a system for general implementation, it does so by persuading or bullying regional or local authorities to purchase that system from their own funds, not by providing the system from central funds. Since regional and local money is always in very short supply, a hospital is in effect encouraged to develop a new system rather than utilize an existing one. Secondly, the evaluation process is likely to prove extremely difficult, especially in such murky areas as "the benefit to patients." At any rate it has not yet been put to the test, at least in the radiotherapy field.

Extent of Dose Computation in the U.K.

The need for wider implementation of computer systems in the U.K. has been examined with information derived partly from Dr. Barber's survey and partly by updating a 1971 survey carried out by the HPA. It seems that in 1973 fewer than 60 percent of British radiotherapy centers were using computers for dose computation, although admittedly the laggards tended to be the smaller centers. But the position may be even worse than this. The 1972 BIR questionnaire yielded a sample of thirty-one centers that gave data on their dose computation activities, both by computer and manually. Only thirteen of these centers were using computers, and of these only five carried out 50 percent or more of their dose computations in this way. Five out of the thirteen centers used the computer for less than 20 percent of the treatment charts. Furthermore, taking all treatment charts, manual as well as computer-produced, for the same thirty-one centers, we find that most centers do not even approach the level of 37 percent in relation to the intake of new patients, especially when we bear in mind that many patients require more than one chart. There is considerable evidence, however, that the volume of charting goes up once a computer system becomes routine, especially if the real-time interactive system is adopted.

Comparison of Dose Computation Systems

I shall now summarize, very briefly, Dr. Barber's analysis of the cost-effectiveness of each system; to be more precise, manual planning versus batch processing versus RAD-8. A study of this kind is based on certain assumptions as to the capital cost of equipment, including software; running costs, including computer time; and staff costs. Most of these factors vary widely from institute to institute, let alone from country to country. For example, one center will buy a dedicated system solely for dose computation and will be content to allow the equipment to sit idle more than half the time, while another institute will use the same system to its full capacity for several different tasks. Again, in the U.K. some radiotherapy centers are able to obtain time on a Regional Health Authority or University computer free of charge, while other institutes have to pay for computing time. Perhaps most important of all, the type and seniority of staff engaged on dose computation varies widely, as does the amount and choice of information demanded by the radiotherapists.

The simplest point to begin is the cost of the hardware, although the equivalent *annual* cost will depend on the method of accounting. Table 2 shows that if a RAD-8 system is amortized over seven years, the annual cost is about £4500, rising to £5700 if additional optional hardware is purchased. (These figures are already somewhat out of date, because of inflation, but the relative costs of different systems will not be greatly in error.) The annual hardware cost for a batch-processing system is, of course, much less—in the range of £200–400.

Table 3 shows the estimated staff costs for treatment-planning. A single technician or physicist will be hard pressed to plan more than 200 patients a year in detail by hand, and our Glasgow colleagues estimate that his productivity is increased by one third by introducing a batch-processing system. Hence the rather odd figure of 267 patients per annum by this method. With the RAD-8 system, if we assume 30 or 45 minutes per patient, a single technician will have no difficulty in coping with even 1000 patients a year. Even at 750 patients a year, the RAD-8 staff costs are considerably lower than those for the manual and batch systems.

Table 4 summarizes the fixed and variable annual costs for the three systems. The only figure not already mentioned is the assumed £1.5 per patient for computer time when a batch system is used. Note that it is also assumed that the interactive system utilizes a technician while the other two require a junior physicist.

The break-even points are summarized in Table 5. The interactive RAD-8 system will pay for itself vis-à-vis either manual or batch processing with 500–600 plans a year, corresponding to a new patient load of about 1500. This applies to a radiotherapy center of medium size, by our scale. The break-even point for manual to batch is more variable, depending on factors difficult to generalize, but should occur well within the patient load of a typical small department.

Conclusions

Dr. Barber produced a list of thirty detailed recommendations which have not yet been endorsed by either the Department of Health or the BIR Task Group. The most important conclusions can be summarized as follows: We wish to ensure that every single radiotherapy center in the U.K. has access either to a dedicated interactive system or to a batch-processing system. We would hope that eventually both systems will be replaced, or will develop into, a time-sharing interactive graphical system such as has been developed here in Dartmouth and is being developed in the Middlesex-Addenbrooke's project in the U.K. We would recommend strongly that any implemented system needs to be maintained and developed, and that a suitable organization needs to be set up and funded for this. Finally, we would like to see some organization set up to enable the very expensive equipment and expertise required for the measurement of basic radiation data to be utilized more fully than is often the case at present.

Table 1.
Size of Radiotherapy Centers in England and Wales

Category	*New Patients p.a.*	*Number* *OP + IP Basis*	*OP Only Basis*
Small	<1000	20 (34%)	33 (56%)
Medium	1001–2500	27 (46%)	19 (32%)
Large	>2500	12 (20%)	7 (12%)

Table 2.
RAD-8 Annual Cost Estimates
(Based on Barber, 1974)

For Amortization Over 7 Years

	£	£
Computer hardware	22140/7	3163
D.E.C. software	750/7	107
Software support (1 man-month)	3375/7	281
Hardware maintenance		700
System implementation (7 man-months/7)		204
Consumables		100
Building		—
		4555
Additional Hardware		
Floating-point processor	4120/7	588
Exchangeable disk	4080/7	583
		5726

Table 3.
Staff Costs for Treatment Planning:
Cost in Pounds per Patient
(Based on Barber, 1974)

	Manual	*Computer*		
		Batch	*Real-Time*	
Patients Planned:				
per year	200	267	500	750
per day	0.75	1	2	3
Staff:				
Junior radiographer *	7.1	5.4	2.9	1.9
Senior radiographer	9.6	7.2	3.8	2.6
Med. Phys. technician middle grade	10.3	7.7	4.1	2.8
Junior physicist	11.5	8.6	4.6	3.1
Physicist - middle grade	16.8	12.6	6.7	4.5

* radiographer = therapy technician in North America

Table 4.
Analysis of Fixed and Variable Costs
(Based on Barber, 1974)

System	*Patients Planned per Man-Year*	*Staff*	*Costs (£)*	
			Fixed (per year)	*Variable (per patient)*
Manual	200	junior physicist	0	11.5
Batch	267	junior physicist	223–427	8.6 (staff) + 1.5 (computer) = 10.1
RAD-8	750	technician	4555	2.8

Table 5.
Break-Even Points
(Based on Barber, 1974)

Manual to batch	159–309 plans/year
Manual to RAD-8	523 plans/year
Batch to RAD-8	565 plans/year

3. A Radiation Treatment Planning System with a Computer/Ultrasound B-Scan/ Interactive Graphics System

W. T. Chu
J. M. Slater
J. E. Chrispens
D. M. Jacobson
I. R. Neilsen

Description of the System

An ultrasound scanner with B-scan and gray scale has been interfaced with a computer to perform a comprehensive task in radiation treatment planning (1). The potential usefulness of diagnostic ultrasound in radiation treatment-planning has been widely discussed (2). The system's planning capability and the usefulness are greatly enhanced by handling the complex graphic input/output data through a multicolor video monitor and two sonic pen digitizers.

A schematic diagram of the system is shown in Figure 1. The patient data, including the body contour, cross-sectional anatomy, and sometimes the treatment volume, are obtained through the B-scan ultrasonography. The echogram data are stored in a scan-converter storage tube and concurrently displayed on a multicolor video monitor. The computer digitizes these data with or without operator interventions. Radiation parameters are graphically entered by the operator with the computer assistance. Based on the patient data and the radiation parameters, the computer calculates the radiation dose distribution, which is stored in a second scan converter and displayed in a contrasting color superimposed on the patient cross-section. When a modification in a plan is necessary, only the calculated distribution is erased in one of the two-scan converters, while the patient data in the other scan converter is kept undisturbed, and new radiation parameters are entered for an alternate plan. Upon production of an acceptable plan, the radiation parameters are displayed superimposed on the patient body contour. The ultrasound scanner probe is moved over the proposed area of radiation on the patient body, and its position is tracked on the video screen. When the probe is localized exactly at the beam port, the patient is marked accurately and quickly.

The system is used for planning of radiation therapy using various external beams, including irregular fields as well as interstitial and intracavitary implant dosimetry.

Hardware

A commercially available ultrasound B-scan unit provides noninvasive imaging of a patient cross section. Recent development in gray scale ultrasonography (3) further assists in delineating tissue inhomogeneities. The computer used in the system is a 32K, 16-bit words machine with a memory cycle time less than approximately one microsecond. The longest delay while waiting for computer responses is on the order of half a minute when a dose distribution is computed and the graphical output is plotted on the video monitor. The sonic-pen digitizers are commercially available units for communicating the x,y coordinates of a hand-held stylus to the computer. A series of sound pulses are generated by a small spark gap in the stylus when it is pushed against a screen and are detected by two long strip-microphones placed in an L shape bordering the video screen or the view box. These units are used not only to enter manually the graphic information into the computer, but also for the operator to interact with the computer.

The interactive graphics is based on the Scan Converter Graphics Terminal (4) which, in its basic form, accepts graphic codes from the computer and translates them into x,y signals directing an electron beam in drawing the desired image (as an electrostatic charge distribution) on the target of a miniature scan-converter storage tube. By scanning the target of the storage tube, the image can be continuously displayed on a video monitor.

Hardware has been organized to perform the following tasks in three distinct modes:

1. **Ultrasound B-scan and its visualization.** When "write" mode in the ultrasound unit is selected, the x,y coordinates and z-pulse (the amplitude of an echo) are written in the scan converter-1. On terminating the scan, the selector in the ultrasound unit is switched to "view" or "computer control," and the image in the SC1 is displayed on the video monitor in green.

2. **Computer-controlled "write" in either SC1 or SC2.** In this "write" mode, computer-generated information is written in either SC1 or SC2. The selection of scan converters is done by software, and the selector in the ultrasound unit must be switched to "computer control." In this mode the "write level" (z-pulse) is written at x,y coordinates reached through digital-to-analogue converters (x D-A and y D-A, respectively). On termination of "write," the image in SC1 is displayed in green and that in SC2 in red, superimposed on the video

monitor. Manually generated graphic data using the two sonic pen digitizers are stored in the computer and can be similarly "written" in either of the two scan converters as the computer-generated data.

3. Computer-controlled search mode in SC1. To digitize graphical data automatically it is necessary to interrogate data in SC1. In computer-control mode with SC1 selected by software, the storage-tube image level is read at x,y coordinates reached by the x,y digital-to-analogue converters. The 12-bit digitized image level and the x,y coordinates are transferred to the computer for further processing. It is noted that for our application it is adequate to use six bits on the image level digitization.

The uses of these three modes are illustrated in the following. Suppose that the patient anatomy has been written in SC1 and displayed in green (mode 1, above). The body contour is digitized (mode 3), and the results are written in SC2 (mode 2) and displayed in red superimposed in the patient anatomy in green for an operator evaluation. Next the critical organs and treatment volume are traced on the patient anatomy displayed on the video screen, using a sonic-pen digitizer mounted on the video monitor. These data are first digitized then written in SC2 (mode 2) and displayed in red. When all computer-generated and manually drawn figures are accepted, they are transferred into SC1, and SC2 is cleared to make room for subsequent procedures. The beam parameters are now entered (mode 2) into SC2 (red) and are evaluated against the patient data in SC1 (green). When the beam data is specified, it is stored in the computer and SC2 is again cleared. Next the computed dose distribution is written into SC2 (mode 2) and displayed in red superimposed on the patient data in green. If the radiation plan requires modification, new beam data is generated from the patient data remaining intact in SC1. When the plan is accepted, the beam data is rewritten (mode 2) together with the patient-body contour in SC2 (red). For the purpose of marking the patient, the ultrasound scanner probe is moved over the patient's body, and the position of the probe is continuously recorded in SC1 (mode 2) and displayed in green superimposed on the body contour and the beam data in red. When the probe position is at the beam entry point, for example, the patient can be marked accurately.

Software

Computations of dose distribution are performed by programs developed elsewhere. For fixed and rotational external beam calculation, a Memorial program (5) is used. A modified version of a program from the Ontario Cancer Institute (6) is used for the irregular field planning. And for the implant dosimetry, the M. D. Anderson program (7) is used. These programs were developed primarily for processing with *digitized* input data and *tabulated* output. As *graphic* input data and *video* output are used in the system, considerable modifications have been made in software to handle graphic input/output data. Pertinent factors entered in developing software are discussed below.

Throughout the entire planning procedure, each step proceeds in an interactive way between the operator and the computer. Specific functions the computer is to perform are selected by the operator: when a decision is sought the computer displays a list of alternatives and the operator makes the choice simply by pointing the desired course, using the sonic pen on the video screen. A similar technique is used to enter numerical data. First the computer displays a list of numbers or a graduated "ruler," then the operator simply chooses an appropriate numerical value, using the sonic pen. Conversely, when specific functions are expected from the operator, the requests are displayed for an operator response. This eliminates much tedium of numerical data entry and keyboard responses which normally require strict formats. It also allows one to operate the system without memorizing the sequence of procedures.

The patient contour is obtained by moving the ultrasound scanner probe over the area of interest and displayed on the video monitor by continuously recording the probe position in one of the scan-converter storage tubes (SC1). The center of the contour is found through a successive approximation, and the contour is digitized by finding intersections with radial lines drawn from the center. The outlines of critical organs and treatment volume are traced, using the sonic pen on the video screen, and the resulting loci of the moving pen are digitized, recorded (in SC2), and displayed. Radiation parameters are entered in the following manner. The operator touches a beam entry point using the sonic pen on the patient's body contour on the video screen. The proposed beam angulation is computed, joining the beam-entry point and the center of the treatment volume; its lateral size is obtained from the projected dimension of the treatment volume on a plane orthogonal to the beam direction. The beam's transverse dimension is simply specified by the operator based on radiographic or other information. This datum is displayed on the video screen and can easily be modified, using the sonic pen until accepted by the operator.

For irregular-beam planning, the port is first drawn on a radiograph then traced, using the sonic pen directly on a view box and storing the image of the port in a scan-converter storage tube. The points of interest, such as lymph nodes, are simply located by using the sonic pen, and their positions are similarly stored. The sector integration for computing scattered radiation is performed on this stored image by finding sectors subtended by segments of the irregular port at each of the points of interest. The patient body contour and anatomy within the entire irregular field is obtained through multiple ultrasound scanning at various intervals. It is planned to incorporate the nonplanar characteristics of the patient body in the calculation of scattered radiation.

In this system the computed dose distribution is displayed superimposed on the cross-sectional anatomy of a patient. For this reason, programs have been developed to search points lying on isodose lines rather than to compute doses at matrix points. The latter method is commonly adopted in available programs as it is suitable for tabulated output.

Other Remarks

The radiation treatment-planning system developed by integrating an ultrasound unit and a computer is more useful and accurate than when the components are used separately. Software has been developed to simplify the operator interaction with the system. This encourages, and enables, radiation oncologists to perform the planning firsthand while the patient is present. The capability of the system in planning based on the patient's cross-sectional anatomy rather than on its planar projections on radiographs makes the system particularly suitable for planning for heavy-particle beam therapy, such as heavy ions or negative pions. The system will be of great value in research, for example, in accurately assessing tissue tolerance in radiation therapy. Its on-line capability and visual presentation render a heuristic quality in training radiological personnel.

REFERENCES

1. Slater, J. M., Neilsen, I. R., Chu, W. T., Carlsen, E. N., and Chrispens, J. E., *Cancer*, *34*, 96-99 (1974).
2. Brascho, D. J., *J. of Clinical Ultrasound*, *1*, 320-329 (1973).
3. Carlsen, E. N., *J. of Clinical Ultrasound*, *1*, 190-195 (1973).
4. Neilsen, I. R., *SIGBIO Newsletter*, *4*, 4-6 (1972).
5. DeClemente, A., Mohan, R., Reddy, M. T., and Holt, J. G., 1971. Memorial Hospital, New York, N. Y., November 1971.
6. Cunningham, J. R., Shrivastava, P. N., and Wilkinson, J. M., Dosimetry Workshop, Hodgkin's Disease, Chicago, Ill., September 1970. Radiological Physics Center, The University of Texas, M. D. Anderson Hospital and Tumor Institute at Houston, Texas (1970).
7. Shalek, R. J., and Stovall, M., *Am. J. Roentgenol.*, *102*, 662-687 (1968).

QUESTIONS

SILER: Can you give us the cost of your system?

CHU: The ultrasound unit is about $25,000. The color video monitor is $3000, and the two sonic-pen digitizers with all the associated electronics are about $3000. The scan converters are about $2500 each. You can use almost any computer—this is a 32K, 16-bit computer, and we don't use all the memory, so it could be smaller.

Supported in part by National Institute of Health Biotechnology Resource Grant RR00276.

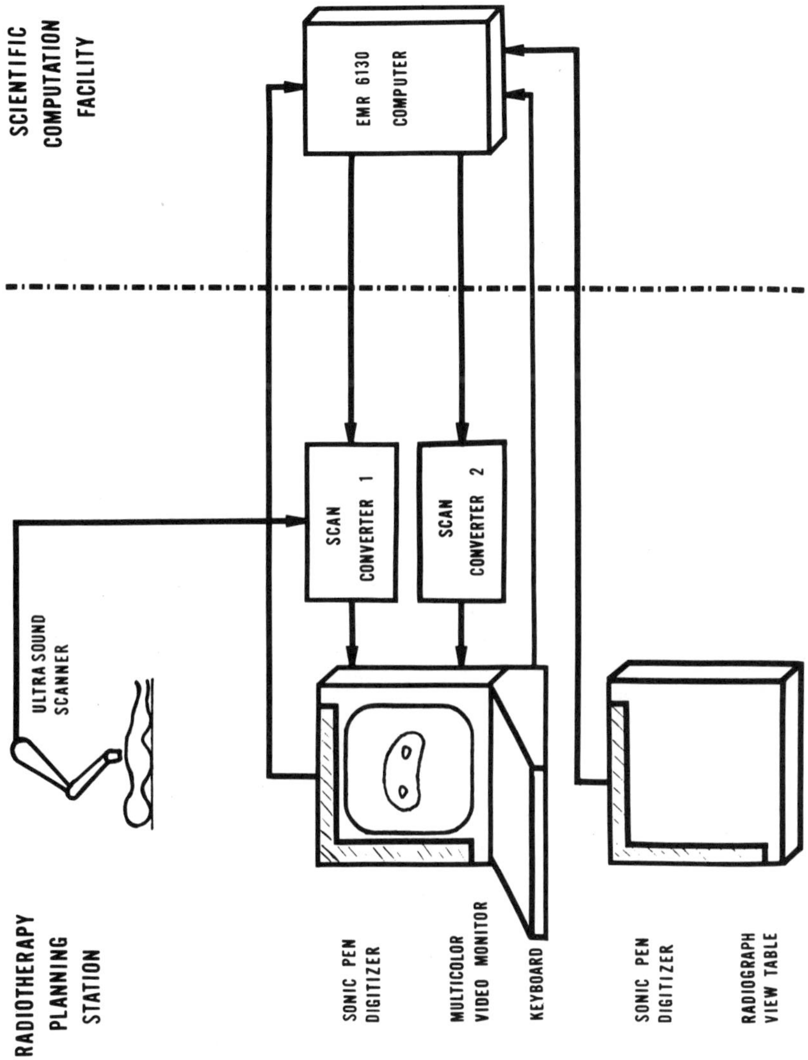

Figure 1. A Schematic Diagram of the Radiation Treatment Planning System

4. Calculation of Dose Distribution for Electron Depth Therapy Paying Regard to Inhomogeneities

D. Fehrentz

Depth therapy with electrons up to about 40 or 50 MeV energy, alone or in combination with megavolt X rays, in many cases produces more suitable dose distributions and a lower integral-dose than with megavolt X rays alone (1). This paper is concerned with the philosophy of a planned computer program for calculation of electron dose distribution and the mistakes involved.

For the mathematical description of dose distributions of electron beams in a homogeneous medium, some of the procedures used for photon beams are also suited, for example, the semianalytical method. For the electron depth dose curve in water, Czaikowsky (2) has given a formula (42 MeV Betatron):

$$D(z) = D_p \cdot e^{-\alpha \cdot \left(\frac{z}{R_p}\right)^{\beta}} + D_s \cdot d_s \left(\frac{z}{z_m}\right)$$

where z is the depth and z_m the depth of the dose maximum. D_p and D_s are the dose contributions of primary and secondary electrons in the dose maximum. The term $d_s\left(\frac{z}{z_m}\right)$ is a function of depth for the dose distribution of the secondary electrons; d_s is independent of primary energy, field size and type of scattering foil in contrast to the coefficients α and β and the practical range R_p. In the above formula, however, the contribution of the Bremsstrahlung and the dependence of the source-skin-distance is missing.

As to the dose distributions perpendicular to the central ray, one can calculate them with a comparatively small number of numerically or analytically described transverse distributions for some field widths, energies, and depths interpolating between them for intermediate values. In the upper part of Figure 1, transverse distributions in polystyrene for electron energies of 10, 20, and 30 MeV are compared at a cone diameter of 4 cm and a depth corresponding to 20 percent relative dose respectively; below in Figure 1, for 30 MeV and cone diameters of 6, 10, and 15 cm in the same depth of 20 percent relative dose. In each case the curve was normalized to the same field width. Obviously, even at the end of depth dose curves the forms of the transverse distributions do not strongly depend on energy and field width.

Because of the large influence of tissue inhomogeneities on the electron dose distributions, they have to be regarded in irradiation planning. A simple approach to correct for inhomogeneities takes the dose in homogeneous water $D'(z')$ for the "equivalent depth" z' and multiplies with a factor according to the quadratic distance law. The virtual source point is seen as the origin of the electrons, which is usually nearer to the body surface than the nominal source point or the scattering foil. In Figure 2 the resulting algorithm is given. This procedure was described by Laughlin (3) and a similar one was recommended by the ICRU (4). But instead of the "coefficient of equivalent thickness" CET (AET with Laughlin) here the respective average relative density of the inhomogeneous layer ρ_i/ρ' is used.

In the characterized correction procedure, the different slowing down of electrons is regarded as if the inhomogeneity were to be extended infinitely perpendicular to the direction of primary electrons and as if the inhomogeneity had no influence on the angular distribution of electrons (rays 1 and 2 in Figure 2). The different scattering of electrons and its influence on the dose distribution are neglected, especially in bone tissue and behind cavities (rays 3 and 4). What errors can result from this?

In a phantom of polystyrene and corklike chest wall and infinitely extended lung tissue behind (density of cork 0.38 g/cm^3) there was a good congruence between calculated and measured depth dose curves for large field sizes of 16 cm × 16 cm and a less satisfying congruence for field sizes of 6 cm × 6 cm. Using electron cones with diameters of 12 cm and 4 cm respectively we obtained the same results.

However, the real lung is not extended infinitely. Particularly, the thickness of lung tissue between chest wall and tumor is not greater than about 12 cm. Also the averaged density of an affected lung is frequently higher than 0.38 g/cm^3 (5). Therefore, the influence of the field edges at smaller field sizes will not affect the depth dose curves to a great degree. In looking at the depth dose curves of 20 and 42 MeV electrons in an irradiated thorax phantom, at a field size of 6 cm × 6 cm, there is a satisfying congruence between calculated and measured dose values.

Transverse distributions for equivalent depths in a thorax phantom and a phantom of pure polystyrene show that the difference at the field edges by electron scattering is not very great within the normal thicknesses of lung tissue. A comparison of measurement and calculation for 42 MeV electrons at a more deeply situated (8 cm), larger cavity in soft tissue (gas-filled intestine) in form of a hollow cylinder of 6 cm diameter and 6 cm height in polystyrene showed a satisfying congruence as well.

To get better knowledge about the effect of electron scattering on the dose distribution at the lung edge, it was measured along the border of a phantom consisting of half cork and half water. Depth dose curves were taken in distances of 1, 3, and 5 cm from the border at an irradiation direction parallel to the border of media. At a distance of 3 cm from the border, the depth dose curves in water and cork are almost identical with the depth dose curves in homogeneous medium. Thus the electron scattering takes effect only up to a distance of about 2 cm along the border of an inhomogeneity and therefore also along a beam edge. Therefore, the described procedure regarding inhomogeneities for the dose calculation in electron depth therapy seems to be applicable.

In order to obtain isodose curves for calculated dose distributions at the edges of inhomogeneities or in their shadow areas (in spite of neglecting electron scattering), an additional smoothing procedure can be used. For example, this may consist of a subsequent averaging each of the calculated dose values with two values of lateral adjoining points seen in the direction of primary electrons. The distances of these points to the point of interest may increase with depth from zero at the surface to about 2 cm in the depth of practical range.

Inhomogeneities of smaller dimensions like bones and cavities (perhaps without the superficially situated cavities in the anterior head-neck area) and the normal inhomogeneities of the lung (bronchia, blood vessels, etc.) produce only little displacements of the depth dose or isodose curves (5, 6). Also in more deeply situated cavities using 42 MeV, electrons produce no significant dose peaks or valleys by scattering.

Whereas single, smaller inhomogeneities, like ribs or bronchia, may be fully neglected or, as in the lung (7) or abdomen, need merely be regarded by a suitable average-tissue density, larger inhomogeneities like thick bones and tumors in the lung ought to be regarded more accurately. The anatomical relations can be received for irradiation-planning by suitable radiographs or ultrasonographs. For determination of the average lung tissue density, transmission measurement with a needle beam of hard gamma-radiation is the most simple method (3).

What differences exist between real and calculated depth dose curves, if an average lung density is used which has been obtained by transmission measurement? The smallest differences naturally result from ultrahard X rays. The differences are also small with electron radiation, if only the central ray through the tumor center is viewed. At the lateral tumor periphery, however, where the average tissue density may be between 1 g/cm^3 in the mediastinum and 0.3 g/cm^3 in the tumor free part of the lung, considerably larger discrepancies of depth doses may occur with electrons than with ultrahard X rays. These differences are smaller with 42 MeV electrons than with 30 MeV electrons. This is a strong reason for using the highest possible energy in irradiating lung tumors with electrons (7).

Small mistakes resulting from not knowing precisely the densities of irradiated tissue layers result in displacements of the depth dose curve of approximately 2 cm at most in one or the other direction. Yet this is not of major importance if the tumor receives the necessary dose by applying a sufficiently high electron energy. With photon radiation the whole tissue lying behind the tumor is always irradiated.

REFERENCES

1. Fehrentz, D., *Electromedica 2*, 68 (1973).
2. Czaikowsky, P. M., *Strahlentherapie 143*, 416 (1972).
3. Laughlin, J. S., *Brit. J. Radiol. 38*, 143 (1965).
4. ICRU, Report 21, Clinical Dosimetry, p. 49, National Bureau of Standards, Handbook 87, United States Department of Commerce, Washington 1973.
5. Breitling, G., Vogel, K. H., *Strahlentherapie 122*, 321 (1963).
6. Heuss, K., *Strahlentherapie 141*, 25 (1971).
7. Starchman, E. D., Chao, J. H., *Radiology 98*, 432 (1971).

QUESTIONS

H. DAVIS: We're using a number of electron radiation transport computer programs in our work at the Jet Propulsion Laboratory. They also include the effects of inhomogeneities and secondary *Brehmstrahlung*. Although they were originally developed, and are being used, in the space program, I believe that they could be modified and used in radiation therapy.

TING: Could you address yourself to the problem of scattering from small inhomogeneities such as ribs?

FEHRENTZ: We have measured at ribs and other bones, too, and the scattering effects are so small that they can be neglected.

PRASAD: Did you use computers to arrive at these figures, or are they experimentally measured?

FEHRENTZ: I used for my expression a desk-top computer. We have a program for photons, and now we want to bring in the program for electrons.

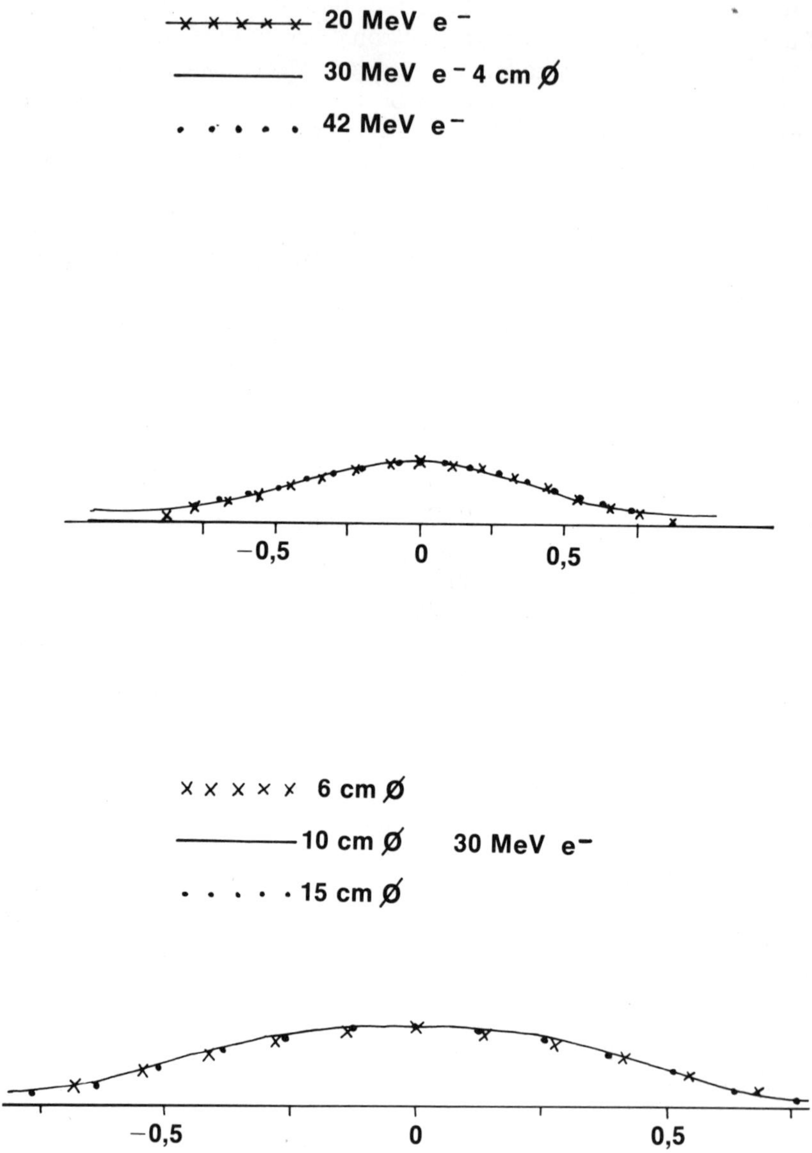

Figure 1. Transverse Dose Distributions (Film Density) of Electrons in a Polystyrene Phantom at Depths with 20 p.c. Relative dose, Normalized to the Same Half Value Width. Nominal SSD (f_n) 100 cm

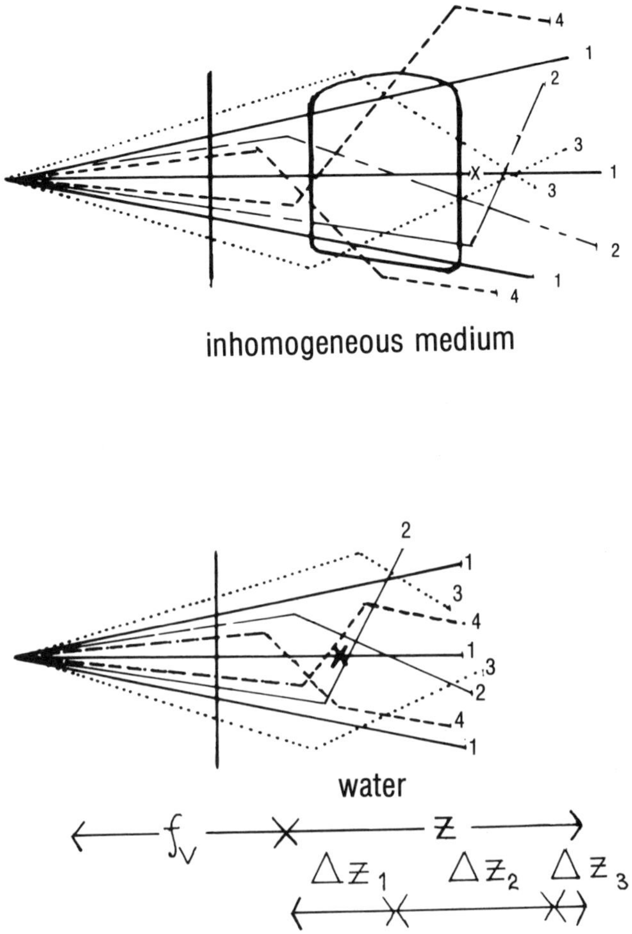

$$z' = \sum_{1}^{n} \frac{\rho_i}{\rho'} \cdot \Delta z_i$$

$$D(z) = D'(z') \left(\frac{f_v + z'}{f_v + z} \right)^2$$

Figure 2. Dose Calculation in Inhomogeneous Tissue (Here — Cavity). Out of the Layer Thicknesses z_i and the Relative Densities ρ_i/ρ' the "Equivalent Depth" (to z) in Water z′ is Calculated. Out of the Dose in Water D′(z′) the Dose in the Inhomogeneous Tissue D(z) is Calculated According to the Quadratic Distance Law Using the Virtual SSD (f_V)

5. A Method for the Automatic Recording of Patient Outline Information

J. Milan
S. C. Lillicrap

For a number of years computer systems have been used with considerable success in radiotherapy to calculate radiation dose distributions. The potential accuracy of the results produced by these systems is, however, often limited by the poor accuracy of input data concerning patient outline and internal structures. This paper is concerned with a method for obtaining patient-outline data with improved accuracy; the principle is described and the most satisfactory way of incorporating it in the treatment planning process is discussed.

The conventional and most simple method of obtaining outline information is to use a piece of lead wire or similar device which is bent around the patient's skin to form a profile, which is then traced to produce hard copy on paper. When a computer is used for dosimetry calculations, this information must be digitized by a manual or automatic method to allow it to be used by a computer program. In situations where a simulator is used in the treatment-planning process, the lead-wire method is convenient, because it allows outline data to be recorded while the patient is in the simulated treatment position. However, the method has shortcomings: it has poor accuracy, and digitization of the outline after it has been transferred to paper can be laborious, although in practice this is of less importance if a suitable digitization device is incorporated in the design of the computer system. A number of devices have been developed to record the patient's outline with greater accuracy, such as formulators, which utilize a number of sliding pins whose tops are moved to follow the skin's surface, or the Newcastle "scope" system, which uses wide-angle television cameras, which view a band of light projected onto the body and display it on a television screen (1). The shortcoming of of these methods is that because they usually require the patient to be positioned on a couch which is separate from that of the simulator, the patient must be moved between couches for the outlines to be recorded, and this makes outline-recording a lengthy procedure when compared to the lead-wire method. An outline-recording device that avoids this problem has been developed at the Royal Marsden Hospital. The method, which has been found to give accurate results, employs an optical device that is attached to the simulator. The device is sufficiently compact not to interfere with the normal working of the simulator, and it is mounted in such a way that outlines may be recorded while the simulator gantry is being rotated about the patient. A schematic diagram of this device is shown in Figure 1. The operating principle is as follows:

A lamp (L), mounted on the simulator gantry, projects a spot of light onto the patient's skin. The spot is viewed by the telescope (T), which is also mounted on the gantry and which projects an image of the light spot through a collimator (C) onto a photomultiplier (P). The light path between the light spot and photomultiplier is completed by a mirror (M) driven by a motor (S). If the mirror angle is adjusted until the output from the photomultiplier is at a maximum, then the distance (D) of the light spot from the gantry may be determined from

$$D = L \times \text{Tan}\,(2 \times (90 - \theta))$$

where L is the distance between the light source and the mirror axis and θ is the angle between the surface of the mirror and the horizontal. L is fixed, therefore D may be calculated directly from θ. The distance (D′) of the patient's skin from the simulator axis will then be given by:

$$D' = R - D$$

where R is the distance from the light source to the simulator axis. In order to make the device lock onto the light spot and track the outline as the simulator is rotated, the motor driving the mirror and the output from the photomultiplier must be incorporated in a servo mechanism. In our prototype system we have used our PDP 8/I treatment-planning computer to act as the intelligence required by the servo. The output from the photomultiplier is digitized and fed into the computer, which controls the angle of the mirror by means of a stepping motor. The computer is programmed to make the mirror oscillate about the angle which produces the maximum output from the photomultiplier. The change in angle for each step of the motor is such that the mean effective change in D is about 0.3 mm. A typical plot of photomultiplier output against angle is shown in Figure 2. Logarithmic signal compression is applied to the photomultiplier output in order to make the device insensitive to changes in the reflective properties of different patients' skin, with the result that significant photomultiplier output is detected several steps from the position of peak intensity. In spite of this, however, the peak is well defined and may be used to determine θ with a high degree of repeatability. The gantry angle (ψ) of the simulator is monitored by means of a potentiometer the output of which is digitized and input to the computer. As the gantry is rotated, coordinates of points on the patient's outline are calculated from:

$$X = D^1 \cos\psi$$
$$Y = D^1 \sin\psi$$

and these data are plotted onto an X—Y plotter connected to the computer. Although a number of outlines have been taken from volunteer subjects, it has proved impossible to check the accuracy of the system, because of the inadequacies of our existing techniques for taking outlines and because of patient movement (breathing, etc.). Figure 3 therefore shows the output obtained from a flesh-textured thorax phantom using the device compared with a tracing of the cross-section of the phantom at a distance of 1 cm from the position of the outline. The discrepancies of up to ±3 mm between the two outlines is consistent with those corresponding to different cross sections of the phantom. Tests on other objects have shown the accuracy of the device to be ±2 mm.

Originally it was envisaged that outline data would be stored in the computer directly in a form ready for use by the treatment planning program and thus avoid the necessity for plotting the data out and then re-digitizing it. In practice, however, there are two major problems with this approach: Small dedicated treatment planning systems such as the Royal Marsden's RAD 8 system (2) can be dedicated to only one task at a time, and it is unlikely that the overall treatment-planning process can be organized so that the computer would not be required for dosimetry calculations and outline recording at the same time. Secondly, the input data required by treatment-planning programs is rather more complex than the basic data produced by the outline-recording device. Apart from the patient outline, other details, such as tumor volume, lungs, sensitive organs, etc. must be added. This information, which must be supplied by the clinician, is generally not available at the time the outline is taken. Also, if the outline itself is a composite outline derived from two partial outlines when patients are treated in both the prone and supine positions, optimum accuracy is obtained only if outlines in both positions are recorded and combined in such a way that the distance of the tumor from the skin along the line of each beam is registered correctly. The manual procedure used to do this is complex, and it would be difficult to devise a systen that would allow partial outlines, having been input to the computer directly, to be combined by computer program. For these reasons a free-standing outline-recording device which produces hard copy on paper is of more practical value than one which inputs data directly into the treatment-planning computer system. In principle a free-standing device based on the principles described above could be constructed at minimum cost using purely analogue techniques. However, fairly complex algorithms are used in out prototype system for locating the light spot, distinguishing it from noise, and correcting for the rare cases in which the light spot may be lost. Since it would be difficult to duplicate these algorithms in an analogue system, our routine system, now under development, will use a digital system. Functionally it will be similar to the prototype system but will employ a microprocessor to keep the cost to a minimum.

REFERENCES

1. Clayton, C. B. and Thompson, D. J., *British Journal of Radiology*, *43*, 489-492 (1970).
2. Bentley, R. E. and Milan, J., *British Journal of Radiology*, *44*, 826-835 (1971).

QUESTIONS

ROSENOW: I wonder if you know the work we did in my department in 1972 which I presented to the Madrid Radiological Conference. This is essentially the same system, I think, as far as the geometry is concerned, and especially the rotating mirror. There are some differences, though. We use a laser beam which enables a daylight use of the machine and we use a photodiode and use the spatial resolution of the photodiode, which is sufficient to detect the position of the light spot.

JAMESON: When you take a continuous outline and it comes to actually computing the dose computations, you work with points rather than with continuous lines. How often do you relate the line to the actual point which you're going to use in your computation? I ask this question because it has an enormous bearing upon the cost and speed of calculation. You can put in a large number of points, or you can put in a relatively small number of points; it affects the accuracy, it affects the cost, it affects the speed.

MILAN: We effectively do take a continuous outline. We sample every three millimeters approximately. It appears to be a continuous outline.

STEBEN: Were there any difficulties in modifying the RAD-8 software?

MILAN: The RAD-8 was a problem insofar as time-sharing the outline taken with the treatment-planning process. That consideration was minor compared with the problems of combining the outline with internal structures, and in particular, combining two partial outlines. That was the biggest stumbling block, which decided us to abandon that approach.

HUGHES: Can you tell me what the viewing angle is?

MILAN: It's about 45 degrees.

HUGHES: 45 degrees? One problem that would present is that you don't see certain areas on the body if you're in the neck region, or down low in the pelvis. What are your comments?

MILAN: Use lead wire in those cases.

HOUDEK: I want to comment on the use of the transverse axial layergraph which not only can give a full contour in one slice plus anatomical structure, but the result is in machine readable form. And on top of that, you can have a simulator in a combined installation and you can simulate and do the cut simultaneously with the transverse tomogram. Our work on this system appears in the August 1974 *Radiology*.

LINDSKOUG: We learned at the last computer meeting in Uppsala that 2-D multiplanar distribution calculations are preferable. This certainly calls for a lot of transversal outlines of the patient along the entire body. I think that the only system that can accomplish this now is the SCOPE system by David Thompson in Newcastle. We are going to use this approach in a framework hanging over the patient's body, and scan along the body of the patient, feeding the contour line of the patient into the computer every centimeter or every second centimeter. The time required for one transversal contour of the patient to be fed into the computer is .2 seconds, and it is very reliable.

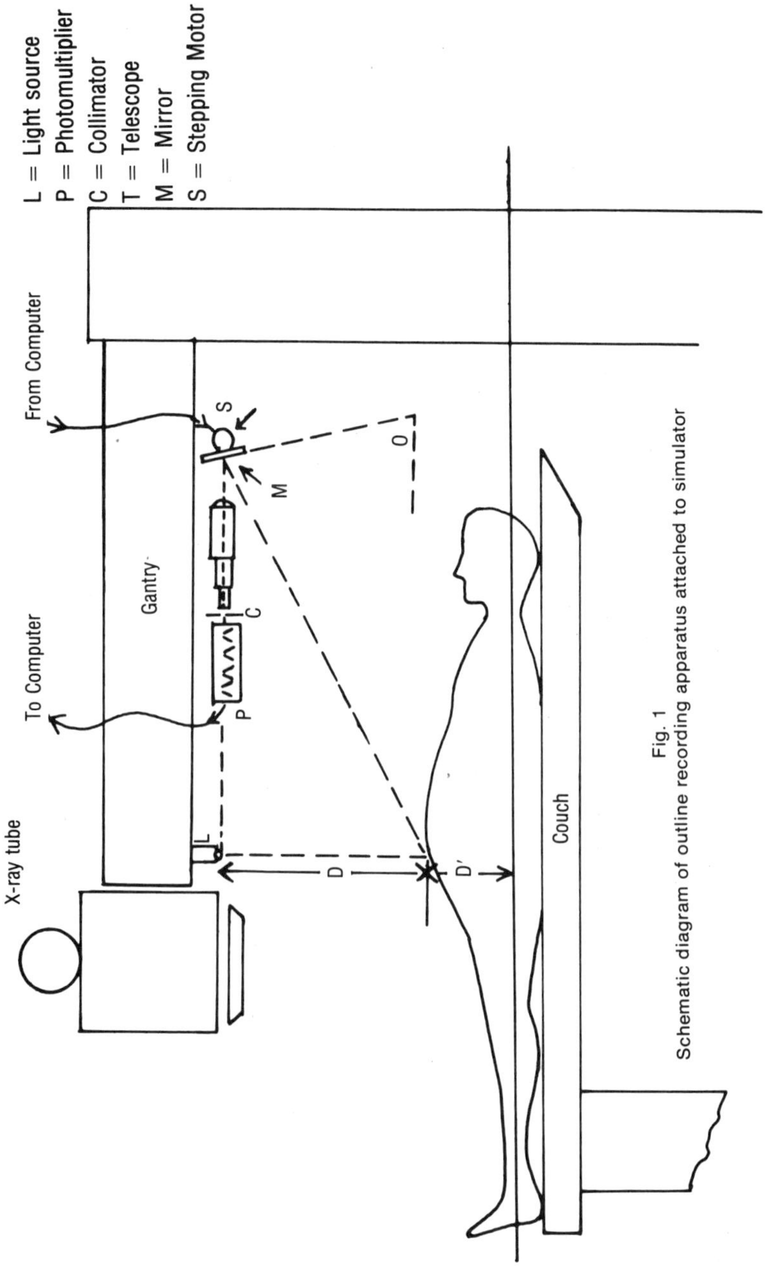

Figure 1. Schematic Diagram of Outline Recording Apparatus Attached to Simulator

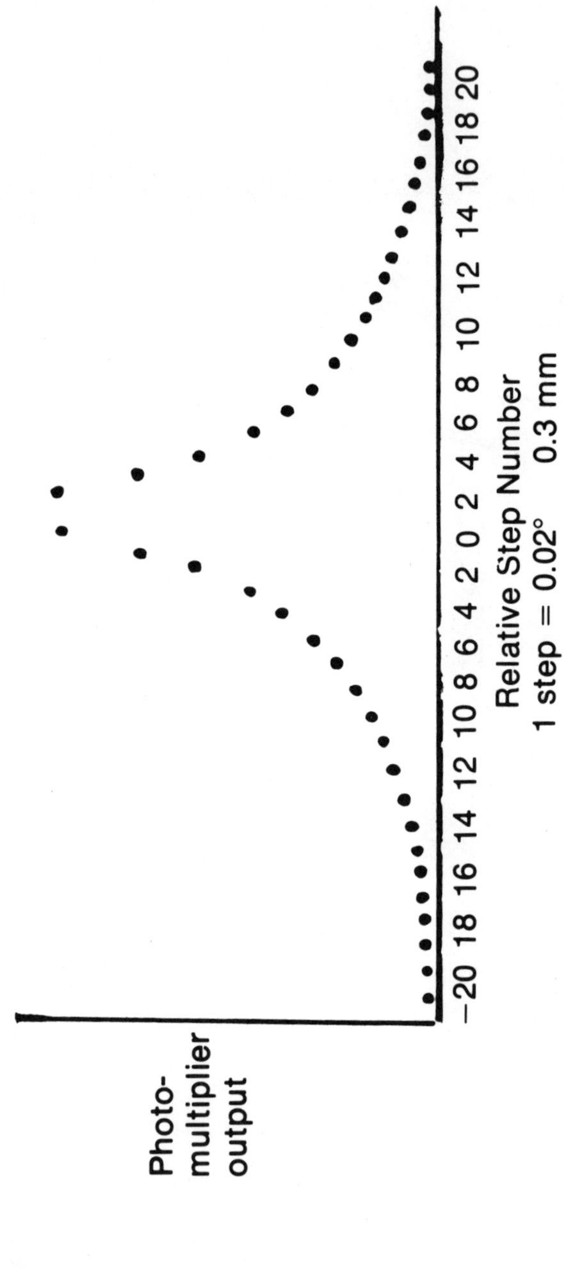

Figure 2. Graph of Photomultiplier Output Plotted Against Mirror Angle

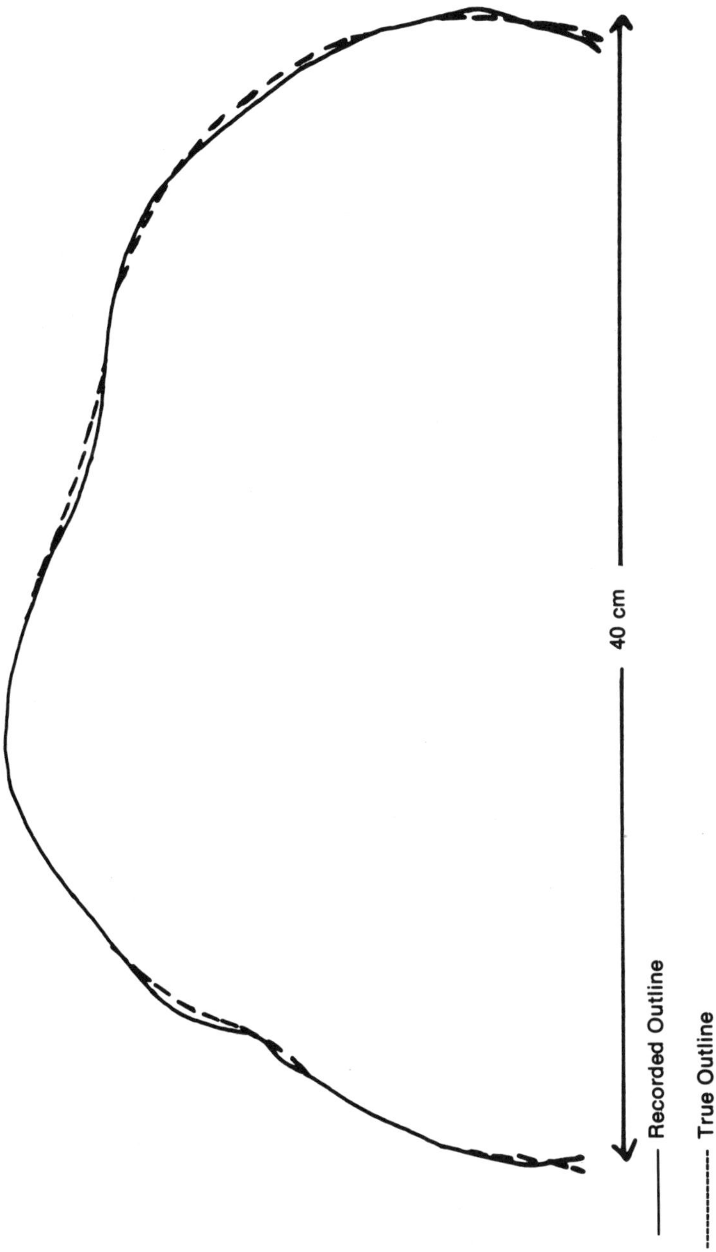

Figure 3. Comparison Between an Outline Traced Directly from Thorax Phantom and One Recorded by the Outline Recording Device

Session VI: Contributed Short Papers

1. A Fast Neutron Treatment Planning System Based on a Real Time Multiprogrammed Mini-Computer

R. E. Pengilley

Introduction

The M.R.C. cyclotron at Hammersmith Hospital produces a beam of fast neutrons having a mean energy of 7.5 MeV. This fast neutron beam has been used for treatment of advanced tumors since 1967, and currently a clinical trial is being undertaken to compare the results of fast-neutron therapy with those of supervoltage X-ray therapy on a number of selected head and neck sites. However, the low mean energy of the beam results in a 50 percent depth dose at only 7.5 cm for a 5 × 5 field compared with 11 cm obtainable with a ^{60}Co beam or 15 cm with 8 MeV X rays. Furthermore, the skin-sparing effect is less pronounced than with supervoltage X rays, the maximum dose falling at 2 mm. In order to obtain the best possible mode of treatment using this beam it was felt that it would be advantageous to study a wider range of plans for a particular treatment than a radiographer could reasonably be expected to create manually and that this requirement could be fulfilled by an interactive computer-based planning system, for which a suitable computer was already in routine use within the unit.

Real-Time Computer System

The basic feature of a real-time computer system is its ability to handle simultaneously several time-dependent physical events. In addition, a real-time system can usually process batch-type computational jobs, according to a priority structure, in one part of the machine while concurrently providing the required fast-access real-time response elsewhere.

The Cyclotron Unit system is depicted in Figure 1. It is based on a

Hewlett-Packard 2116B computer with 32K of core together with a 2.4 Mwd disc which holds the master copy of the Real-Time Executive operating system, all user programs and most data files. In order to service the on-line laboratories with the required facilities, the manufacturer's software was supplemented by a Remote Access system. Thus normal use of the computer comprises adjacent program development, along with users at remote terminals acquiring data, storing it in disc files and scheduling calculation programs (which may be automatically timed to enable repetitions of this sequence).

Radiotherapy Planning in Real-Time

The principal consideration in implementing a neutron therapy-planning system was to ensure that its design structure would be compatible with the existing real-time configuration without rendering the system too impracticable and unnatural to use. This meant eliminating, so far as possible, transfers of large amounts of data to or from slow peripheral devices while retaining sufficient input/output interaction for the user to feel he is steering the planning process. The way in which this is done, using a separate program for each stage, is described below under Input/Output Techniques.

Also, the Real-Time system is completely disc-based and has no magnetic tape. This places a limit on the amount of immediately accessible data storage that can be tolerated. Since exchanging a cartridge in the interchangeable disc drive to provide more storage temporarily disables most of the computer system, this operation could not be performed as often as would be required for planning facilities to be available at any time.

The data-storage limitation could be a serious hindrance to expansion in the real-time situation if it was planned to examine depth-dose distributions by interpolating from tables. The Cyclotron Unit system overcomes this by computing depth doses directly from a mathematical formula rather than by dose table interpolation. This way, the only large amounts of permanent mass storage required are archival and can be filed on a cartridge offline at a time of minimum load on the computer. The calculation system offers additional benefits in that three-dimensional planning can be effected with no increase in on-line data storage. Moreover, the system becomes easily adaptable for treatment-planning for other therapy machines by generating the small sets of parameters required to describe each beam and notifying the calculation program of the available treatment machines.

The Computational Algorithm

The basic formula used to compute the percentage depth doses for the fast neutron beam has evolved in several stages. It takes the form

$$D(T) = D(C) \cdot k(d,z) \cdot \exp(SW + SO)$$

where D(T) is the percentage depth dose at the point T within the treatment region relative to the central axis point of maximum dose,

D(C) is the corresponding percent depth dose at the central axis point C at the same depth below surface as T,

k(d,z) is a modifying off-axis factor,

and SW, SO are correction factors for wedge filters and obliquity of beam incidence.

The Central Axis Model

Let C = (0,0,z) be a point at depth z on the central axis of a beam. In an initial attempt to describe the dose at C the method of Sterling, Perry, and Katz (1) was tried. This suggests that, for ^{60}Co radiation, the central axis percentage depth dose D(C) is related to the ratio field area/perimeter A/P by the equation

$$\log D(C) = h(z) - m(z) \log (A/P)$$

where h(z) and m(z) are linear functions of z. Figure 2 shows this relation at nine depths for the six basic neutron field sizes for which measured depth-dose data have been obtained by Bewley and Parnell (2). This showed some prospect of conforming to the ^{60}Co situation. A linear least-squares fit was applied to the measured data at sixteen depths to determine values of h and m, and these were then plotted against depth (Figure 3). The m graph exhibits rather less linearity than the h graph, but to complete the investigation the two graphs were treated by least-squares fits to yield the four constants required to describe the percentage depth dose in terms of depth and field size. These constants were used to regenerate the dose tables, but the results differed fairly significantly from the measured data, especially near the surface. Figure 4 shows a comparison for a 9.5 × 9.5 cm field and indicates the fundamental difference between the nature of the model and that of the neutron dose distribution. The data were then divided into two sets at around 3–5 cm, and each region was fitted separately. Although this resulted in a slight improvement of fit to the lower region, the upper region could not be fitted at all satisfactorily by this method.

To cope with the initial "shoulder" of the distribution, an expression due to Atwood and Norman (3) was examined. This represents D(C) as

$$D(C) = 100 \cdot [1 - (1 - \exp(-z/D_0))^M]$$

The empirical constants D_0 and M were found for the six measured fields by least squares analysis. Using Atwood's equation to express depth in terms of percentage depth dose, the depths of the principal percentage depth doses (10, 15, 20, 25, 30, 40, 50, 60, 70, 80, 90) were obtained for the six measured field sizes. At each principal percentage depth dose it was possible to fit a straight line to the graph of depth vs. log (area). These lines were then used to interpolate central axis data for all 25 field sizes used. Finally, Atwood's expression was fitted to this new data to obtain values of D_0 and M for all the used field sizes.

The results showed that the values of D_0 plotted against log (area) lie very close to a straight line. The values of M do not seem so closely correlated. However, most of the measured depth doses were for square fields, and the implicit assumption that all nonsquare fields behave as square fields of the same area may not be valid. For example, at 250 kV a 20 × 5 cm is equivalent to a 60 sq. cm square field. The effect of this with neutrons is as yet unknown. Meanwhile, the values of D_0 and M for a particular field size are being retrieved from a look-up table.

The Off-Axis Model

In order to compare the dose D(x,y,z) at the point T = (x,y,z) with the corresponding dose D(0,0,z) at C = (0,0,z) (See Figure 5), the model formulated in the General Field Equation by Sterling, Perry, and Weinkam (4) was tested:

$$k = 0.5 - 0.5 \text{ erf } \frac{l/L - 1}{\sigma\sqrt{2}}$$

where l/L are as indicated in Figure 5 and σ is a parameter dependent on the therapy unit. This is derived directly from the cumulative probability function[1]

$$k = 1 - \int_{-\infty}^{l/L} \frac{1}{\sigma\sqrt{2\pi}} \exp \frac{-(x-\mu)^2}{2\sigma^2} dx$$

To determine a value or values for σ, D(T)/D(C) was plotted in probability against l/L for various field sizes at different depths, and the points falling between 80 percent and 30 percent probability were used to estimate a value for σ. For the fast neutron beam this parameter was found to be highly dependent on depth and field size. From this and from the nonstandard nature of the decrement lines, it was concluded that the cumulative normal probability theory would not provide a satisfactory model for neutrons.

The off-axis ratio from the Extended General Field Equation developed by Weinkam, Kolde, and Sterling (5) has been applied. This has the more general form

$$k(d,z) = 0.5 - 0.5 \operatorname{erf} \left[\frac{u-1}{A|u-C|+B} + D\right]$$

$$\text{where } u = \frac{s\sqrt{(x^2+y^2)}}{(s+z)\cdot L}$$

$$s = SSD$$

$$L = \frac{\sqrt{(x^2+y^2)}}{2 \max \left(\frac{|x|}{w}, \frac{|y|}{H}\right)}$$

and $A = A_0 + A_1 s + A_2 z + A_3 L$, etc. for B,C,D.

For each field size, using only principal plane data determined from either isodose charts or decrement lines, the dose D(x,0,z) was obtained at a number of off-axis points (typically 36). The model was fitted to the data one field at a time using a simplex minimization procedure (6,7) minimizing on the parameters $A_0, \ldots, D_3$. The error function was evaluated using Hastings' (8) approximation:

$$\operatorname{erf}(t) = \operatorname{sign}(t) \left[1 - (1 + a_1|t| + a_2|t|^2 + a_3|t|^3 + a_4|t|^4)^{-4}\right]$$

where the a_i are known numerical constants. This model appears to give a reasonable representation over the majority of the field, although errors at the edge are in the region of 10 percent of measured dose. This is felt to be acceptable, however, in view of the difficulty of measuring the depth dose in this area.

Input/Output Techniques

For input of patient structure a television system is used which consists of a TV camera and circuitry to generate a binary representation of the image as 256 lines of 512 bits each from the video signal. In order to achieve a fast transfer rate and high resolution in real time, the signal is sampled at a predefined intensity level using an 8 MHz crystal. The information is converted to parallel form in groups of sixteen bits and this is loaded into sixteen 512 bit shift registers. When the shift registers are full, they are sent to the computer, sixteen repetitions of this process transmitting an entire image in 1.3 seconds.

In routine use, the patient's outline, tumor and vital organs are drawn on three melinex sheets, placed on a light box under the camera, and transmitted to the computer for filing.

For entering details of the beam configuration and output of results, a Tektronix 4010-1 video terminal is used. The graphics capability enables this device to be used for echoing the patient data and for superposition of the desired isodose contours of the completed plan. These are drawn within the patient outline using Crane's algorithm (9). Beam entry and exit points are located on the screen, using the thumbwheel-controlled cross-hair cursor, after the outline, tumor and vital organs have been displayed. Field sizes and wedge angles are entered via the keyboard in the usual way. A T-bar and optional wedge symbol appear to indicate the presence of a beam.

All the input data is stored in temporary disc files. The isodose distribution resulting from the defined treatment plan is then computed and, on completion, the operator requests display of up to twenty selected isodose contours. If the plan is found to be unsatisfactory, or if a general investigation study is being performed, the beam data entry program can be rescheduled to modify the configuration and the process repeated from that stage. At any time, the current values and results may be transferred to intermediate length storage for subsequent recall. A Hard Copy Unit attached to the terminal is used to make a permanent record of the plan as required. This is done via a console switch which initiates a raster scan of the screen; the copy is then delivered in eighteen seconds. The copying process is completely independent of the computer, thus eliminating a potential output bottleneck in the real-time system.

System Status

Transfers have been made from the TV system via disc files to the 4010 terminal, and software to analyze the patient structure into coordinate form is under development. Meanwhile, all input data is from paper tape while the calculation routines are being tested. Attention is being focused on the off-axis model, since it is being found necessary to sample measured data at a fairly large set of points in the interior of the field in order to avoid vacuous predictions. The program for displaying patient structure and labeled isodose contours is already operational.

Negotiations are in hand for extension of the system, when completed, to other sources of radiation within Hammersmith Hospital. The software should largely be directly transferable, the main effort involved being in obtaining the sets of eighteen parameters necessary to describe each beam.

Conclusion

A nondedicated mini-computer-based treatment-planning system for fast neutron therapy has been described. By use of graphical input/output facilities, the system aims to give the radiotherapist a helpful plan representation. Dose values are computed from a formula with minimal data storage to ease disc-accessing requirements in a real-time multi-user environment and to render the system more easily expandible for use with other treatment machines.

APPENDIX

The Cyclotron Unit Computer System

Figure 1 shows a block diagram of the entire system, which is based on a Hewlett-Packard 2116B computer with 32 K of 16 bit word core. The main mass storage device is the 2.4 Mwd HP 7900A moving head disc drive consisting of one fixed platter and one exchangeable cartridge. The fixed platter contains a core image of the operating system together with user programs, while the cartridge is used for development work and for data files.

Seven remotely situated laboratories are linked to the computer, the primary equipment in each case being connected via specially developed optically isolated long line interfaces and the terminal by direct cable.

The manufacturer's system software is centered on a disc-based Real Time Executive. This features multiprogramming with unlimited numbers of tasks, high and low level languages, and a File Management Package. The system divides the user area of core into two partitions, foreground and background, and subdivides each into core-resident and disc-resident. Programs are assigned priorities and are queued on this basis. Uncompleted foreground disc-resident programs may be swapped out to disc in favor of those of higher priority. This area is used when fast access is required, for example in collecting online nuclear data from a multichannel analyzer handling short-lived isotopes. Simultaneously, the background area can be used for data-processing and calculation and for program development. Such programs, once initiated, must nominally run to completion before freeing the partition.

The manufacturer's software has been augmented by a remote access system. This runs in foreground and enables laboratory users to dump or recall data to disc files or paper tape, schedule programs, alter parameters, plot spectra, etc.

It should be emphasized that the combined software does not constitute a time-sharing system; only a limited amount of user interaction is allowable to avoid holding the background area.

ACKNOWLEDGMENT

The author wishes to acknowledge the work done by Mr. Y. Kutsutani of the National Institute of Radiological Services, Chiba Shi, Japan, in developing the prototype calculation program during his stay at Hammersmith in 1972.

REFERENCES

1. Sterling, T. D., Perry, H., and Katz, L., *British Journal of Radiology*, *37*, 544-550 (1964).
2. Bewley, D. K., and Parnell, C. J., *British Journal of Radiology*, *42*, 281-288 (1969).
3. Atwood, K. C., and Norman, A., *Proc. Nat. Acad. Sci., U.S.*, *35*, 696-709 (1949).
4. Sterling, T. C., Perry, H., and Weinkam, J. J., *British Journal of Radiology*, *40*, 464-468 (1967).
5. Weinkam, J. J., Kolde, R. A., and Sterling, T. D., *British Journal of Radiology*, *46*, 983-990 (1973).
6. O'Neill, R., *Applied Statistics*, *20*, No. 3 (1971).
7. Nelder, J. A., and Mead, R., *Computer Journal*, *7*, 308-313 (1965).
8. Hastings, C., *Approximations for Digital Computers* (Princeton University Press, 1962), p. 186.
9. Crane, C. M., *Computer Journal*, *15*, No. 4 (1973).

QUESTIONS

SILER: Could you briefly describe again the algorithm that you're using?

PENGILLEY: The algorithm we're using at the moment falls into basically three parts. It consists of a product of three factors to describe the central axis dose at a given depth, and a modifying off-axis factor, and another exponential factor for wedge filters and oblique incidence. To describe the central axis dose, we use a formula due to Atwood. In fact, it was developed for use in analyzing multi-hit survival curves about thirty years ago. To describe the off-axis ratio, we use an expression developed by Weinkam which is based on an error function together with sixteen parameters that are to be fitted to the data. This takes quite a long time to run on the computer because we don't have any floating point hardware. It can take up to five hours to obtain the necessary data for the equation we need.

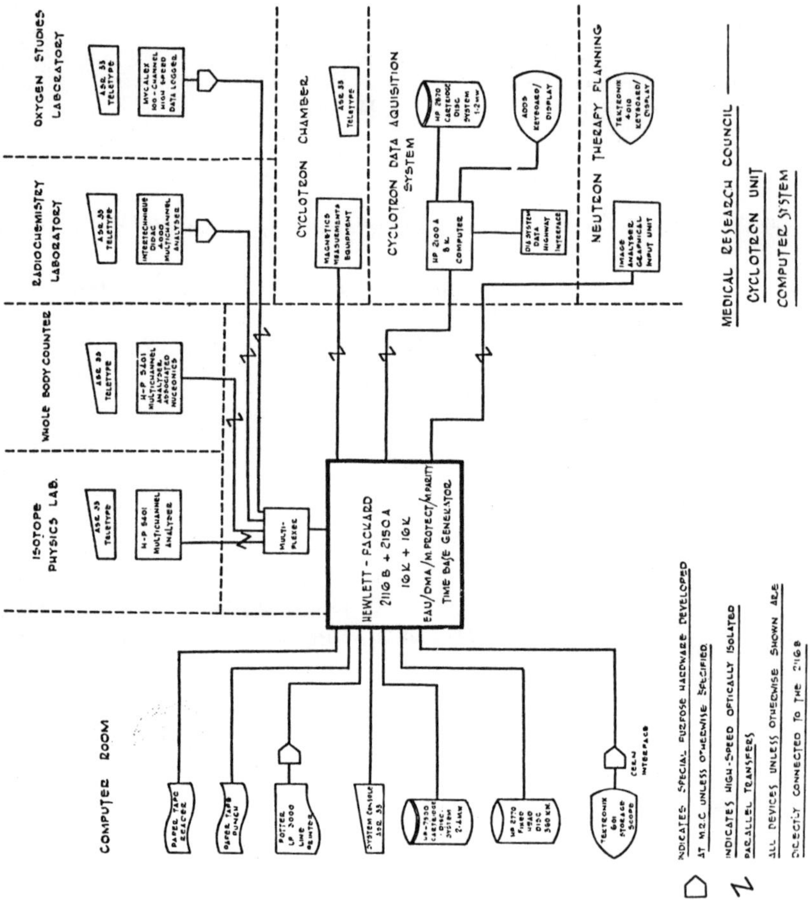

Figure 1. The M.R.C. Cyclotron Unit Computer System

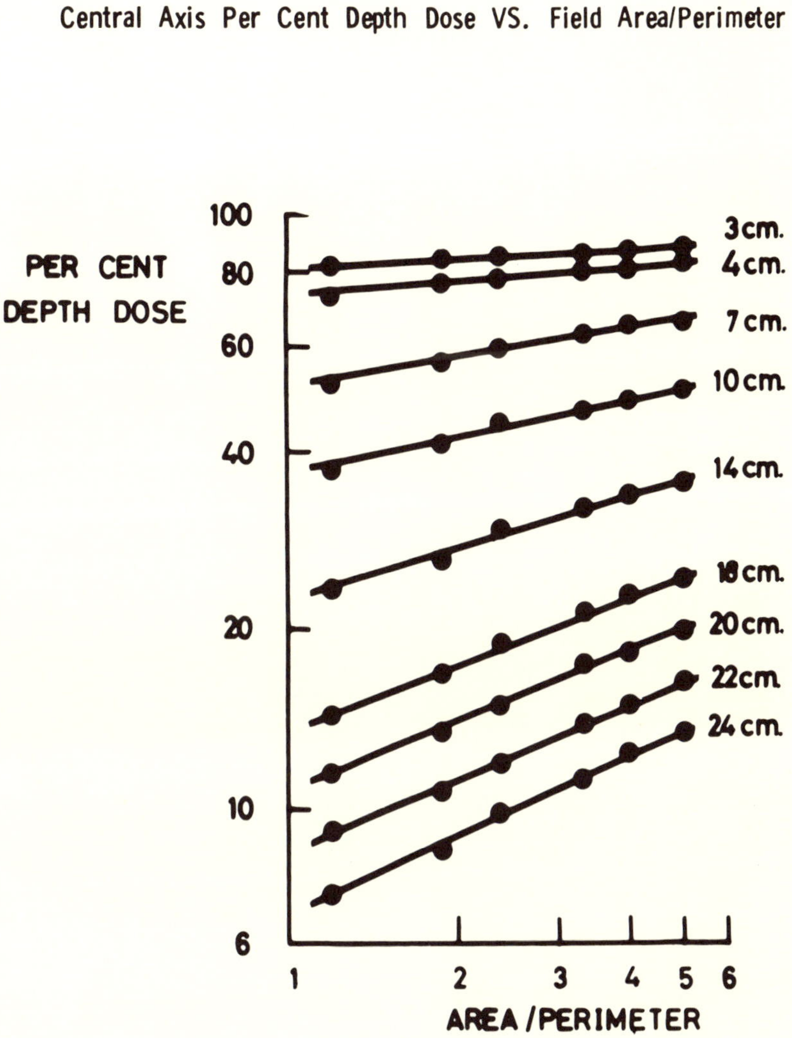

Figure 2. Change in central axis per cent depth dose with field area perimeter (both logarithmically) at nine depths below su face for the six measured neutron field sizes

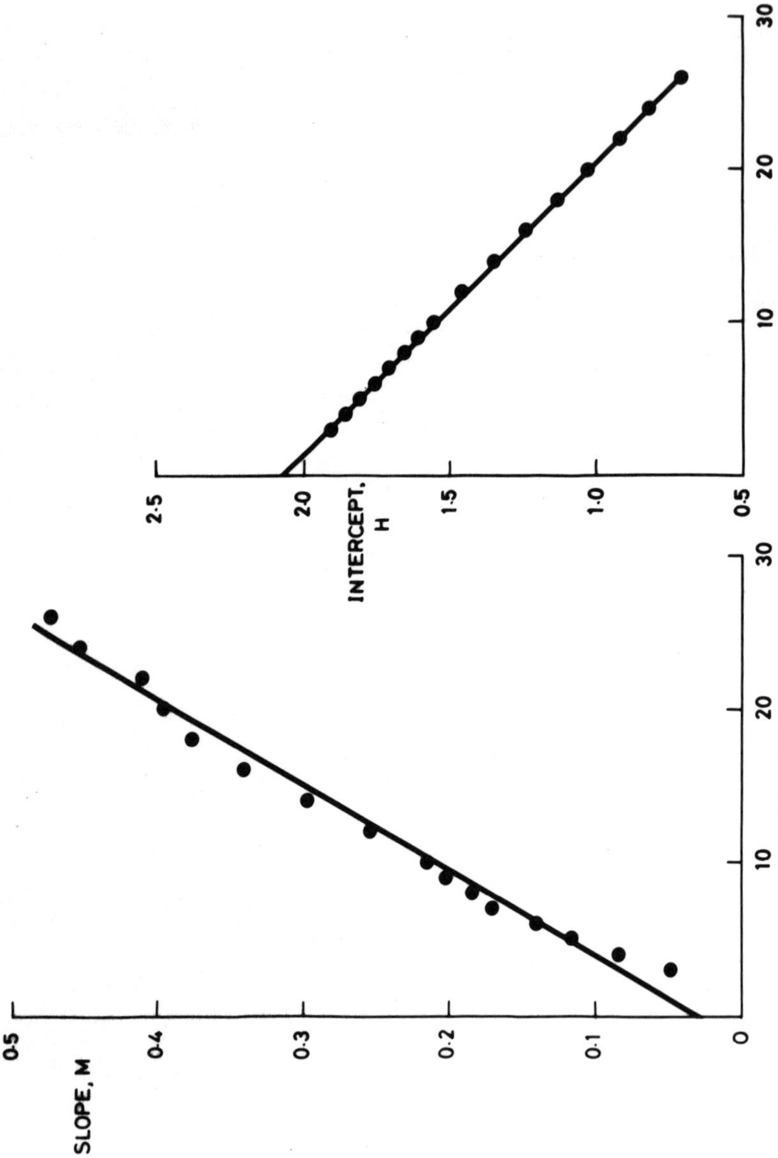

Figure 3. Log D(C) = h(z) − m(z) log (A/P). Change in slope, M(z), and intercept, h(z), with depth, z

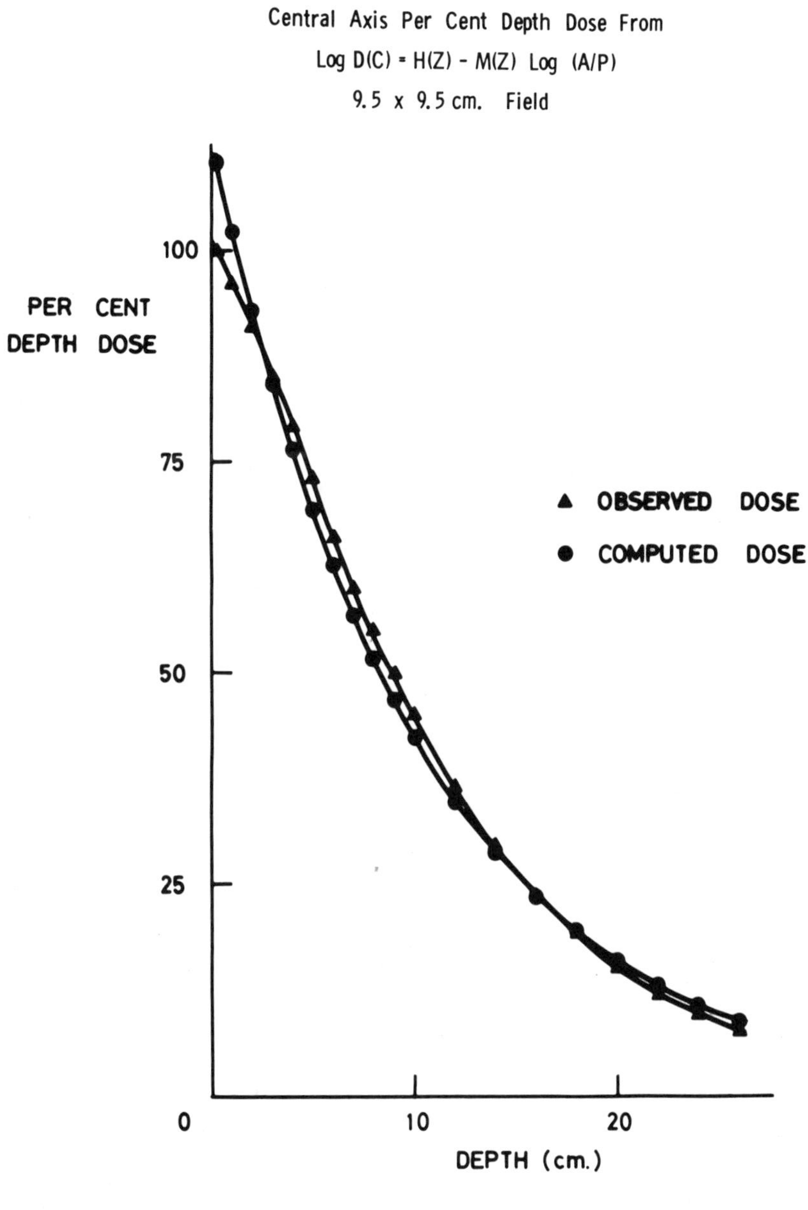

Figure 4. Comparison of computed central axis per cent depth dose using log D(C) = h(z) − m(z) log (A/P) with observed neutron dose for 9.5 × 9.5 cm. field at 120 cm. SSD

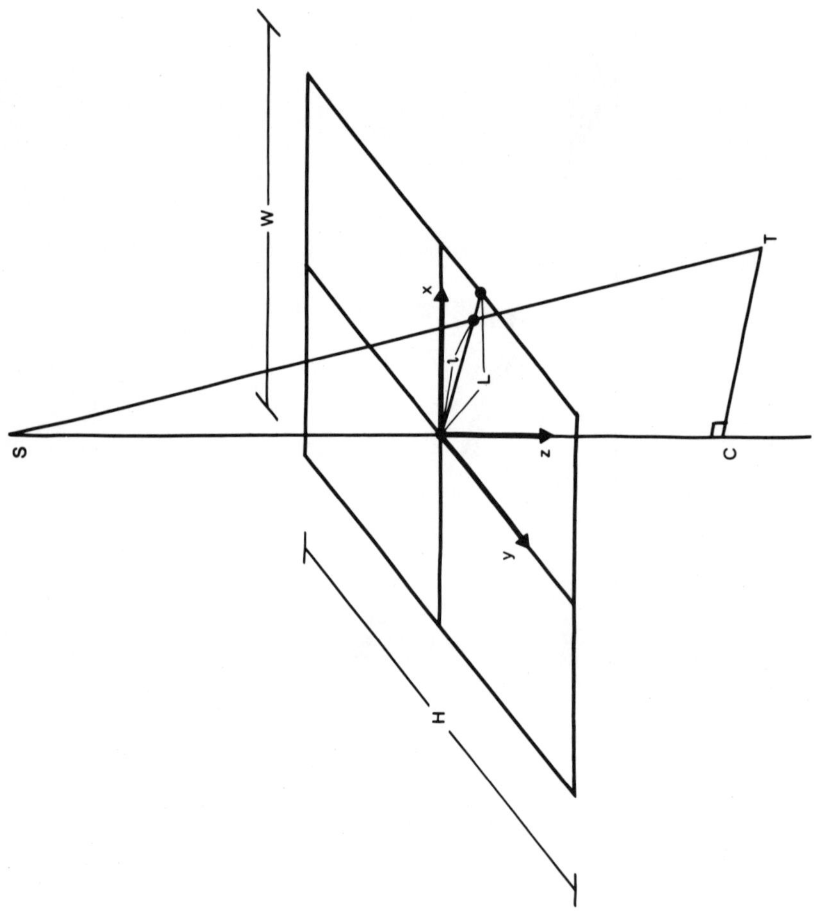

Figure 5. Off-axis notation (see text)

2. Computer Modeling of Neutron Dose at Various Locations within the Body during Pion Radiotherapy

M. E. Schillaci
D. L. Roeder

Introduction

Since negative pions were first proposed for use in radiotherapy more than a decade ago, several experiments and calculations have been carried out with encouraging results. Now, with the completion of facilities such as exist at the Clinton P. Anderson Meson Physics Facility in Los Alamos, clinical trials will begin shortly. A brief review of the basic physical mechanism involved in negative pion radiotherapy is, perhaps, in order. As with all charged particles, a negative pion has a definite range, exhibiting a Bragg peak in the dose distribution which depends on the pion mass. The depth in matter at which the pion beam comes to rest, then, is determined by its initial energy. Upon stopping, the negative pion becomes captured into an atom, cascading down to lower energy levels. Eventually, the pion is absorbed by the atomic nucleus, and its rest mass is transformed into energy, causing the nucleus to disintegrate—a reaction called a "star." Many of the star fragments are highly ionizing particles, such as heavy ions, alphas, protons, etc. It is these particles—the charged star fragments—that deliver the therapeutic dose, resulting in a large (~2-3) radiobiological effectiveness (RBE) and a low (~1.6) oxygen enhancement ratio (OER) in the stopping region. In addition, since the star is produced at the end of the pion's range, the entrance dose is relatively low (RBE~1).

Besides these highly ionizing, short-range particles, photons and (more importantly) neutrons are also produced in the star, delivering their dose outside the treatment volume as well as within. The dose delivered by these long-range particles to nearby vital structures as well as the resulting whole-body dose is of obvious importance in developing a treatment plan, and constitutes the subject of this paper. In our initial study of this problem (1), we found that the dose delivered by star photons was negligible compared to that of star neutrons; consequently, we shall deal with the latter only in this report. However, photons produced as a result of neutron interactions are included in the determination of dose.

The transport of neutrons and photons through tissue is computed using ANDY (2), a multi-energy-group, general geometry, Monte Carlo transport program. In principle, ANDY can handle neutrons and photons with any energy, provided the relevant cross-sections are contained in the code's library. In practice, however, for the chemical elements needed to describe tissue and bone adequately, the library restricts the energy ranges to 17 MeV and below for neutrons, and 10 MeV and below for photons. The cross-section library utilizes both experimental and theoretical input and is constantly being updated and expanded; however, the present restrictions on energy required an approximation scheme to deal with the higher energy (>17 MeV) star neutrons. The geometry of the problem must be specified in terms of five kinds of surfaces: planes, spheres, circular cylinders, ellipsoids, and cones. Also, inhomogeneous media, consisting of regions with different elemental compositions, can be accommodated. Very complex systems can, in principle, be modeled using ANDY, but the size and speed of the computer impose practical limitations.

Human Model and Neutron Source

The human model used for this problem is illustrated in Figure 1. The simplifications of body and organ shapes were necessitated by core and running time limitations. Arms and legs were left out for these same reasons. Three different elemental compositions were used for lung, bone, and remaining soft tissue, with total densities of 0.3, 1.5, 1.0 g/cm (3), respectively, and these are listed in Table 1. The coordinate system has its origin at the base of the trunk on the central axis, with the z-axis directed upward, x-axis to the left, and y-axis to the rear. A short description of the various components of the model is given below:

Trunk - a circular cylinder of radius $r = 14.15$ cm and $0 \leqslant z \leqslant 70$ cm. Volume = 37,834.3 cm^3.

Ribs - a circular cylindrical shell with $13.45 \leqslant r \leqslant 13.70$ cm and $35 \leqslant z \leqslant 70$ cm. Volume = 746.3 cm^3.

Pelvis - one half of a circular cylindrical shell with $13.45 \leqslant r \leqslant 14.00$ cm and $0 \leqslant z \leqslant 25$ cm, sectioned by the x-z plane. Volume = 529.9 cm^3.

Spine - a circular cylinder with $r = 2$ cm, axis parallel to the z-axis and passing through (x,y,z) = (0, 11.45 cm, 0), divided into four sections: (1) $70 \leqslant z \leqslant 80$ cm; (2) $35 \leqslant z \leqslant 70$ cm; (3) $25 \leqslant z \leqslant 35$ cm; (4) $0 \leqslant z \leqslant 25$cm. Volume = 1005.3 cm^3.

Heart - a sphere with r = 5.25 cm and center located at (0, - 8 cm, 51 cm). Volume = 606.1 cm^3.

Lungs - upper half of ellipsoids with semi-axes (5 cm, 7 cm, 23 cm) parallel to (x,y,z)-axes, respectively, and centers located at (±7 cm 0, 43.5 cm), sectioned by the plane z = 43.5 cm. Volume = 3372.0 cm^3.

Neck - a circular cylinder with r = 6.25 cm, axis passing through (0, 7.90 cm, 0), and containing spine-1. Volume = 1101.5 cm^3.

Skull - a segment of spherical shell with $9.2 \leqslant r \leqslant 10.0$ cm and common center located at (0, 6.15 cm, 86 cm), sectioned by the plane z = 80 cm. Volume = 753.0 cm^3.

Brain, together with mouth, eyes, auditory system, etc., constitutes the interior of the skull. Volume = 3000.1 cm^3.

Admittedly, this model is crude; however, it is an improvement over the simple spherical model with uniform composition used in our previous calculation.

Two treatment volumes were chosen to illustrate two rather different cases: (1) a large tumor located deep within the body; and (2) a small tumor located close to the surface of the body. In the first case, a spherical 1-liter treatment volume (r = 6.20 cm) was located in the abdominal region, with center at (0,0,30 cm). In the second case, a spherical 0.01-liter treatment volume (r = 1.33 cm) was located just under the surface of the neck, with center at (4.91 cm, 7.90 cm, 75 cm). Neutrons were randomly distributed both in location within the treatment volume and in direction of motion.

Although several experiments are being done at Los Alamos to determine the charged particle and neutron spectra resulting from pion stars, these data are not yet available, and other data which do exist have large errors and are often contradictory. Thus we have chosen to use a theoretical spectrum from average tissue (1) based on a Monte Carlo intranuclear cascade and evaporation model (3). In our previous work, we described two alternative approximation schemes for dealing with star neutrons with energy greater than 17 MeV. In the first approximation scheme we placed the number of neutrons with energy $E_n > 17$ MeV into the last energy bin (15–17 MeV) of the ANDY code. In the second scheme, we placed all of the excess energy (from neutrons with $E_n > 17$ MeV) into this last energy bin. We label these schemes Approximation I and Approximation II, respectively. The star neutron spectrum used here is identical to that used in our previous work and is illustrated in Figure 2.

Dose Calculation

The dose delivered to a region is determined by simple summing the net neutron and photon energy crossing each bounding surface of the region and dividing by the mass of the region. This procedure ignores any energy transferred by charged particles from one region into another. Since charged particles produced by star neutron interactions have a range $\lesssim 1$ cm, the error resulting from this neglect is small for regions with dimensions much greater than 1 cm.

As mentioned in our previous work, we made a comparison of the results of our earlier calculation with those of another calculation (Hamm and Turner, private communication) which used the full star neutron spectrum up to $E_n = 100$ MeV and a completely different code. That comparison indicates that our two approximation schemes bracket the more accurate treatment. Approximation I is slightly favored at short distances and Approximation II favored at greater distances. For simplicity, we have averaged the present results from the two approximations, introducing an error in the 1-liter case of about –40 percent for distant (>20 cm) regions. In each case, 2×10^4 stopped pions were assumed, resulting in statistical errors ranging from a few percent for the largest doses—i.e., in the region containing the treatment volume and regions closest to the treatment volume, to $\sim$80 percent for the smallest doses—i.e., the most distant regions.

It should be noted that a random distribution of stars such as was assumed in this calculation will not produce an exactly uniform dose distribution within the treatment volume; nevertheless, we shall assume this distribution is approximately constant. It has been estimated (Huston, private communication) that for treatment volumes greater than the peak region of a single pion dose distribution, the energy deposited within the treatment volume by all star products (expressed in convenient units) is $\sim 10^{-6}$ rad/π^- stop/cm^3). Thus, the treatment dose for a 1-liter treatment volume is $\sim 10^{-9}$ rad/π^- stop and for a 0.01-liter treatment volume, $\sim 10^{-7}$ rad/π^- stop.

The results for the two cases considered here are shown in Tables 2 and 3, respectively. We express the neutron dose for each region as a fraction of the treatment dose. In the first case, where the 1 liter treatment volume was located in the abdominal region, the trunk tissue (including the treatment volume) and the nearby section of spinal column received an average dose of $\sim$1 percent of the treatment dose. All other regions received only a small fraction of 1 percent of the treatment dose. The whole-body dose is almost 1 percent of the treatment dose. In the second case, where the 0.01 liter treatment volume was located just under the surface of the neck, all regions received much less than 1 percent of the treatment dose. This is not too surprising, since many neutrons can escape the body without interaction because of the proximity of the treatment volume to the surface.

Finally, as an indication of the neutron hazard to nearby personnel, we present in Figure 2 the neutron leakage spectrum from the body for our first case. This curve is certainly not reliable above 10 MeV due to the nature of the approximations made. It should be noted that other sources of radiation—e.g., gamma rays and neutrons produced at the target or along the pion channel—may also be significant.

Conclusions

The whole-body dose calculated for our first case is consistent with results obtained in our previous calculation for a 1-liter treatment volume. The dose reported here includes the neutron dose within the treatment volume, whereas the dose reported in our earlier example is the average *external* dose. Nevertheless, the numbers obtained are in substantial agreement (7.9×10^{-12} rad/π^- stop here vs. 6.8×10^{-12} rad/π^- stop earlier). For our second case (0.01 liter) we here obtain only 60 percent of the whole body dose reported for the 0.01 liter treatment volume studied previously. This difference can be understood in terms of the location of the treatment volumes in these comparative examples; the earlier calculation corresponding more closely to a tumor located deep within the body, and the present calculation corresponding to a surface nodule. In both cases, we can conclude that the neutron dose is very small and does not constitute a significant hazard during pion radiotherapy. Experiments measuring the neutron dose at various locations within a phantom will be carried out at Los Alamos, thus providing a test of these calculations.

Some obvious improvements that can be made in this calculation are: (1) extend the cross-section library so that neutrons with energies up to 100 MeV can be included; (2) replace the theoretical star neutron spectrum with good experimental data; and (3) include RBE factors in the calculation of dose. The cross-section library is being continually updated and extended, so that number 1, above, may soon be satisfied. Experiments are now being planned and carried out at Los Alamos, thus meeting number 2, above. Since the dose is calculated for each energy group, it is a trivial matter to include an RBE factor as required by number 3, above, provided reliable RBE data for neutrons can be supplied for the energy range $0 \leqslant E_n \leqslant 100$ MeV.

The calculations described here required 66 minutes of time and the full 58K core of a CDC 7600 computer. Increasing the complexity of the model would require a larger core and, possibly, a longer running time.

REFERENCES

1. Schillaci, M. E. and Roeder, D. L.: *Phys. Med. Biol. 18*, 821 (1973).
2. Harris, D. R., "ANDYMG3, the Basic Program of a Series of Monte Carlo Programs for Time-Dependent Transport of Particles and Photons," Los Alamos Report LA-4539 (1970).
3. Guthrie, M. P., Alsmiller, R. G., Jr., and Bertini, H. W., *Nucl. Intrum. Meth. 66*, 29 *and 91*, 669 (E) (1968).

Table 1.
Elemental Mass Densities (g/cm³)

Element	*Lung*	*Soft Tissue*	*Bone*
H	.031	.106	.106
C	.030	.232	.345
N	.008	.024	.059
O	.230	.638	.735
P			.105
Ca			.150

Table 2.
1-Liter Treatment Volume-Abdominal Region
(treatment dose ~ 10^{-9} rad/π^- stop)

Region	*Dose (10^{-9} rad/π^- stop)*
Trunk (ex. Bone and lung)	.010
Neck (ex. bone)	.00013
Heart	.0019
Brain	.000049
Lungs	.0024
Spine-1	.000050
Spine-2	.0020
Spine-3	.011
Spine-4	.0023
Skull	.000033
Ribs	.0015
Pelvis	.0022

Whole-Body Dose = .0079 Treatment Dose
Average Bone Dose = .0018 Treatment Dose

Table 3.
0.01-Liter Treatment Volume-Neck Surface
(treatment dose ~ 10^{-7} rad/π^- stop)

Region	*Dose* (10^{-7} rad/π^- stop)
Trunk (ex. bone and lung)	.000014
Neck (ex. bone)	.0012
Heart	.0000070
Brain	.000087
Lungs	.000018
Spine-1	.00035
Spine-2	.000031
Spine-3	.00000036
Spine-4	~ 0
Skull	.000074
Ribs	.000019
Pelvis	~ 0

Whole-Body Dose = .000054 Treatment Dose
Average Bone Dose = .000043 Treatment Dose

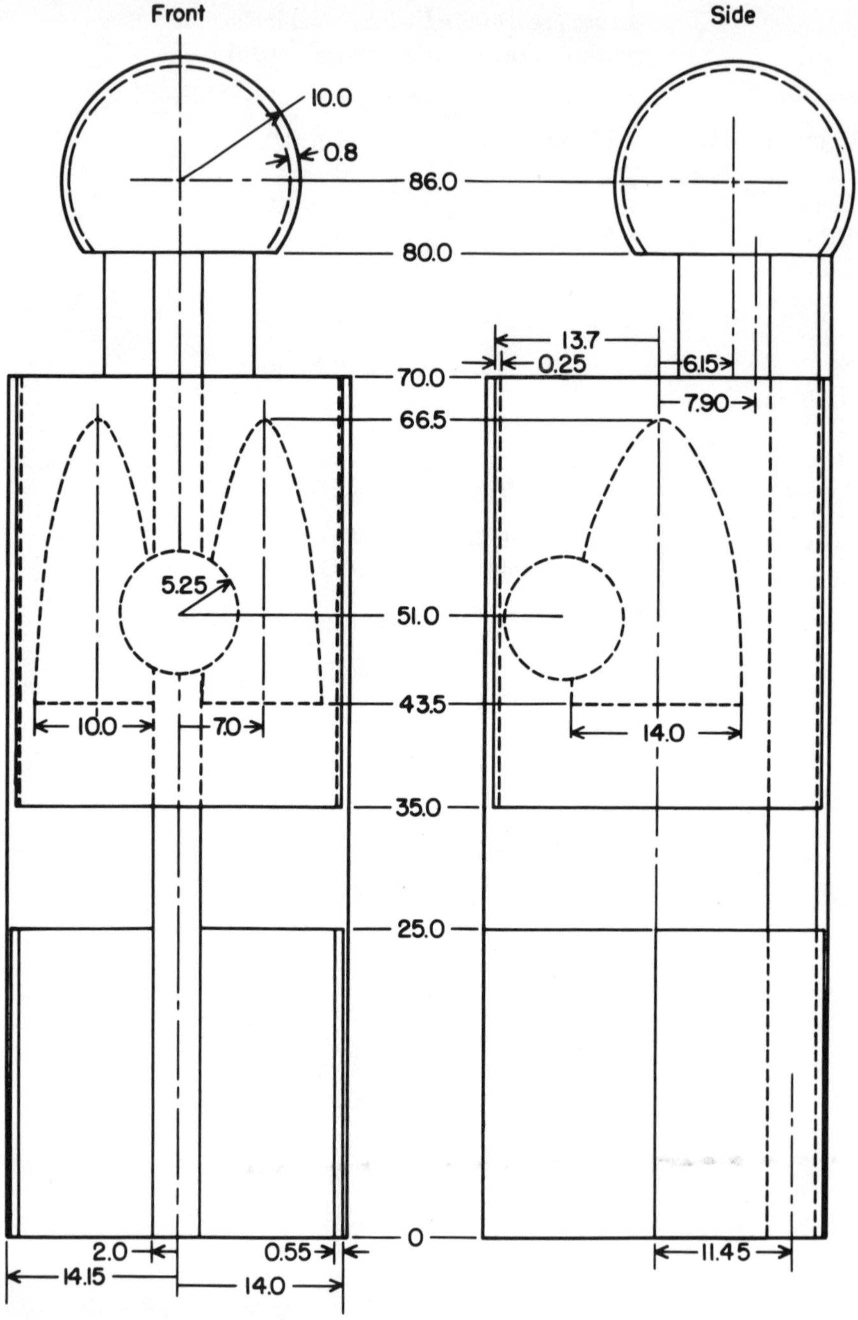

Figure 1. Human Model Specifying Geometry for ANDY Program (all Dimensions in cm)

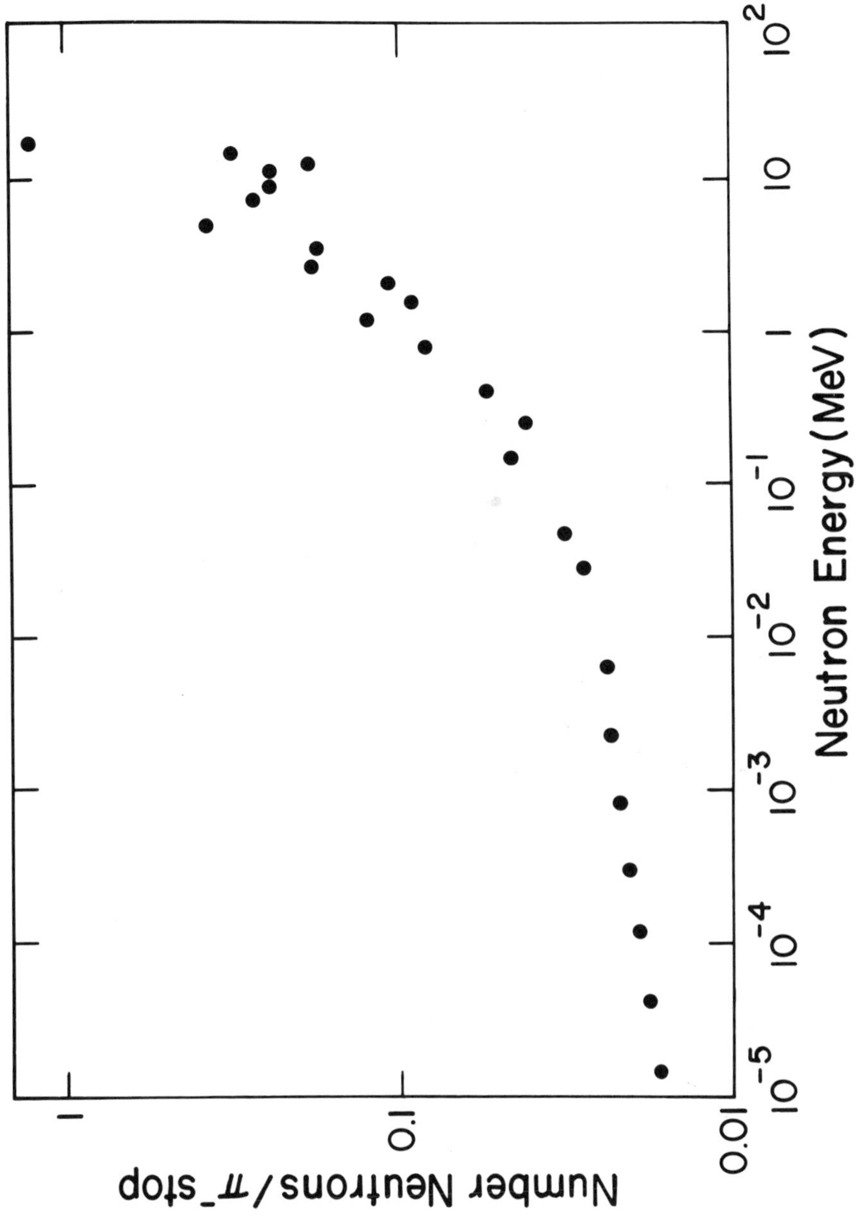

Figure 2. Energy Spectrum of Neutrons Leaving the Body for the Case of a 1-Liter Treatment Volume in the Abdominal Region

J. Clemens
B. Bjarngard
A. L. Boyer
M. Goitein
R. Larsen
G. K. Svensson

3. Computer Automation of Compensating Filter Design

The use of compensating filters is a well established method in radiation therapy to counteract the distortion of the dose distribution that occurs when the photon beam enters the patient's body through an irregular surface. The purpose is to insert along each ray from the focus enough material so that the beam again has the dose distribution that it would have if it were incident upon a flat surface. The compensating filter is inserted in the beam at a distance from the patient to preserve the skin-sparing effect of the beam, as was originally done by Ellis et al. (1). The proportions of primary and scattered radiation vary with depth and field size, and the filter therefore cannot be made to compensate at all points in a volume (2, 3).

To build a compensating filter is a time-consuming process which requires (a) that an "elevation map" be constructed of the area of the patient where the beam is to enter, (b) that this map is put in exact geometrical relation to the direction and position of the beam, and (c) that a filter be manufactured using this correctly oriented map. Several methods have been developed for this purpose (4, 5). The objective of the development work reported here has been to use a digital computer to produce the elevation map. From this information, the compensating filter can be manufactured in many different ways. Stacking lead sheets cut to fit the elevation curves as described by Wilks and Casebow (6) is one method, below called a terrace filter. The assembly of small aluminum, copper, or other metal blocks of different thicknesses on a tray or in a frame (a block filter) is a technique introduced by Ellis et al. (1).

The production of the elevation map requires the gathering of the data describing the patient's surface and the transformation of these data to the correct beam orientation and to the position of the filter during treatment. Several devices can be used to measure the patient's surface. The well-known rod box (2, 5) consists of a number of parallel pins in a frame. The rods are slid down to make contact with the patient's skin. The vertical positions of the rods are then measured, and these data describe the patient's surface. We have used this device and entered the measured data either manually, through the keyboard, or automatically, using the computer's analogue and digital input devices to read the specially constructed sensor which digitizes the rod lengths. We have also used an ultrasonic scanner to produce polaroid films of the patient contours. For this application the ultrasound transducer was replaced with a pointer. By using a graphic input device, such contours in parallel planes were entered into the computer. The most elegant solution to the problem of entering the patient's surface contour is probably to read the coordinates directly from the ultrasound arm or a similar device into the computer. This requires a special interface, which is commercially available.

Details of the orientation of the beam in relation to the patient's contour are entered into the computer via the keyboard. These data include gantry angle, collimator opening, rotational angle, and distance from source to target. The program then proceeds to design the desired filter.

Figure 1 shows some details of the calculational procedure. The computer first correctly orients the surface, represented by 41 × 41 points with respect to the beam center line. The compensating filter is also represented by 1681 points in one plane. A plane is located perpendicularly to the center line through the point on the surface closest to the source.

Through each point in the compensating filter plane, the computer projects a ray from the source to the patient's surface and finds the missing tissue by an interpolation routine. This value is converted to the thickness of compensating material required. In the present implementation, a preset ratio h/d of filter-to-tissue thickness is used. We do not, at the present time, vary this ratio with the depth at which we want optimum compensation. This approach is desirable, since the depth of the tumor varies from case to case (2, 3). It is, however, a trivial modification to allow the h/d ratio to be selected depending on this depth and the area of the field.

The program offers the user a choice between block type filters and terrace filters. In the first case the output is a scale drawing of the rectangular array of blocks with the thickness of each block indicated. This is shown by Figure 2. For terrace filters a scale drawing of the contours of the lead sheets is produced, Figure 3. Additional information, such as beam geometry and patient identification data, are given on a line printer.

The program described here was written on a PC-12 computer, primarily in FORTRAN. It requires 12 K of memory. Filter data are stored (on magnetic tape) and edited separately from the patient contour data, as schematically indicated by Figure 1.

This presentation is indeed a progress report in that many improvements can be made to simplify further and extend the capabilities of compensator manufacture. Our experiences indicate that the use of a computer to produce the filter specifications in a simple form for manufacture represents a great simplification. The program allows the use of a variety of ways of measuring the patient contours and of producing compensating filters. For instance, the rod box is very convenient for design of compensators for the head and neck region, while other methods might be more suitable for large treatment areas.

Since the raw data from the measurement are stored in the computer, modifications to the original treatment scheme can easily be made, for instance when it is desired to change the relative orientation of the contour and the therapy beam. An important physical advantage is offered by the possibility of adjusting the amount of compensation to the depth of the tumor. It is also possible to let the ratios of h/d change with the lateral position in the field. This provides a method to more accurately take the varying proportion of scattered photons into account. Finally, since the geometric transforms are general and the input and output segments are modular, the program can be adapted to solve other problems, such as shaping the isodose curves for individualized wedges.

REFERENCES

1. Ellis, F., Hall, E. J., and Oliver, R., *Brit. J. Radiol.*, *32*, 421 (1959).
2. Van de Geijn, J., *Brit. J. Radiol.*, *38*, 865 (1965).
3. Khan, F. M., Moore, V. C., and Burns, D. J., *Radiology 96*, 187 (1970).
4. Sorenson, N. E., *Phys. Med. Biol.*, *13*, 113 (1968).
5. Khan, F. M., Moore, V. C., and Burns, D. J., *Radiology*, *90*, 593 (1968).
6. Wilks, R., and Casebow, M. P., *Brit. J. Radiol.*, *42*, 452 (1969).

QUESTIONS

BLINICK: The factors you seem to have incorporated are strictly due to the primary attenuation through the thickness of the filter. Have you taken into account in the program what happens to scatter radiation underneath?

BOYER: No, not at all. That has to do with the fact that we're using a linear relationship between missing tissue thickness and block height. As I pointed out, we can add a functional relationship based on the scatter-defined parameters. This is something we plan to look at in the very near future.

M. COHEN: You cannot compensate completely for every depth. If you compensate for a 5 cm depth in tissue, you will be out at 2 cm and

10 cm, etc. I didn't see anything in your program that said, "We want to compensate at a particular depth in tissue in any given case."

My other question deals with the rationale of this approach. I'm a compensator man, myself, but when you're using a computer to calculate your treatment plans, although you may get a different distribution without the compensator, you still can optimize it. So why bother with the compensator? I thought the whole idea of using computer calculations is that you get rid of this dreadful chore of making compensators for every patient.

BOYER: As to your first question—I do realize you can only compensate at one depth. Where you compensate is again a function of this relationship of the missing tissue depth to filter thickness. As the program stands now, it's up to the discretion of the person putting that number in as to what depth you compensate.

As to the rationale—it appears to us that if you use compensating filters to turn all of your patients into square blocks, then it radically changes the way you use a computer in treatment-planning. You're now able to treat simply square blocks of tissue rather than patients with curvature.

ELLIS: Is there any intention of bringing heterogeneities into this compensating system?

BOYER: We have thought about a very elegant system in which irregular field shapes, tissue heterogeneities, etc. were taken into consideration in order to give a perfectly uniform distribution at some optimal depth.

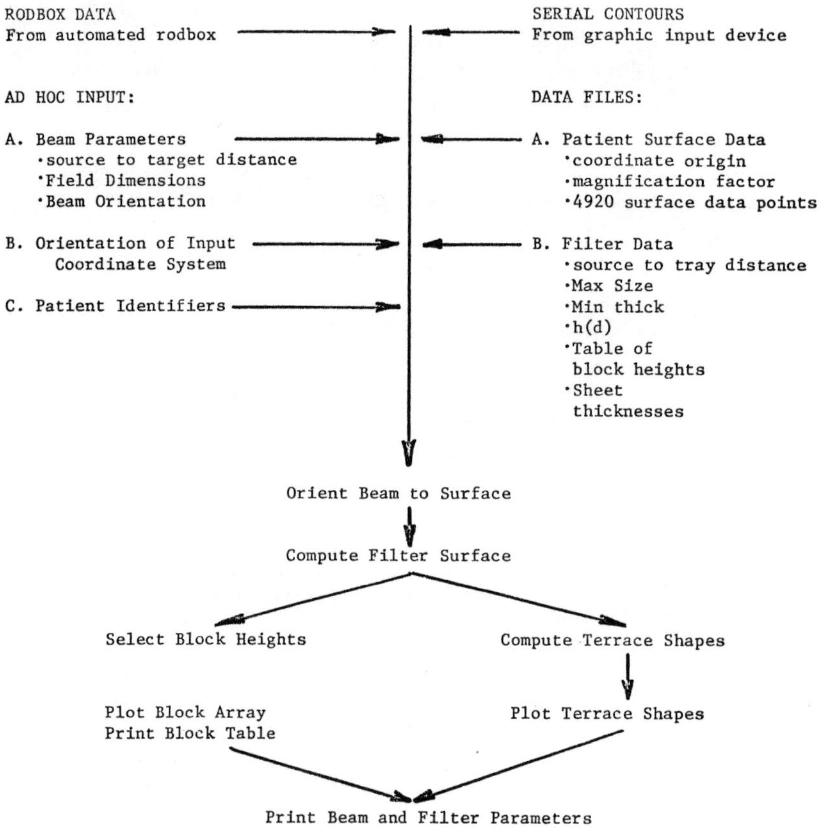

Figure 1. Outline of the Program

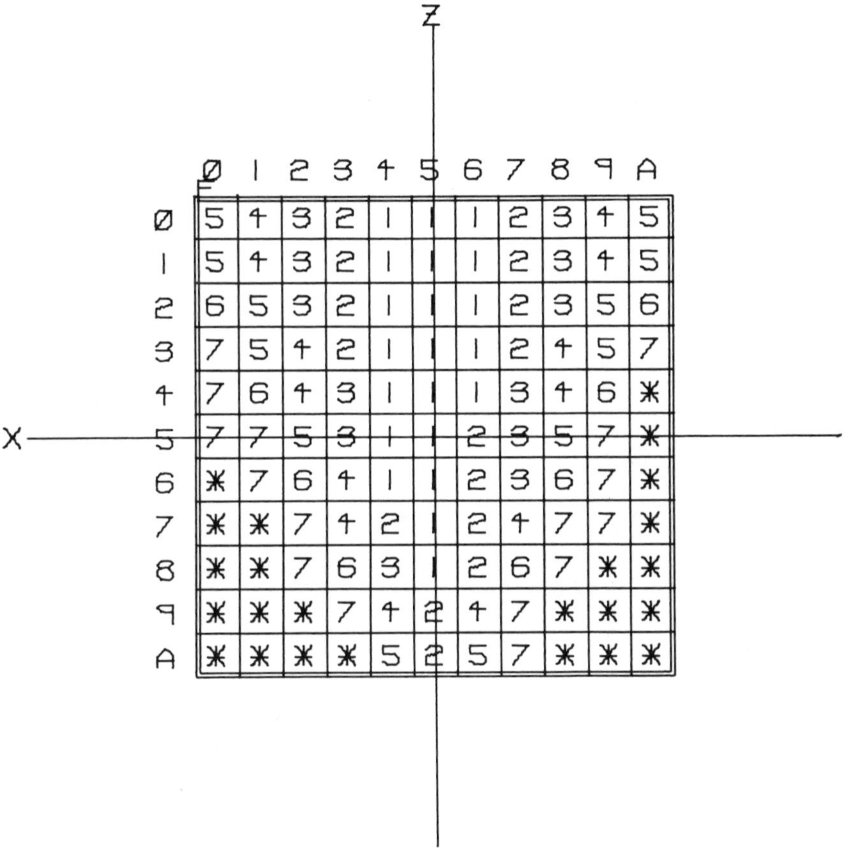

Figure 2. This Example of Computer Output Shows a Drawing of the Rectangular Array of Blocks in a Block Filter. The Symbols Indicate Standard Thicknesses of Blocks Corresponding to the Compensation for 1 cm, 2 cm . . . of Missing Tissue. The Original Drawing is to Scale (1:1)

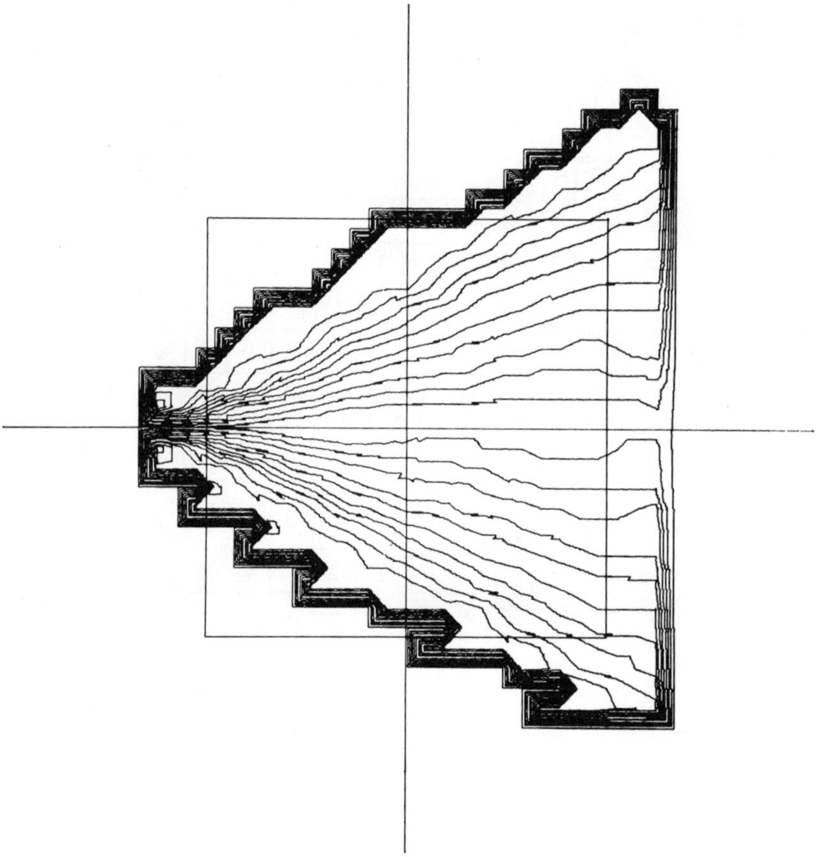

Figure 3. The Computer Output for a Terrace Filter Consists of a Drawing Showing the Profiles of Sheets of Standard Lead Thicknesses. The Original Drawing is to Scale (1:1)

4. A Pilot Program for True Three-Dimensional Dose Calculations in External Beam Radiotherapy

H. Frey
D. Chapman
D. Freida
A. Miller
R. Vokoff

All current "3-D" programs are basically serial 2-D programs. Doses are calculated in a plane as though the plane were a section of an infinite cylindrical phantom. A large inhomogeneity just outside the plane of calculation cannot be taken into account.

Everyone knows what must be done, i.e., calculate the scatter dose to each point from every other point in the phantom, but they have not implemented this method because of the supposed excessive computation time.

In order to determine whether this potentially most accurate method was economically feasible, the author gave the problem as a class project to a small class of graduate students in a course entitled "Computer Applications in Radiology." The usual pretty front and hind ends of a complete dosimetry program were dispensed with, i.e., the input and plot routines, and the bare bones of the dose calculation routines only were written.

The algorithm chosen was an extension of the method of scatter-air ratios used to such good effect by Cunningham. The calculation was performed in two parts. First, the primary dose was calculated to each point of the volume under consideration by straightforward calculation of inverse-square, absorption in slant tissue distance, and an air dose modification factor which could be used to account for penumbra, blocks, tissue compensators, field-shaping, wedges, etc.

Once the primary dose is known for all points, we must make reference to a table of scatter functions which tells us the scatter dose to any point for one rad of primary at any other point. This scatter function can be derived from standard SAR tables by fairly simple operations.

Let us define a scatter function S(d,r) as follows:

$$SAR(d,r) = \int_0^d TARZ(x)S(d-x,r)dx \qquad (1)$$

Thus, the SAR can be defined as the convolution of the zero area TARZ, which is the primary dose at each depth, and a scatter function S which is the scatter dose received at a point from a disc of radius r, d cm above the point, which disc is uniformly irradiated with 1 rad of primary. This convolution can theoretically be solved by the use of Laplace or Fourier Transforms, viz.,

$$F(S) = \frac{F(SAR)}{F(TARZ)}$$

A program to use this approach resulted in an excessively oscillating function, so due to the pressure of time we temporarily retreated to the discrete case:

$$SAR(d,r) = \sum_{n=1}^{d} TARZ(n)\, S(d-n,r) \qquad (2)$$

When solved for S this yields:

$$S(n,r) = \frac{SAR(n+1,r) - \sum_{i=0}^{n-1} S(i,r)TARZ(n+1-i)}{TARZ(1)} \qquad (3)$$

e.g. $S(0,r) = SAR(1,r)/TARZ(1)$; $S(1,r) = \dfrac{SAR(2,r)-S(0,r)TARZ(2)}{TARZ(1)}$

$$S(2,r) = [SAR(3,r)-S(0,r)TARZ(3)-S(1,r)TARZ(2)]\,/TARZ(1) \qquad (4)$$

Given this scatter function, we can easily recalculate the scatter-air ratio for any depth and radius by the use of equation 3. This still, however, presupposes a uniformly irradiated field.

In order to allow for noncircular nonuniform fields, we would like to have a scatter function for a point rather than a disc. We thus define a new scatter function:

$$DS(d,r) = [S(d,r+\epsilon)-S(d,r-\epsilon)]/4\pi r\epsilon \qquad (5)$$

Here we have taken the *increase* in scatter caused by an additional thin ring of tissue, and divided by the area of the ring to obtain the scatter dose to a point for 1 rad of primary irradiating 1 cc of unit density tissue, d cm above and r cm lateral to the point in question. The scatter dose at any point can now be calculated by integrating over the entire volume above the point.

$$SCATTER(X_0,Y_0,Z_0) = \int_0^z \int_0^y \int_0^x PRIMARY(X,Y,Z)DENSITY$$
$$(X,Y,Z)DS(Z-Z_0, \sqrt{(x-x_0)^2 + (y-y_0)^2})dxdydz \qquad (6)$$

Note that several factors are still not taken into account in this approach:

(1) Scatter from below. This could be added relatively easily but

would probably require additional measurements rather than simple reference to published tables.

(2) Absorption of the scatter by inhomogeneities. The calculation of DS has assumed unit density material between the two points in question, and the absorption term enters implicitly rather than explicitly. If this tabular function can be fitted with an analytic function, and if this function can be chosen to have absorption enter explicitly, then this factor could also be handled.

(3) Scatter of scatter. I assume that this is a small fraction of the total dose, at least for supervoltage at normal depths, but if it were shown to be significant, could probably be approximated by a simple percentage increase in all the DS values.

To test this concept, a small pilot program was written. Doses were calculated in a $10 \times 10 \times 10$ volume which could be scaled. Only Cobalt 60 was considered. The source could be placed anywhere with respect to the irradiated volume. A 10×10 air dose modification array allowed for any arbitrary function to be applied to the incoming beam. This is to be used for blocks, wedges, tissue compensators, penumbra, irregular field borders, etc.

The irradiated volume is represented by a density matrix, containing the density at each point. For calculating the primary dose, the inverse square factor is straightforward. Absorption is handled by summing the densities along the ray from the source to the point. The point of intersection with the air dose modification array is then determined, and the appropriate factor applied.

Once these primary doses have been calculated, equation 6 is used to calculate the scatter at every point. Any plane through the volume may then be selected for conventional 2-D printout.

This whole approach is very obvious and straightforward, and if it has not been done before by twenty people in this room, it is undoubtedly because they thought it would take too much computing time to be practical.

This program was written in G level Fortran without optimization and run on the IBM 360/91 at HSCF at UCLA. Calculation of primary dose at a point took 0.6 msec. Calculation of scatter-dose integrating over the $10 \times 10 \times 10$ array took 24 msec./point. Thus the total calculation was only approximately $25 \times n^6$ microseconds for the whole array. Note that this is for unoptimized FORTRAN. If the scatter calculation routine were hand-coded, I have no doubt that a factor of 5–10 improvement could be made. This is well within the range of practicability. The $10 \times 10 \times 10$ array took only 25 sec. in the unoptimized version. Since this is potentially the most accurate method available, it could be calculated on a relatively coarse grid to check the results of faster but less accurate calculations, or interpolations could be carried out. This algorithm could also be used to provide accurate spot doses at a few critical points in the treated field.

I have been asked how one would enter the thousand density values required. In the final program I plan to be able to enter contours in two or more planes, with the value of the density inside it, and have the program interpolate the contours of intervening planes. Thus relatively little extra data input would be required.

What is the actual status of the work at this time? The scatter functions S(d,r) for discs have been derived and working backward generate the SAR's with an accuracy of 3–4 percent. The scatter functions DS(d,r) for points still yield errors of scatter of up to a factor of two, though this is clearly a programming rather than a conceptual problem. The timings obtained are, of course, independent of the accuracy of the scatter functions. Perhaps I should have told the students that their grades would be dependent on the accuracy of the final program.

QUESTIONS

CUNNINGHAM: We did similar work involving volume elements in 1969, and it was presented at the Madrid Radiological Conference last year with comparison with experimental measurements for this sort of semigeometrical setup. The approach is not identical, but it's analagous.

BJARNGARD: I think for those of us who have been involved in reactor shielding calculations, it might be worth pointing out that your approach is very similar to the calculation with build-up factors.

RENNER: In numerical analysis one often runs into the situation where, in order to attain a number, as you decrease the size of the little pieces you add together to get you to a final number, your error may decrease and then may take off and increase. This poses a natural limitation on how much you can cut things down into little sizes. Have you run into this yet?

FREY: Yes, we took this into account in designing the program and figured we'd be adding so many small numbers that we might well have them falling off the end in the round-off error, so we've prepared a routine that will actually add numbers of comparable dimensions until they've become an order of magnitude bigger, at which time you add them into the next dimension, and that way when you're all through, you add them together, and you don't lose them in the round-off. So far, we haven't found it necessary to do it, but this is part of the plan.

5. The Future Role of the Computer in Radiotherapy Treatment Planning

J. M. Wilkinson

External beam treatment planning is a process that results in a decision to use a particular configuration of beam and machine parameters in the treatment of an individual patient. The process is flow-charted in Figure 1. Although this may not represent an accurate description of the process for every center, it will be sufficiently general to form a basis for the current discussion. The intention is to start at the point where the target volume has been decided on and then look at the subsequent stages in the process where the computer could have a possible role.

The Choice of Treatment Parameters

Decisions are required concerning the following parameters:

(1) Type and quality of radiation
(2) Number of beams
(3) Beam directions
(4) Beam dimensions
(5) Shielding
(6) Source to surface distance
(7) Beam weighting
(8) Beam modifying filters

The tumor dose and time fractionation scheme have been omitted from the list, as it is assumed that a prescription policy will be decided independently of any individual patient, and that the relative dose-distribution will be the criterion on which the plan is judged. That restricts the definition of treatment-planning, but it is within this context that the comments made in this paper apply.

It is desirable that all treatment plans for a particular kind of tumor in a particular site be very similar, because it is only by standardizing the technique that one can start to evaluate the treatment and obtain a sound basis on which to consider possible improvements. Hence, in the vast majority of cases the first six parameters in the list will be decided on the basis of what was done last time, modified only slightly in accordance with measurements made during the localization procedures. This automatically takes into consideration practical limitations and many of the dose distribution requirements—for example, avoiding certain tissues. Only the last two parameters require any form of calculation, and, indeed, with experience in using a standard technique it is possible to make a good guess at each of these. It can be said that such treatments virtually plan themselves. This firmly implies that a treatment-planning philosophy, such as that adopted by the RAD-8 and P.C. computer systems, which encourages a free choice of such parameters as the beam directions and the number of beams for each new patient, is undesirable. Only very rarely, when new equipment becomes available or when it is thought possible to improve on a treatment technique, will it be necessary to consider the parameters individually, and even then the practical limitations may reduce the choice of some to the level of triviality. Furthermore, as none of the parameters are completely independent of one another, there is by no means a completely free choice. This is illustrated by a technique used in Manchester in the 1940's for treating carcinoma of the middle ear. Orthovoltage X rays were used because that was what was available at the time, which in turn influenced the choice of the number of beams. This is a complicated technique, using five non-coplanar beams, and the dosimetry was done adequately without a computer. Today megavoltage X rays would be used, and the technique would be a relatively simple wedged pair. Generally, the choice of the type and quality of radiation will be influenced by the location of the tumor and, in the absence of any unequivocal radiobiological evidence, by the prejudices of the radiotherapist or physicist concerned!

Beam directions will be those taking the shortest route from skin surface to tumor center that is compatible with sparing critical tissues; beam dimensions will be chosen so that they enclose the target volume within the field; shielding will be positioned to protect critical areas after the beam directions have been chosen; and nonstandard source-surface distances will be chosen only if practical limitations force the issue. Again it is only in the choice of beam weightings and beam-modifying filters that dose calculations are called for in arriving at a sensible proposal.

Dose Calculations

Dose calculations are done for one of two reasons: either to provide the necessary information for making adjustments to certain of the parameters (and it has just been suggested that ideally one should need to adjust only beam weightings and beam modifying filters), or, finally, to confirm that the dose distribution requirements have been met.

It should be possible to calculate the dose at any point of interest within the irradiated volume, and a system that restricts the calculation points to lie in a single plane or restricts the beams to being coplanar is inadequate. This again is a criticism of some of the commercially available systems. To perform calculations with non-coplanar beams the coordinates of the dose-calculation points, expressed in a patient-reference system, must undergo a three-dimensional transformation and be expressed in the coordinate system of each beam in turn. This also removes the restriction to calculating in a single plane.

An important consequence of lifting the coplanar beam restriction is that a two-dimensional patient contour is no longer useful input information. Instead, for each beam it is necessary to know the shape of the entry surface, and for lung and oesophagus treatments, the shape and location of lung tissue, expressed in the beam-coordinate system. If the beam direction is determined prior to the dose calculations, this anatomical information may be restricted to areas that lie within the geometric limits of the field. This is a further argument in favor of predetermining beam directions.

Adjustment of the Parameters

It is sometimes useful to make small adjustments of beam direction to achieve dose homogeneity within the target volume. However, if, as suggested, this parameter is predetermined, the same effect may be achieved by adjustments of beam weightings and beam-modifying filters. This implies a need for a very flexible system of filters, and if no suitable wedge filter is available, it will be necessary to design and manufacture an additional compensating filter. The normal concept of a compensating filter is that of a device designed to correct for surface curvature. In this case it would have three purposes: first, to correct for surface curvature; second, to correct for changes in thickness of any regions of inhomonogeneity; and third, to give a fine adjustment of wedge angle superimposed on that obtained from available wedge filters. The design of the additional compensating filter, starting from the desired shape of the isodose surface at the tumor depth, is a suitable job for the computer. Better still, the computer could drive the equipment used for manufacturing the compensator. There is one major objection to using compensators: they cannot readily be interlocked, and without a sophisticated computer checking system, they enhance the possibility of execution error. An adequate treatment plan well executed constitutes better radiotherapy than a perfect plan erroneously executed!

The other parameter that cannot be determined finally before dose calculations are made is beam weighting. Again the computer can be of help in making this choice by quickly investigating the effects of changes in the weightings and returning with the most appropriate values—that is to say, values that result in the homogeneous dose-distribution within the target volume, while, at the same time, not exceeding tolerance levels at the beam entrance surfaces.

The Isodose Display

The isodose display is a method of presenting the results of the dose calculations for an assessment of the dose distribution. If non-coplanar beams are used, it is not possible to assess the dose distribution by looking at an isodose display in a single plane. Alternatives would be to have plots in a series of parallel planes, or in three orthogonal planes, or we can look to some kind of 3-D imaging system. The end point of this exercise, however, is not to produce an isodose display but to assess the dosage distribution. In particular we are interested in the dose at the tumor center, the dose around critical organs and near to the beam entry points, and the dose homogeneity in the target volume. This represents a relatively small fraction of the information available in an isodose display. The remaining information is not relevant to the assessment of the proposed treatment. It would be much more efficient to perform the dosage calculations only in and around the regions of interest. The computer could be programmed to search for hot spots or cool spots by following dose gradients, and hence reduce the number of dose-calculation points to a minimum. The output would then be an objective statement of the dose and dose homogeneity, or perhaps the range of doses, in the regions of interest. The size of the treatment volume is determined by, and bears a direct relation to, the field dimensions chosen. The radiographic checks will provide the evidence as to whether the tumor lies within the treatment volume. Is this not sufficient information, without any isodose displays at all, for the radiotherapist to assess the proposed treatment?

Summary

The points made in this paper are as follows:

(1) The computer has no role to play in the choice of most of the treatment parameters, particularly the number of beams and the beam directions, and computer systems that encourage a free choice of these parameters for each new patient are based on a

bad treatment-planning philosophy.

(2) The computer system should allow dose calculations for techniques that use non-coplanar beams, and indeed should allow for the inclusion of all possible choices of treatment parameters. Any that does not is inadequate.

(3) With non-coplanar beams, a two-dimensional patient contour is not useful input information. If the beam directions are predetermined, it should be replaced by information about the patient surface and internal structures that lie within the geometric limits of each beam.

(4) The computer has a possible role in determining the most appropriate beam weightings and in designing and manufacturing compensating filters. Such filters should be designed on the basis of the desired isodose shape at the tumor depth, and not solely to correct for surface irregulatities. And, finally,

(5) The question is raised: With standardized techniques, good radiographic verification procedures, and knowledge of the dose levels at the surface, near critical organs, and in the target volume, are isodose displays really necessary?

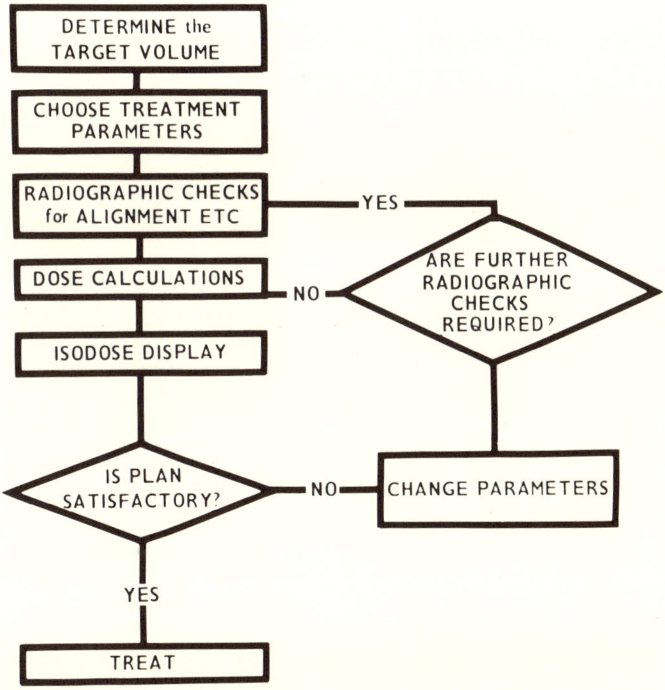

Figure 1. Flowchart of External Beam Treatment Planning Process

6. RADGRAF Progress Report and Projections for the Future

C. M. Newton
J. W. Johnson

RADGRAF, our remote graphics radiation treatment-planning system, was described to you at the Uppsala Conference. At that time it could be reported that response times were surprisingly good but that noise problems were not yet entirely overcome on the ordinary dial-up telephone link between the IMLAC graphics terminal and its host IBM 360/91 computer. Subsequently, additional software developments for both the host and the IMLAC's minicomputer resulted in solid communications support that circumvented all but the rarest line noise problems and further sharpened response times by efficient handling of graphical data. Except for very infrequent local hardware problems, this system has been stable for well over a year for Richard Nelson's terminal in New Jersey, as well as a number of terminals for this and other applications in the Los Angeles area.

Rather than jumping into new endeavors, we have invested the past two years in efforts such as the foregoing to ensure system and program reliability, and in investigating what features are desired by people engaged in radiotherapy.

We have worked in close cooperation with the Departments of Radiation Therapy at UCLA, Cooper Hospital in New Jersey, and Huntington Memorial Hospital in Pasadena, California. By listening, we have learned.

Interim Program Developments

The major change in the external beam program was the incorporation of a later version of the Memorial program called EXTREP. The new program provides better computing efficiency and improved output. The graphics input/output routines are completely separate from the computation section, giving us the option of utilizing different computation routines with a minimum of effort. Also, a substantial savings in the core requirements was achieved by overlaying all the graphic routines with the Memorial program. From an operational point of view, many small detail changes have been made. These were in response to specific comments and observations from the departments using the system. Some of the more significant of these changes were the continuous light-pen tracking routine, which supplements the GRAF/pen data tablet; the rewriting of the beam-definition frame; and display of numerical output for the Memorial program.

Experience with Use of the Program

We have had an opportunity to monitor the system as it was being used by a number of individuals of varying levels of experience. We can say with some confidence that our system is easy to use. Persons with no prior computer exposure are able to run it successfully after very little assistance. The cost of treatment plans seems to be within reason. For example, a plan with rotational beam and five contours of varying density, costs between $2.00 and $4.00, depending on the coarseness of the matrix and the step size of computation. This does not include connect charges, which are $3.00 per hour during prime time, or telephone charges. Time to plan a treatment may run from 10 minutes to 30 or 40 minutes, depending on the number and complexity of plans tried and the number of anatomical contours to be specified.

Recent Resumption of New Program Development

Having reached the point where it is now possible to recommend wider use of this system, we have very recently resumed the development of new programs. Several interesting aspects of this uncompleted work may be worth mentioning.

(a) **Representation of iridium wires.** Two years ago a program facilitating the three-dimensional specification of wire location from stereo pairs was well under way and tested satisfactorily for a variety of theoretical curves. Interpolation subsequent to curve fitting enabled the user to indicate points along the wire's curve without regard to their stereo correspondence in Z, or close and even spacing. However, these functions and the method of fitting have not worked well on the curves typical of the U-shaped afterloaders recently introduced by our Department of Radiology. Several fitting approaches (e.g. exact, variously weighted regressions) were explored for five different functions. A graphics program written for this investigation now is being included in the Iridium Wire Program. Basically, the wire is fitted piecewise with different functions, the computer negotiating a satisfactory fit to each segment initially. If the user believes he can improve the fit in one segment, he can indicate the points on which the fit is to be based. These may include displayed interpolated points, permissible in such an application and sometimes enabling iterations to a far better fit. He may choose, then, from among a variety of simple functions and fitting approaches. The well-known hazards of polynomial curve-fitting are portrayed effectively by graphics visualizations, as are the trade-offs between regression and exact fits. Although in most cases the automated fitting of the entire wire seems to be satisfactory, the therapist probably will want the power to override the computer's decisions in some.

(b) Faster and more reliable input of needles or U-shaped implants. We have worked on some strategies for advising users about possible implant exchanges or (for U-shaped implants) end reversals for a single implant, in situations where there may be a number of errors and where there are allowable uncertainties. The computer responds with all suggestions it can offer, together with a statement on whether these would suffice to explain the whole problem. The user may interact with the display to try out some of these changes.

A subsequently developed three-dimensional rotating display of the implants performs very nearly as well as the foregoing, more elaborate program. Rotation is about Z, the axis of rotation for the paired views. Instead of computing an average Z value for each point, one alternately contributes Z from one projection and then the other. Properly identified implants move smoothly, assuming the well-known illusion of three-dimensionality. U-shaped implants with reversed ends do a tight little dance, and exchanged implants hop back and forth. Speed of motion (recall the low-bandwidth communications to the remote terminal) is accomplished by sending a sequence of display frames to the terminal, thereafter rapidly running through them locally to produce the sensation of movement.

(c) New graphical output displays. A cubic "viewbox" can be moved about in a 3-dimensional field, with contours appearing where its walls intersect the field. It is effective for moderate-gradient fields, but perhaps log transforms should be tried for fields in the immediate vicinity of implants. Other graphical outputs, such as dose-volume histograms, maps that call especial attention to hot and cold areas, etc., are pretty standard. We await evaluation of all of these in actual use by therapists.

Future Plans

We shall continue to modify existing software in response to the needs of our users. It is our intent to complete the design and implementation of a patient record-keeping system. With respect to the external-beam program, we shall add the capabilities of producing iso-effect curves based on user's choice of model (CRE, ret), etc.

Our next major phase of software development will proceed with the delivery of the PDS-4. At this time a number of software packages will be developed to exploit the standalone capabilities of the PDS-4. The radium-needle and iridium-wire implant programs are being designed to permit crude, inexpensive explorations followed by higher-quality confirmatory treatment plans. The former will be moved as far as is possible to standalone execution on the IMLAC's minicomputer.

The variety of graphical outputs also seeks economy. When the novelty wears off, as one hopes it will, it is likely that users will rely on simple outputs, such as dose-volume histograms, for much of their work, using more sophisticated displays for more difficult cases.

We are keeping ourselves informed of developments in networking and are awaiting next year's inauguration of the satellite-based TELNET commercial system. One anticipates a substantial economy in communications costs, as well as an adequate bandwidth for graphics. Backup reliability by virtue of being able to access a number of computers on the system is especially attractive for medical applications.

There is room in radiotherapy for a variety of approaches. Larger centers can afford a substantial mini-computer, and the capabilities of these continue to grow. Centers with small patient loads probably will do best to access a time-shared service by way of an inexpensive typewriter terminal. But the IMLAC graphics terminal enables a moderate-sized radiotherapy center to obtain a very sophisticated level of support for a moderate initial cost. If the center grows, the terminal's standalone capabilities can be expanded.

ACKNOWLEDGMENTS

We would first like to thank Karl Ryden and the others at the Health Sciences Computing Facility for their development of the IMGRAF system. The UCLA Department of Radiotherapy has provided much of the feedback necessary for making improvements in RADGRAF. We would like to give special thanks to Richard and Mary Nelson for technical advice, and for their courage in being our first truly remote graphics users.

IV. Cell Population Models and Parameters

Chairperson: L. Cohen

Session VII: Invited Papers

1. Clinical Data and Biological Parameters in Relation to Optimization of the Treatment Schedule

L. Cohen

Optimization of a radiotherapeutic treatment schedule implies the selection, from among all practicable fractionation schemes, of that giving the maximum differential response between the tumor and the associated normal tissue. For this purpose the clinical response expected with various dosage schedules is standardized by using graphical plots relating dosage to treatment time, equations for estimating the position and slope of iso-effect lines, empirical power functions (NSD) relating dosage to fractionation and time, or cell population kinetic models yielding iso-effect boundaries that differ in origin, slope, and shape for different tissues and tumors.

From two to six parameters, which have to be derived statistically from available clinical data, are required for these various systems together with coefficients for radiation quality (LET) and biochemical factors (OER). Best-fitting parameters are identified by appropriate search programs. These can be used to select an optimal treatment scheme, giving either the highest therapeutic ratio or the maximal probit difference.

1. INTRODUCTION: OPTIMIZATION FUNCTIONS

The concept of an optimal dose requires that two biological systems, the disease process and the normal tissues, be considered. It is not always possible to deliver a dose that is both safe and effective. At best a therapeutic regime having a reasonable prospect of cure with a tolerably small risk of complications must be accepted. The optimal dose may be defined either as that giving the highest probability of uncomplicated cure or that entailing the lowest "cost," in terms of the relative risks of recurrence and of complications, assuming such costs can be evaluated.

These relationships were first recognized by Holthusen (9), elaborated by Strandqvist (15) and Cohen (2) in relation to the changing therapeutic ratios associated with time and volume factors, and redefined in terms of characteristic cost functions by Moore and Mendelsohn (13). Biological effects depend on the size, number, spacing, and sequence of individual dose-fractions, as well as the physical dose, the irradiated volume, radiation quality (LET or RBE), and various physical or chemical environmental conditions (temperature, oxygenation, sensitizing, and protective agents). Attempts to "correct" for uncontrolled variables have led to a variety of iso-effect formulae, from which biologically equivalent standard doses can be derived for any given treatment procedure.

2. ISO-EFFECT FORMULAE

Two approaches to the problem of standardizing the dose, or the associated biological response, have been explored. These are, first, the empirical systems, exemplified by dose-time plots or nominal standard dose formulae, which are essentially interpolative. The second approach is based on inferred or computed changes in the cell population of irradiated tissues, assuming implicitly that similar reactions or responses reflect similar surviving fractions, thus equating iso-effect with iso-survival functions. The cell population kinetic systems are extrapolative, in that response levels or probabilities can be computed.

2.1 Empirical Power Functions

These are designed to relate equivalent doses to the treatment time, number of fractions, and/or treated volume. The total dose (D_t) is related to an equivalent single exposure (D_s), the overall treatment time in days (T, elapsed time + 1) and the number of fractions (W), by the nominal standard dose (NSD) relationship. This is formulated by Ellis (7) as

$$D_t = D_s \cdot W^w \cdot T^t \tag{1}$$

For normal human skin and connective-tissue stroma, $w = 0.24$ and $t = 0.11$. Cohen and Kerrich (6) and Von Essen (17) introduced tumor-volume and/or field size as additional variates with simple corrections for RBE. A more elaborate appraisal of these relationships, leading to the development of the "cumulative radiation effect" (CRE) system has been made by Kirk, Gray, and Watson (12).

The NSD system as defined by Ellis is strictly applicable to a single-tissue type (connective-tissue stroma). Parameters in the other equations are known accurately only for skin, epidermoid carcinoma and mammary cancer. A similar formulation could be developed for other systems if accurate estimates of the parameters required (D_S, w, t) were derived for each of the tissues, organs or tumors studied. This would entail a fairly elaborate statistical analysis of a large number of clinical reports on tumor cure rates and normal tissue reaction rates covering a widely varying range of fractionation schemes.

2.2 Cell Population Kinetic Systems

Iso-effect lines can also be generated by computing the total dose required to achieve a given cellular surviving fraction (S), or iso-survival level, with various fractionation schemes. The absolute log-surviving-fraction (Q = -log S) has been proposed as a standard parameter for measuring biological dosage, assuming or fitting plausible cell kinetic parameters (3).

In contrast to the empirical systems, the cell population kinetic models are well suited to the introduction of radiobiological factors derived from cellular experiments *in vitro* or *in vivo*, for predicting possible effects of new modalities on the clinical iso-effect function. Effects of changing radiation quality—including the use of heavily ionizing particles (LET and RBE), variation of oxygen-tension (hypoxia and re-oxygenation), cell synchronizing or other physical or chemical agents known to affect the cellular lethality curve (heat, sensitizers and protective agents)—can be anticipated and evaluated.

Several formulae have been used for this purpose, employing either the "exponential + dose-squared" cellular lethality model (11) or some version of the single-hit multitarget model with the components for initial slope (irreparable injury), sublethal injury, and repopulation (1, 18). Typical of these models is the formula for the surviving fraction (S) after a single dose (D) of radiation:

$$s_1 = e^{-\alpha JD}\,[1-(1-e^{-\beta KD})^N] \qquad (2)$$

where J is the irreparable initial slope, K the slope for the reparable component, N the extrapolation number, and α and β quality coefficients related to RBE and/or OER. If the same dose is subdivided into W fractions over T days, the final surviving fraction would be

$$S_W = \prod_{i=1}^{W-1} \left[\frac{S_1 \cdot H_i}{S_i+(H_i-S_i)e^{-VL}} \right] \qquad (3)$$

Where V is the average interval between fractions (= T/W days), and L the generation rate of surviving cells with a repopulation capacity limited to a level (H) determined by cumulative effects of irreversible radiation damage to supporting tissues. The seven parameters required for this type of model include the mean cellular lethal dose $D_O = \frac{1}{J+K}$, the extrapolation number (N), ratio of transient to irreparable events (K/J), regeneration rate (L) and regeneration limit (H), field and volume factors (not in Equations 2 and 3), in addition to specific coefficients for LET, OER or other factors (α and β).

3. DATA: RADIOBIOLOGICAL AND RADIOTHERAPEUTIC

The various model systems can be tested, parameters fitted, and iso-effect functions derived, only if sufficiently accurate and comprehensive data on the radiosensitivity of the particular tissue, organ or tumor concerned is available, so that all the unknowns in the equation can be evaluated. There are at least three distinct types of data, each requiring appropriate statistical treatment.

3.1. Defined-Response Data

This type of data is generally obtained in an experimental situation where a carefully graduated range of dosage is studied, determining the effective dose (yielding 50% response or some other predefined level), for each of several treatment schemes. Similar data can be obtained in fractionated radiation therapy when the interval between fractions is long enough for a reaction to a previous dose to be seen before the next exposure is given. For example, skin reactions produced by treatment at intervals of a week or more can be "titrated" by continuing the treatment at a fixed dose-per-fraction only until a minimal dry desquamation is observed.

Defined-response data points effectively constitute an iso-effect line or function and can be used to draw dose-time curves, best-fitting Strandqvist-type lines on logarithmic coordinate charts, or computed iso-survival functions fitted to cell population kinetic models. Standard statistical methods can be used to derive best-fitting (least-squares) estimates for the various parameters concerned.

3.2 Graded-Response Data

In many clinical and experimental systems the exact dose needed to produce a predefined "standard" response is not known, nor easily derived by direct observation, but can be inferred by observing reactions at recognizably higher or lower levels than the standard. If the severity of the reaction can be ranked or graded, then previous data on graduated single exposures would indicate how the dose associated with an observed reaction could be normalized to correspond with a standard reaction. Doses adjusted in this way can then be treated like defined-response data by standard statistical methods.

3.3 Quantal-Response Data

In most of the clinically significant reactions to radiation therapy, and also in many radiobiological animal experiments, the observed end-point is an all-or-none phenomenon that cannot be graded. Examples are the death or survival of an experimental animal, cure or no-cure of a tumor. With these observations, the dosage scheme associated with any one animal or patient has no direct relevance to the observed quantal response. Dosage for a positive reaction or a cured cancer may be just at or well *above* the median effective level, while a negative response or failure to cure may result from a dose quite near or well *below* the median. Several approaches to the problem of identifying a median or other standard response rate have been explored. The objective is to define an iso-effect line or boundary which effectively separates quantal reactors from nonreactors and minimzes the number and magnitude of discrepancies in this discriminatory function. Methods currently in use are presented below.

3.31 Graphical discrimination (by eye). A simple two-dimensional dose-time plot of responders (marked x on the graph) and nonresponders (o) can often be resolved by a freehand or ruled line separating most of the x's above from most of the o's below the line, with very few points on the "wrong" side of the boundary. This method may succeed in defining crude tolerance limits or response levels for different treatment times with well-dispersed data points, but the position and slope of the median line is determined only by the relatively few discrepant observations and could be inaccurate.

3.32 Composite dose-time plots (Strandqvist). Some of the defects of graphical discrimination are obviated by Strandqvist's strategem of recording the separate responses in two systems (tumor and normal tissue) and evaluating the resultant contingencies. Tumor recurrence means underdosage, tissue necrosis is overdosage, and tumor-cure with tissue-recovery represents a narrow zone of acceptable dose-time combinations. This composite zone or boundary is much more sharply defined than that obtainable with any single tissue alone. A disadvantage is that the parameters derived (origin and slope of the iso-effect line) may not belong to either of the tissues irradiated, and probably would not be valid for other tumors in the same site or the same tumor type in other sites. It is also not possible to optimize the treatment scheme by using composite parameters.

3.33 Coefficient of separation (Pearson). This statistical index is used as an objective measure of the separate identity of two data sets. If a "biological dose" is computed for each data point in groups of reactors and nonreactors, the coefficient, for separation of the two groups of doses, becomes a measure of the validity of the model and parameters chosen. Best-fitting parameters are those which maximize this index (10). Unfortunately, the coefficient is sensitive to outlying data points which may be irrelevant (very large doses above the median boundary or small doses well below this line), hence will not remain consistent in replicate investigations. Also, the slope of the best separation lines may differ from the slope of iso-effect lines (16).

3.34 Minimal-deviant search program. This is a computer-operated version of the visual or graphical discrimination process and has the advantage of being objective and also not confined to linear two-dimensional plots. In this program, the iso-effect boundary is identified by minimizing the sum of squares of deviations from the boundary for all *discrepant* data points (reactors below, and nonreactors above, the line). An advantage of this method is its general utility for all quantal-type data sets. A possible disadvantage, as in all "separation" methods, is inaccuracy in defining the position and slope of the boundary if the number of discrepant points is small.

3.35 Multi-probit linear regression. If the effect studied is a median value, then an iso-effect line is a locus of points each being the median position for data in a particular treatment group. Each group would contain reactors and nonreactors, and the relative proportion of reactors would increase with increasing dose, forming a characteristic frequency distribution around the median. Probit analysis of any one group would identify the median dose and variance for that group. Multiple probit analyses, for many fractionation schemes, yields the required iso-effect locus and its confidence limits (8), from which the required parameters can be derived explicitly. While the multi-probit method is the most general, and theoretically the most rigorous search procedure available, it has serious practical limitations in that the data are segmented, hence used inefficiently. A relatively crude analysis requires several hundred entries, and the volume of data needed increases proportionally if the number of parameters or fractionation schemes studied is increased.

3.36 Compound probit search program. Without the mathematical rigor of the multi-probit system, this compromise has the advantage of using all available data efficiently and accepting relatively small data sets. The cell kinetic parameters are initialized (using plausible input values), and all data points replaced by computed survival levels (a convenient parameter is the absolute $\log_{10}$-surviving-fraction), which are then treated as biological "doses." Probit analysis is carried out on the new composite data set, deriving the conventional mean (μ), standard deviation (σ) and chi-squared values for the computed log-surviving-fractions. Parameters are then varied systematically, using either a universal grid search pattern or a sequential ridge search, converging on an optimal combination of parameters which simultaneously minimize the coefficient of variation (σ/μ) and chi-square values.

4. VALID DATA SETS

The set of variates needed to derive parameters for generating iso-effect functions or developing optimization procedures by analysis of clinical data is obviously an important part of the therapeutic record and should be included in any data set or tumor registry designed for evaluation of radiation response. There is also need to identify all tissues or organs traversed by the radiation beam, since each of these systems requires full specification of all treatment factors which may influence local reactions. Certain well-defined variates will be required in each case to resolve specific parameters for the tumor and the various normal tissues involved.

4.1 Primary Dose-Time-Volume-Response Factors

For purposes of analysis of quantal data relating to a specific tumor or organ, a given treatment scheme is sufficiently specified by the following five variates and two statistics:

(1) Dose (minimum tumor dose or maximal dose within organ of interest, total for whole course);
(2) Number of fractions;
(3) Total treatment time (inclusive days from first exposure to last, equals elapsed time + 1);
(4) Size (field-size as equivalent circle or tumor mean diameter);
(5) Gap (interval between split courses if any; a further four entries for dose, fractions, time, and size are needed after each gap).

The *statistical* rates needed are given by:

(6) The number of cases treated with that particular combination of 5 variates;
(7) Number of cases responding (tumor cured or specified quantal reaction observed).

4.2 Secondary Radiosensitivity Coefficients

Effects relating such radiobiological coefficients as RBE and OER to radiation quality (LET), dosage, physico-chemical environment, and cell-type can be evaluated by assigning appropriate coefficients to the parameters in the cell-population kinetic model (5). Technical factors of interest in this respect are:

(1) Radiation quality (LET or the energy and character of the ionizing particles), with either RBE for the system studied or the corresponding coefficients for the various components of the cellular lethality function;
(2) Oxygen and re-oxygenation, the OER and associated coefficients for the cell parameters, the level of hypoxia, and the changing proportion of cells affected;
(3) Other sensitivity-modifying environmental factors: temperature, chemical sensitizers, protective agents, and their associated coefficients;
(4) Intrinsic or cycle-specific changes, radiosensitivity, and corresponding parameters.

A clear understanding of the functional dependence of all the cell population kinetic parameters upon each of these factors is an obvious prerequisite to their use in optimization procedures.

4.3 Follow-Up Data: End Results and Late Effects

The clinical record should contain both graded and quantal data together with the pathogenetic time-sequence of the reactions and of the onset and duration of tumor remission. In this regard the tumor response and the reactions of each normal tissue or organ of interest must be separately annotated.

4.31 Tumor response and cure rates. Regression of the tumor can be observed in relation to either the initial response or the end-result. The immediate response is assessed from a series of dated volume measurements before, during, and after the course of treatment. The end-results are determined by serial follow-up, noting the dates of maintained remission or of recurrence. From this information the following variates and computed parameters can be derived:

(1) Initial tumor volume (at first treatment);
(2) Observed pretreatment growth parameters (doubling times);
(3) Rate of macroscopic regression following treatment;
(4) Period of observation without recurrence (updated annually);
(5) Time to appearance of first recorded recurrence;
(6) Tumor volume at time of observed recurrence;
(7) Observed or inferred postrecurrence growth parameters;
(8) Computed cellular radiosensitivity parameters.

4.32 Normal tissue reactions and late effects. Reactions appear after a latent interval, ranging from a few days to many years, may be transient or permanent, and vary widely in severity. To record this information, reactions are observed at suitable intervals and graded at each visit. As a general guide to grading reactions, the following 10-level ranking procedure has been proposed:

0 = No detectible reaction
1 = Doubtful, suspected, or threshold response
2 = Transient radiation effect
3 = Minimal long-lasting radiation reaction
4 = Permanent radiation injury of limited extent
5 = Marked radiation damage (high-dose effect)
6 = Extensive radiation injury but no necrosis
7 = Extensive damage with limited necrosis
8 = Massive necrosis of irradiated volume
9 = Unknown or data not available

Any response level can be chosen for analysis and fitted to iso-effect tolerances, cell population kinetic models, or optimization studies.

5. OPTIMAL TREATMENT SCHEDULES

The treatment of brain metastases from epidermoid cancer (primary in lung) by neutrons, for example, could, in principle, be optimized by considering the separate sensitivities and parameters (adjusted by high-LET coefficients) of brain and squamous carcinoma, and choosing an optimal treatment scheme. The following four logical steps are implied:

(1) Collection of follow-up data on squamous cancer in all sites, noting in each case the variates as listed in section 4.1;
(2) Examination of these data set by the search program (sec. 3.36) deriving radiosensitivity and cell kinetic parameters for the tumor;
(3) Making a similar collection of available data on radiation injury to the human brain, using the same search program to derive corresponding parameters;
(4) Identification of optima by one of the following procedures:
(a) Generation of iso-effect tables for both systems (for "cure" of the tumor and "tolerance" of the brain), and a point-by-point calculation of the ratio of tissue tolerance to tumor lethal dose (therapeutic ratios); or
(b) Computation of expected response rates (as probits), using previously established parameters for both tumor and normal tissue, for a preselected range of fractionation schemes, estimat-

ing the "best-risk" dose (equal chance of recurrence or necrosis) for each treatment scheme, and selecting that procedure associated with the maximum probit difference.

REFERENCES

1. Barendsen, G. W., *Nature, 193*, 1153-1155 (1962).
2. Cohen, L., *Am. J. Roentgenol., 84*, 741-753 (1960).
3. Cohen, L., *Computer Programs in Biomedicine, 3*, 27-35 (1973).
4. Cohen, L., *Cancer, 32*, 236-244 (1973).
5. Cohen, L., *Radiology, 114*, 213-217 (1975).
6. Cohen, L., and Kerrich, J. E., *Brit. J. Cancer, 5*, 180-194 (1951).
7. Ellis, F., *Clin. Radiol., 20*, 1-7 (1969).
8. Fischer, J. J., and Fischer, D. B., *Brit. J. Radiol., 44*, 785-792 (1971).
9. Holthusen, H., *Strahlentherapie, 57*, 254-269 (1936).
10. Kagan, A. R., Lee, K. H., Wollin, M., and Norman, A., *Brit. J. Radiol., 46*, 354-359 (1973).
11. Kellerer, A. M., and Rossi, H. H., *Radiation Research, 47*, 15-34 (1971).
12. Kirk, J., Gray, W. M., and Watson, E. R., *Clinical Radiology, 22*, 145-155 (1971).
13. Moore, D. H., and Mendelsohn, M. L., *Cancer, 30*, 97-106 (1972).
14. Neufeld, J., Wright, H. A., and Hamm, R. N., "A comparison of two-component models of cellular survival," *Fourth Symposium on Microdosimetry*, 415-436 (1973).
15. Strandqvist, M., *Acta Radiol. Suppl.*, 55 (1944).
16. Szechter, A., and Schwartz, G., *Brit. J. Radiol., 47*, 237-238 (1974).
17. Von Essen, C. F., *Amer. J. Roentgenology, 83*, 556-570 (1960).
18. Wideroe, R., *Acta Radiol. (Ther), 4*, 257-275 (1966).

QUESTIONS

M. COHEN: I wonder whether you could comment on the philosophy that I've heard several radiotherapists express, that far from working to an optimum dose which would give you the peak of that curve relating to tumor control versus reactions, you should work at a tumor dose higher than that, knowing that the number of adverse reactions is thereby going to be increased, but since the hospital is equipped to deal with these reactions, we can cope with them.

L. COHEN: This is taking optimization one step further, which is to apply weighting coefficients relating to the importance of recurrence and of adverse reactions in individual patients. This is not easy because there are psychological, economic, and social implications. If we can ever agree as to what the appropriate weighting ought to be, I would go along with that suggestion.

SHRIVASTAVA: Does the curve that you showed on the normal tissues and the tumor for optimization, take care of the increased repair response of the normal tissues to the insult—the homeostatic response, if you like?

L. COHEN: Yes, indeed, it does. That's not a difficult thing to build into the cell population kinetic program.

FREY: You showed derived curves. You didn't say very much about what the assumptions were upon which those curves were derived or how well they fit other data and why we should accept a curve which shows a changing slope where there are no data points along the line.

L. COHEN: In that particular slide we only looked at a very small segment of the data for clarity. It is important to look at data at both extremes of the time scale. Part of the optimization function relates to the fact that the normal tissue curve becomes flat at long treatment times, whereas the tumor lethal dose increases continually by curving upwards with very long treatment times.

SHRIVASTAVA: When you maximize probit values, the difference between the different probits seem to be very small, and it seems to me that one could have chosen a whole range. Could one really go to the extent of choosing between 1.54 and 1.53 and doses of 908 or 909? Does one really have to go to that extent of optimizing?

L. COHEN: This particular situation happens to describe a neutron procedure where the curves are very flat. It was merely testing the program to see what kind of answers it gave. In other situations, the differences become quite large. For clarity I haven't presented the whole table, merely a segment of it. There's a big difference between probits of 1.40 and 1.55 when it comes to the real probability of complication and control. One may have an optimum where there's a 79 percent chance of controlling the tumor if you're prepared to take a 21 percent risk of normal tissue damage, which means the uncomplicated control rate is somewhere around 50 percent.Now a small change in probit difference will alter these risks quite substantially.

2. The NSD Concept

F. Ellis

Introduction

Previous experience with daily fractionated external-beam radiotherapy suggested a correlation between dose and time. The iso-effect relationship for equivalent dose was given by $D = K.T^n$ where n was about 1/3.

With experience of treating patients 3 times a week instead of daily it became obvious that for the same effect the dose must be reduced by 10-15 percent. Following the work of Puck and Marcus (1) and of Hewitt and Wilson (2) on radiation of cell cultures *in vitro*, it seemed that the dose per fraction as well as the time was important in determining the biological effect.

Therefore, in evaluating Time Dose Relationships it seemed desirable to separate the effect of the fractionation pattern from the time effect. How to do this was not clear. The very different cell survival parameters published and the lack of knowledge of which if any applied to which normal tissues made it impossible to determine any quantitative relationship from radiobiological data. It was decided therefore to attempt this separation of time from fractionation by deduction from clinical experience. This is called an empirical approach. Its essence is the derivation of rules of action from nondocumented evidence without statistical support. It is the way in which most medical practice has been conducted so far.

The N.S.D. Concept

This is an attempt to separate the effects of fractionation and time in clinical radiation therapy.

It applies to normal tissue and rests on four assumptions:

(1) The difference between malignant and normal cells lies in the

failure of the former to respond to the homeostatic control that is an essential feature of normal cells.

(2) The healing of skin reactions depends on the connective tissue.

(3) The squamous carcinoma cell, since it is not hormone sensitive, as some are, is a model for a normal cell without homeostatic control.

(4) Homeostatic control depends on time.

In this regard it should be noted that homeostatic control is a general term for the complex process by which normal cells respond to needs to proliferate when necessary and to stop proliferating when the need ceases, or continue at a certain necessary rate, e.g., the response of bone marrow to hemorrhage or to infection, the healing of wounds and injuries, the continual renewal of desquamating bowel and skin cells.

As a consequence of assumption 2, any ulcer of the skin should heal if the connective tissue of the skin (i.e. the dermis) is in good condition. This applies to any ulcer whether due to trauma, burns, or radiation. If the dermis is destroyed, healing follows by granulation of subcutaneous connective tissue and a scar remains.

Radiation damage to cells is either lethal or sublethal. Recovery of sublethal damage is by two processes: intracellular and extracellular. The intracellular recovery is common to all cells, but apart from nutritional factors, the extracellular homeostatic influences aid only the normal cells.

The response of the body organs to radiation demands a feedback mechanism that takes time to operate. The nature of this response is complex and not well understood. There is evidence that cell cycle time is shortened and that protective mechanisms are activated, e.g. pigmentation of the skin and an increase in the numbers of some blood cells.

There are certain other axiomatic statements which apply to the use of radiation treatment of malignant disease, some of which follow from the above.

(1) The limiting factor in radiating cancer is normal tissue tolerance.

(2) Normal tissue tolerance is connective tissue tolerance.

(3) Apart from bone and brain, connective tissue throughout the body is similar (fibroblasts and capillaries).

(4) No two malignant tumors are identical or will respond identically to radiation.

(5) The effect on tumors is incidental and only partially predictable.

(6) The effect on tumor cell population, dependent only on intracellular damage and repair, is related to dose per fraction if recovery between fractions is complete (with intervals of about 24 hours).

(7) Cell proliferation of both normal and malignant cells occurs as inhibition of mitosis due to radiation ceases. It is impossible to know just when it starts and how quickly it proceeds for either the normal or malignant cells. This is not an essential difference between them. The help which normal cells derive from the homeostatic control is such a difference.

It was decided to use graphs of clinical results to relate an iso-effect dose to the number of fractions and the time based on the essential difference between malignant and normal cells. This seemed to be provided by the composite graphs of normal skin reactions and squamous carcinoma survivals on log-log scales by Lionel Cohen (3, 4).

The squamous-carcinoma five-year-cure graph represents many hundreds of cancers from various sites. It has a regression coefficient of 0.22. The skin reaction graphs, one from patient reactions and the other from clinical experiments, both have the same slope (0.33). That these are the same for different degrees of reaction suggests that the mechanisms of damage and repair are the same for these different degrees. The results also suggested that the total effect (slope 0.33) on normal cells is made up by an intracellular effect (slope 0.22) (dependent on homeostatic control and necessitating feedback) and time-dependence (slope 0.11).

These considerations provided data for the formula.

$$\text{Total Dose} = \text{N.d.} = (\text{NSD})\ \text{N.}^{0.24}\ \text{T.}^{0.11}$$

Where N is the number of fractions of d rads given in time T days for an iso-effect represented by the Nominal Standard Dose (NSD) in rets (Rad Equivalent Therapy). Because treatments in these were given five times weekly, whereas time is seven days weekly, the regression coefficient for N was modified from 0.22 to 0.24.

This description indicates why the concept, through using skin reactions and squamous carcinoma results, is deduced from normal connective tissue cells.

It also provides one figure which can be used for prescription and comparisons.

Volume Effects

The volume effect is considered important by most radiotherapists. It is usually considered in relation to the area of the field in square centimeters or to the volume in cubic cm. treated to a high dose. This is probably unrealistic, since the effect of the radiation will depend on the organ concerned. If, for instance, the arytenoid perichondrium is damaged, the nutrition of the cartilage will be so affected that necrosis may result. This could cause serious laryngeal complications even if the volume treated were very small. On the other hand a much larger field which spared part of this cartilage might not cause similar complications even with the same dose unless it treated the whole of the perichondrium of the thyroid or cricoid cartilages. The important points to consider are the dose and the proportion of an organ absorbing a dose in excess of tolerance. If a dose of radiation to reach a certain NSD of the volume, or the nature of the volume, is such that the acute effects tax the patient's tolerance or that of the organs in the beam, the time should be increased so as to achieve the maximum tolerable NSD as shown by the late effects.

Low Dose Rate Radiation (Brachytherapy)

It is desirable to have for radium and other intracavitary type radiation a similar method of estimating biological effect. Since there are no hard, documented figures to provide the relationship, it is again necessary to use clinical observations as the basis for such an estimate. It then appears that the effect of 1800 rets is produced by a dose of 6000 rads in seven days. For effects on normal tissue irradiated at various dose-rates, a series of doses equivalent to 1800 rets (or a dose of 6000 rads at 35.7 rads/hour) can be derived on the basis of clinical experience, using a table of corrections factor (Table I). The ret dose due to a dose of D rads given at a dose rate corresponding to a correction factor CF is such that

$$\frac{\text{Rets}}{1800} = \frac{\text{D Rads}}{\text{C. F} \times 6000} \quad \text{i.e. rets} = \frac{0.3 \text{ D Rads}}{\text{C.F.}}$$

Rets from beam radiation can be added to rets from continuous radiation to give an estimate of combined biological effect. The biological basis for a dose rate influence on clinical effects is provided by the work of Hall (5). There is an undoubted effect of difference in dose rate on the survival of cells cultured *in vitro*. In the range of dose rates from 10,000 rads/minute to .001 rads/minute for Hela cells in culture, there is a change in D_O from 150 rads at the highest to 270 rads at the lowest dose rate, and the extrapolation number changes from 2 at the highest to 1 at the lowest dose rate. Almost the whole of the change occurs over the range of dose rates used clinically—100 rads per minute to 1 rad/minute.

Relationship to Cell Survival Data

1. Two things suggested that D_O = 160 rads and n = 2 might be the cell survival parameters fitting the connective tissue. Calculations by R. Oliver (6) based on these parameters:

a. Fit the NSD concept better than other parameters do,
b. Fit the iso-effect line for low-dose rate radium treatments surprisingly well. (Assuming the half life for sublethal damage repair to be about 45 minutes.)

2. The values of dose per fraction and number of fractions for a given NSD (2000 rets) and for a certain cell survival (10^{-11}) coincide. The best fit is given by $D_0 = 150$ $n = 2.2$.
3. For different regimes given 1800 rets, the cell survivals based on these parameters are almost identical.

Acute and Late Effects

It has been said (7) that acute effects are paralleled by late effects in animal work. This is probably true of patients for the same time relationships. If the treatment is given in a very short time, however, e.g.—to skin or mucous membrane—the acute effect on the epithelium produces a reaction that is much greater than if the same NSD were given in a much longer time. In that case the acute reaction may be relatively slight, but the late effects will be similar.

The NSD value is considered to refer to cell killing. If a large number of cells are killed in a short time, the clinical effect will be greater than if they are killed in a long time. The NSD concept is related to the late effect because it is a connective tissue (probably endothelial cell) effect and not dependent on the epithelial cells.

If 15 × 200 rads in three weeks is considered a limiting dose because of acute effects and this can be safely increased to 25 × 200 rads if given in five weeks, the number of malignant cells killed is much greater.

Because of these considerations it is thought that volume should not be taken into account to modify the NSD. To give the necessary NSD the time should be increased if necessary. To reduce the NSD is undesirable unless the tumor is growing very rapidly, in which case to prolong the time of the treatment course might be to fall behind the rate of the growth of the tumor, while to reach the NSD desired might be to exceed tolerance to acute effects.

Strandquist Lines

(1) In iso-effect graphs relating log-time to log-dose it is accepted that with conventional treatment schedules, the slope of the resulting straight line is about 0.33.
(2) If the frequencies of treatments are the same for different schedules, the iso-effect lines will all have the same slope.
(3) If the frequencies of treatments are different, the slopes of iso-effect lines will vary.

Support for the NSD Concept has been derived from many sources:

(1) Figures published by Fowler (7) relating dose to fraction numbers for skin reactions but taking no account of time, when used in the NSD formula for various times show a surprising coincidence.
(2) Fraction dose and related number for the same effect on Hodgkin's disease (8) do not correspond to the NSD formula, but if the time factor is omitted (giving results in rens* for tumor effect), they show almost exact coincidence. This fits the principle behind the concept that for a malignant condition, the time factor, related to homeostatic control, should not apply.
(3) Patients treated by various schedules to about the same clinical level of effect on normal tissues in Oxford apparently received doses corresponding to similar ret figures.
(4) Patients treated at Hammersmith (10) and at Manchester (Eason, personal communication) by different schedules seem to have similar ret doses for techniques that have been discarded and for the modified techniques adopted.
(5) The graph relating probability of cure to ret does for supraglottic carcinoma (11) suggests that cure is closely related to ret dose. The probability of cure increases from 15 to 95 percent with an increase in ret dose from 1760 (= 30 × 200) to 1970 (= 36 × 200 rads).
(6) The table relating tumor and normal tissue effects for carcinoma of the larynx (12) suggests that the margins between failure, cure, and necrosis are relatively narrow.
(7) Similar margins are shown for carcinoma of the anus (Ellis, unpublished).
(8) The relationship between rets and complications and the way in which they parallel rens (tumor effect) by eliminating the time factor from the formula is shown by Hilaris and Tokita's data (13) relating complications and cures for carcinoma of the cervix uteri at the Memorial Hospital, New York.
(9) It proved possible using the NSD concept to correlate complications with radiation schedules when it proved impossible to do so from physical doses in rads (14).
(10) Philips and Buschke related late spinal cord injuries to ret doses. Fifteen hundred rets seems to be a critical level.
(11) Philips and Margolis (16) showed the relationship of ret dose to pneumonitis both clinically and in mice, and the sensitizing effect of using actinomycin D on this complication.
(12) Stewart and Fajardos (17) investigating cases of carditis in patients treated for Hodgkin's disease and breast carcinoma, showed that at values above 1500 rets the incidence of this complication mounted steeply.

*ren = rad equivalent neoplasm.

(13) From clinical results as shown by long-term cures of many skin cancers in various sites it seems that the NSD concept and the associated formula provide a satisfactory method of relating dose per fraction and number of fractions for treatments given daily, four times weekly, three times weekly, twice weekly, or once weekly in total times varying from four to seven weeks.

In general, (a) there seems to be no need to produce a marked reaction, and (b) an NSD value in a short time will produce a greater acute reaction than the same NSD over a long time, although the late effects will be the same. The rad dose will of course be greater with the smaller acute effect over a long time.

(14) *For high extrapolation numbers* tumors (in animals) in which D_0 and n are known, cell-survival calculations indicate that *for the same NSD* the cell survival is decreased as the number of fractions is decreased and larger fraction doses used. These (fibrosarcoma, malignant melanoma, etc.) have the same resistance to radiation as human tumors of similar nature, and a *clinical* trial of weekly or daily fractions in the same total time is indicated.

(15) The use of this concept (18, 19) explains the deficiencies in clinical radiotherapy of not treating all fields at each treatment session. In the case of a parallel opposed pair of fields, for instance, the biological effect if only one field is treated at each session is greater than if both are treated at each session even though the total physical doses are the same.

Conclusion

The NSD concept based on deduction from clinical experience provides a formula that facilitates:

(a) The comparison of radiotherapy schedules relative to their effects:
  (i) within the same center
  (ii) between centers
(b) The elucidation of the causes of complications
(c) The safe variation of radiotherapy schedules in clinical work
(d) The same correction of errors detected during a course of treatment
(e) The combination of low dose rate (interstitial and intracavitary) radiation and high dose rate (beam) radiation
(f) Teaching of radiotherapy
(g) The devising of schedules to meet radiobiological characteristics of the tumor when they are known

It must be emphasized

(a) that the NSD concept applies to late effects (acute effects can be expected to be the same only if the same NSD is reached in the same total time)
(b) that the partial tolerance principle must be used (20)
(c) that an R.B.E. adjustment is necessary for other radiation than cobalt
(d) that since the effect of radiation is to kill cells, there is no volume correction used in the NSD concept. Indeed, a larger volume requires a larger rather than a smaller dose, and a longer time should be taken to avoid exceeding acute tolerance. The proportion of an organ treated may be a more realistic criterion than volume.

REFERENCES

1. Puck, T. in *Cytogenetics of Cells in Culture*, ed. R. J. C. Harris, London Academic Press (1964).
2. Hewitt, H. B. and Wilson, C. W., *Br. J. Cancer*, *13*, 675 (1959).
3. Cohen, L., Ph.D. thesis, Univ. of Witwatersrand (1960).
4. Cohen, J., and Kerrich, J. E., *Br. J. Cancer*, *5*, 180 (1951).
5. Hall, E. J. "Cell killings at very low dose rates," in *Time and Dose Relationships*, N.C.I.-A.E.C. Conference, Carmel, Calif., Brookhaven Nat. Lab. Pub. 50230 (C-57) 1970, 308-317 (1969).
6. Oliver, R., personal communication, Hammersmith Royal Post-Grad. Hosp., London.
7. Fowler, J. F., *Br. J. Radiol.*, *38*, 365 (1965).
8. Friedman, M., Pearlman, A. W., and Turgeon, L., *Am. J. Roentgenol.*, *99*, 483 (1967).
9. Strandquist, M., "Studien uber die kumulative wirkung der Rontgensirahlen bei Fraktionierung," *Acta. Radiol., Suppl.*, *55*, 1 (1944).
10. Morrison, R., and Deeley, T. J., *Clinic. Radiol.*, *13*, 145 (1962).
11. Shukovsky, L. J., *Am. J. Roentgenol.*, *108*, 27 (1970).
12. Aristizabel, S. A., and Caldwell, W. L., "Radiation tolerance of the normal tissues of the larynx," *Radiology*, *103*, 419-422 (1972).
13. Hilaris, B., and Tokita, N., personal communication (1974).
14. Buchler, Dolores A., Kline, J. C., Peckham, B. M., and Ellis, F., *Radiology*, *110*, 687 (1974).
15. Ellis, F., and Sorensen, A., *Radiology*, *110*, 681 (1974).
16. Phillips, T. L., and Margolis, L., "Radiation Pathology and the Clinical Response of lung and esophagus," *Front. Rad. Ther. Onc.*, *6*, 254-273 (1972).
17. Stewart, J. R., and Fajardos, L., *Radiol. Clin. N. Amer.*, *9*, 511 (1971).
18. Wilson, C. S., and Hall, E. J., *Radiology*, *98*, 419 (1965).
19. Ellis, F., Sorensen, A., and Lescrenier, C., "Schedules for opposite parallel fields," *Radiology*, *111*, 701-707 (1974).
20. Winston, B. M., Ellis, F., and Hall, E.J., *Clinic Radiol. 20, 8* (1969).

GENERAL REFERENCES ON NSD

1. Ellis, F. The Relationship of Biological Effect to Dose-Time and Fractionation Factors in Radiotherapy in *Current Topics in Radiation Research*, vol. 4, ed. M. Ebert and A. Howard Amsterdam, North Holland Publishing Co., 357-359 (1968).
2. Ellis, F. Dose Time and Fractionation: A Clinical Hypothesis, *Clinic Radiol.* 20, 1 (1969).

QUESTIONS

SCHULZ: We could probably spend the remainder of this conference dissecting the NSD concept. One point I'd like to make is that this concept tends to indicate that the time/dose relationship is of no importance as long as you give the right number of rets, and I was wondering if Dr. Ellis really subscribes to this.

ELLIS: I don't see how you get that conclusion.

SCHULZ: If you're going to describe the treatment solely in terms of the number of rets, you don't know what time the treatment took, and you don't know how many fractions were used, and you don't know the dose per fraction. All you know is the number of rets. If I say someone got 1800 rets, you can't tell me how many fractions that patient received.

ELLIS: I see what you mean, but one thing I've *never* said is that you shouldn't specify the dose and the number of fractions, the time, and the interval between fractions, and any variation there is.

SCHULZ: I think you should make this clear to your disciples, then, because there are an increasing number of papers occurring in the literature with doses just specified in rets. You showed us a slide of Shukovsky which indicated that the treatment of carcinoma of the larynx had a very steep dose-response curve—dose expressed in rets. If you go back to what he actually gave, that curve doesn't have anywhere near the steepness that was implied.

ELLIS: I said right at the beginning that the dose and the physical factors must be stated. The ret dose is a thing to be tested, and it provides something to test treatment schedules against. If you've got a figure for comparison, you know whether you're above or below it.

SCHULZ: I'm afraid your disciples don't adhere to that—

ELLIS: That's not my fault. Many people use the formula without bothering to read the paper.

Table 1.

Dose Equivalent to 6000 Rads in Seven Days = Fx 6000 Rads

Dose Rate in Rads/Hr	*Dose Factor F*	*Dose Rate in Rads/Hr*	*Dose Factor F*
25.0	1.06	70.0	0.780
27.0	1.051	75.0	0.758
30.0	1.033	80.0	0.737
32.0	1.019	85.0	0.717
35.0	1.001	90.0	0.702
35.7	1.000	95.0	0.687
40.0	0.967	100.0	0.672
45.0	0.931	110.0	0.642
50.0	0.897	120.0	0.622
55.0	0.864	130.0	0.602
60.0	0.832	140.0	0.584
65.0	0.805	150.0	0.567

3. A Brief Review of the CRE System

J. Kirk

Introduction

In a series of papers (2, 3, 4, 5, 6, 7) the concept of the Cumulative Radiation Effect (CRE) has been presented as a scale of accumulative subtolerance radiation damage. The biological effect generated in normal connective tissue by fractionated or continuous radiation therapy is described by the CRE on a unified scale of assessment. In these papers the CRE system has been presented in considerable detail, and it is the purpose of this contribution only to summarize the salient features of that system.

The CRE system has its basis in the hypothesis proposed by Ellis in his development of the NSD (1). The NSD serves to designate any fractionated course of radiation which achieves normal tissue tolerance and is defined only at that point. Ellis showed that the biological effect of tolerance could be described by one figure, which could be evaluated from an empirical equation in which effects of dose, number of fractions, and time were separable. However, although the CRE system and the NSD share the same basis for fractionated radiation, there are important fundamental differences in concept.

Since most identifiable effects in normal tissue (tolerance, erythema, etc.) are described within observable clinical limits by lines of the same slope on a graph of log D against log T as shown in Figure 1 (where D and T are the total dose and treatment time, respectively), the intercepts of these lines on the log D axis completely characterize these effects and can be used as numerical descriptions of them. The numerical values of these intercepts, CRE's, are monotonically increasing with the severity of the effect. This is the basis for a scale of measurement of biological effect as described by the CRE for all subtolerance levels of damage.

The CRE System

Before describing general properties of the CRE system, it would be helpful to define the use of the terms "schedule" and "regime." A "schedule" of treatment is the repetitive application of fractions of equal doses at equal time intervals over a specified treatment time. A "regime" is a course of treatment comprising one or more schedules. These schedules can be fractionated or continuous in nature and may be separated by intervals when no treatment is given. The main properties of the CRE system are summarized below.

Fractionated treatment regimes. The basic equation for the assessment of fractionated schedules is:

$$R_F = D \,.\, N^{-0.24} \,.\, T^{-0.11},$$

where R_F is the CRE for fractionated radiation (reu),
D is the total dose (rads),
N is the number of fractions, and
T is the total treatment time, inclusive of the first and the last days of treatment (days).

An alternative form of this equation which is most useful is

$$R_F = \rho \,.\, d \,.\, N^{0.65},$$

where ρ is the repetition parameter $\left[= \left(\frac{T}{N}\right)^{-0.11}\right]$, and
d is the dose per fraction.

It can be seen from these equations that at tolerance, the CRE and NSD have the same numerical value.

It is frequently necessary to combine the effects of different schedules with different repetition parameters and doses. Since the CRE equation is nonlinear in the number of fractions, it is necessary to develop the concept of equivalent conditions at the junctions between schedules. Suppose that some schedule A, identified by subscripts, a, achieves a CRE,

$$R_a = \rho_a \,.\, d_a \,.\, n_a^m, \text{ when } m = 0.65.$$

Suppose also that a schedule B were to follow schedule A and that N_b fractions were to be given on this latter schedule. Had schedule B been given from the commencement of radiation, n_b fractions would have been given to achieve the CRE, R_a;

$$R_a = \rho_b \,.\, d_b \,.\, n_b^m.$$

The equivalent condition at the junction between schedules when the CRE is R_a is:

$$\rho_a \cdot d_a \cdot n_a^m = \rho_b \cdot d_b \cdot n_b^m,$$

as shown in Figure 2.

From this equality, n_b can be found. The final CRE achieved after schedule B is then

$$R_F = \rho_b \cdot d_b (n_b + N_b)^m.$$

The equivalence conditions are extremely important in the evaluations of CREs and can be applied to fractionated or continuous radiation or any combination of them. The above analysis is essential to an understanding of equivalence conditions, but simpler methods for special cases can be adopted in practice, as has been pointed out by Wara et al. (9). On his suggestion, the above analysis reduces to

$$R_F^{\frac{1}{m}} = R_a^{\frac{1}{m}} + R_b^{\frac{1}{m}},$$

where $R_b = \rho_b \cdot d_b \cdot N_b{}^m$.

Frequently, in the interests of machine economy, not all fields are given every day. A typical practical result of this could be that on alternate days a point in tissue could receive doses d_a and d_b. It is assumed that the same number of fractions of each dose is given, with the same repetition parameter for both. From a CRE analysis, the effective dose given each day to obtain the same effect would be

$$\left[\frac{\left(d_a^{\frac{1}{m}} + d_b^{\frac{1}{m}}\right)^m}{2}\right]$$

This effective dose is always greater than the mean of the doses d_a and d_b and leads to an enhancement effect with important consequences in patient treatment. This enhancement is demonstrated in Figure 3 for parallel-opposed fields. As a corollary to this, it is also found that the temporal ordering of these fractions is of no consequence and, for example, all the doses, d_a, could be given first and all the doses, d_b, second, achieving the same enhancement.

This could be important for patients who, perhaps following surgery, could only be treated in one position initially.

Continuous radiation: Long-lived sources. The total doses (D) and times (T) of various treatments with radium which achieve tolerance can be plotted on a graph of log D and log T as shown in Figure 4. From a consideration of this graph, in an analogous way to that for fractionated therapy, a CRE equation describing the biological effect achieved by continuous radiation, R_C, of constant dose rate can be developed and is of the form

$$R_C = k \,.\, q \,.\, D \,.\, T^{-0.29},$$

where q is a factor for the RBE of the radiation, and
k is a parameter combining a normalization factor between fractionated and continuous radiation and a parameter to allow for varying areas and volumes.

The form of this equation is such that both fractionated and continuous radiations are linearly dependent on dose and are thus compatible. Another useful form of this equation is

$$R_C = k \,.\, q \,.\, r \,.\, T^{0.71},$$

where r is the dose rate in rads per day.

Equivalent conditions can also be applied at the junction between schedules of continuous radiation, and this allows the assessment of the CRE from more complex regimes. Such regimes could result from adding or removing needles from implants and so on.

When the dose rate from an implant differs from that intended, it is usual to apply a biological correction to the modified time of implantation found by multiplying the intended time by the ratio of the dose rates. On the CRE system, it is a simple and natural calculation to compare different dose rates and times which are equivalent in achieving the same biological effect, and the customary "biological correction" can be deduced by linear approximation.

Continuous radiation: Short-lived sources. By considering the rate of change of CRE with time for long-lived sources, a generalized differential equation can be developed for arbitrarily varying sources. A particular application of this differential equation is the development of an expression to determine the CRE achieved by a source whose dose rate varies considerably during the course of treatment in an exponential manner. There are two ways in which short-lived isotopes such as ^{198}Au are frequently used.

One is the use of ^{198}Au seeds in moulds for surface application when the mould is left in place for a finite time, t. The CRE equation for a finite time of application is

$$R_C = k \,.\, q \,.\, r_o \,.\, \left[\frac{Z.L}{0.693} \,.\, \left(1 - e^{-\frac{0.693.t}{Z.L}}\right)\right]^Z,$$

Where L is the half-life of the isotope,
r_o is the initial dose rate, and
Z = 0.71

The total dose, D, given in the course of this treatment is given by

$$D = \frac{r_o \cdot L}{0.693} \cdot \left[1 - e^{-\frac{0.693}{L} \cdot t} \right].$$

The situation where isotopes such as ^{198}Au grains are permanently implanted is a special case of the above equations and can be written as

$$R_C = k \cdot q \cdot r_o \cdot \left[\frac{Z.L}{0.693} \right]^Z.$$

The total dose, D, given in the course of this treatment is

$$D = \frac{r_o \cdot L}{0.693}.$$

When proper allowance is made for the various parameters in the equations for long-lived and short-lived continuous radiations, comparisons can be made between various possible schedules with different isotopes designed to achieve the same CRE. Some examples of the predictions of the CRE system are shown in Table 1.

Area-volume factors, normalization, and RBE. To determine the value of the parameter k in the continuous equations for the CRE, which is composed of a normalizing constant, μ, and an area or volume factor, Φ, and can be written as

$$k = \mu \cdot \Phi,$$

it is necessary to evaluate μ. This can be done by considering fractionated and continuous schedules which attain the same biological effect, for example, tolerance. But to do this, since no schedules are available for comparison for the same areas or volumes, area and volume correction factors must first be established. Following the practice of Paterson of using separate area and volume factors, since no reliable data are available to combine them, the following area and volume factors have been developed:

$$\Phi_a = \left[\frac{A}{100} \right]^{0.24}$$

$$\Phi_v = \left[\frac{V}{1000}\right]^{0.16}$$

where the factors, Φ, are defined to be unity for an area of $100cm^2$ and a volume of $1000cm^3$. Evidence suggests that the factors should both be unity for these reference areas and volumes.

With these correction formulae established, schedules of fractionated and continuous radiation can be compared, and it is found that the normalizing constant is

$$\mu = 0.77.$$

An empirical relationship for the RBE, q, can be found which relates the absorbed dose of ^{60}Co for a given effect to that of any other radiation for the same effect. This equation has the form

$$q = \left[\frac{E}{E_o}\right]^{\omega},$$

where $\omega = -0.05$, and E is the equivalent single energy for a bremsstrahlung radiation or the mean energy for an isotope.

With these relations established, the CRE can be assessed for any regime consisting of any combination of fractionated and continuous radiation—providing no gap occurs in treatment.

Gaps in treatment. The CRE system, in common with the NSD system and others based directly on it (8), is a scalar description of effect, since any level of damage is uniquely described by one number. The CRE value for a level of damage is independent of the way in which that level was reached. An excellent analog is found in the scale of temperature where the numerical value of the temperature is a complete description of the thermal state of a body, and the way in which heat is given to or removed from that body to achieve that state is of no consequence. As a corollary, the way in which that body returns to the ambient conditions from a perturbed state is completely independent of the way in which the state was reached. Thus for biological effects assessed on such scalar systems as the CRE the same is true, and the decay of CRE during a gap must depend only on the CRE achieved before it and not on the time taken to reach it.

The original form of the CRE equations does not contain explicitly a term for decay, but these equations can be reformulated. A gap formula can then be obtained. Since the CRE scale of assessment is scalar, the gap formula must be exponential, although not necessarily of simple form. However, the simple form is compatible with what little information is available on the effect of gaps and is found to be

$$\gamma(G) = e^{-0.008.G},$$

Where G is the time of the gap and

$$\frac{R_g}{R_o} = \gamma(G),$$

Where R_o is the CRE achieved previous to the gap, and
R_g is the CRE remaining after the gap.

The functional dependence of the gap formula is shown in Figure 5.

The facility of assessing intervals in treatment, in addition to the properties of the CRE system already described, allows the assessment of complex regimes, such as those encountered in the treatment of carcinoma of the cervix, to be readily carried out.

Applications. Present applications of the CRE system in practical radiotherapy fall into three broad categories: routine CRE evaluations of treatment plans, such as absolute assessments or determining equivalent schedules or modifications of plans for gaps occurring in regimes; retrospective and prospective surveys, to establish better treatment strategies or restrictions in levels of dosage; and iso-effect treatment-planning. Many of these applications can be time-consuming and computer programs have been developed for CRE evaluations.

Two classes of programs have been written. For a PDP-8 computer, a package of programs has been produced which is especially convenient for simple CRE calculations, determination of equivalent schedules, and the routing of planning modifications. For iso-effect (iso-CRE) treatment-planning, where the CRE has to be assessed at many points and where a considerable amount of data on depth doses for plain and wedge fields, etc., must be stored, a program has been written for an ICL 1900 series computer. The CRE system is particularly appropriate for treatment-planning, since its formation as an absolute scale of assessment enables distributions to be generated without stipulating tolerance levels for tissues. As an example, an iso-CRE computer plan for treatment of carcinoma of the bladder is shown in Figure 6. Iso-effect planning, which takes full account of the temporal aspects of treatment, has great potential and could help to eliminate possible complications, such as high dose effects resulting from volumes of tissue where the biological effect could be high even though the dose is not, as a result of the temporal ordering in the application of fields.

Future applications of the CRE system of a more speculative nature must inevitably include efforts to establish treatment regimes that have an optimal curative effect on tumors whose kinetic properties are known for the same biological effect (or CRE) on normal tissues. It is certain that investigations into the effects of time on radiation and other treatments for cancer in the search for improved or time-optimal therapy regimes have much more to offer than the pursuit of further refinements in the spatial distribution of dose.

Conclusions

In the above necessarily brief and superficial description, the fundamental properties and equations of the CRE system have been presented. Many points of interest have had to be omitted but are fully discussed in the papers already cited. In summary, the CRE system is a unified scale of assessment of biological damage from complex regimes composed of both fractionated and continuous radiation therapy given in any temporal arrangement.

REFERENCES

1. Ellis, F., "The Relationship of Biological Effect to Dose-Time Fractionation Factors in Radiotherapy," in Ebert, M. and Howard, A., eds., *Current Topics in Radiation Research*, North Holland Publishing Company, Amsterdam (1968), *4*, 357-397.
2. Kirk, J., Gray, W. M., and Watson, E. R., *Clinical Radiology*, *22*, 145-155 (1971).
3. Kirk, J., Gray, W. M., and Watson, E. R., *Clinical Radiology*, *23*, 93-105 (1972).
4. Kirk, J., Gray, W. M., and Watson, E. R., *Clinical Radiology*, *24*, 1-11 (1973).
5. Kirk, J., Gray, W. M., and Watson, E. R., *Clinical Radiology*, *26*, 77-88 (1975).
6. Kirk, J., Gray, W. M., and Watson, E. R., *Clinical Radiology*, *26*, 159-176 (1975).
7. Kirk, J., Cain, Olive, Gray, W. M., and Watson, E. R., *Clinical Radiology* (in press).
8. Orton, C. G., and Ellis, F., *British Journal of Radiology*, *46*, 529-537 (1973).
9. Wara, W. M., Phillips, T. L., Margolis, L. W., and Smith, V., *Cancer*, *32*, 547-552 (1973).

Table 1.

The Relative Dose Rates and Doses Required on Several Treatment Strategies in Common Usage to Achieve the Same Biological Effect (a CRE of 1800 reu.).

Treatment Strategy	*Initial or Constant Dose Rate (rads/day)*	*Total Dose (rads)*
(a) Radium (7 days)	836	5850
(b) Radon (infinite)	1260	6960
(c) Gold (infinite)	1560	6050
(d) Radon (7 days)	1440	5700
(e) Gold (7 days)	1650	5350

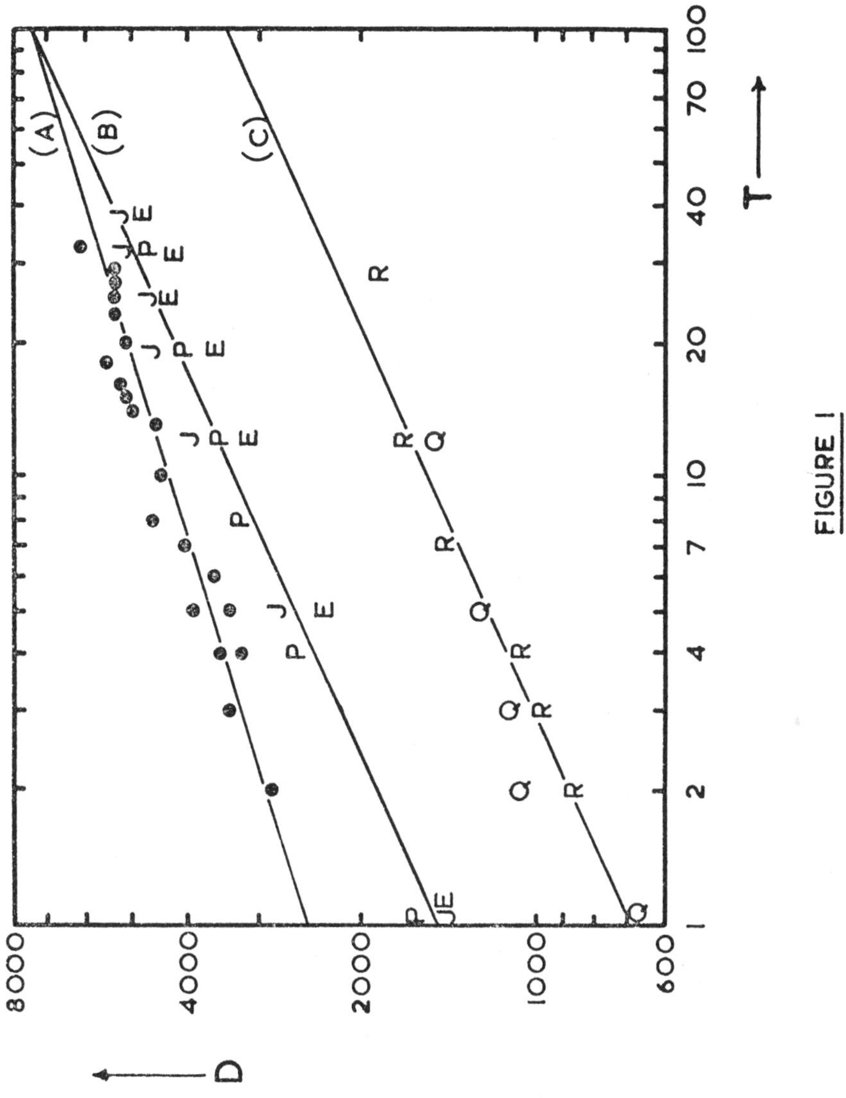

Figure 1. Iso-effect Curves for Different Fractionation Schedules Shown as the Dependence of the Total Dose (D) in rads on the Total Treatment Time (T) in Days for the Following Effects: Squamous Cell Carcinoma (A), Normal Connective Tissue Tolerance (B) and Skin Erythema (C)

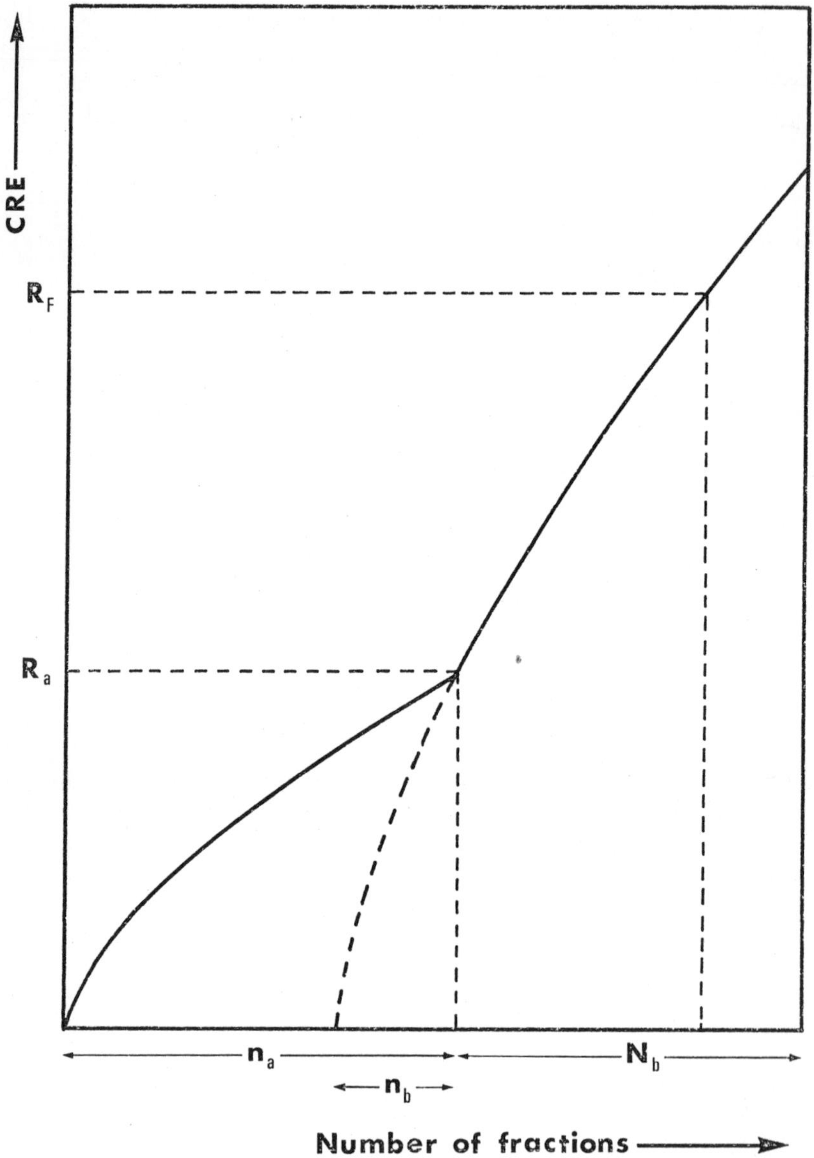

Figure 2. Diagrammatic Representation of the Equivalence Conditions Existing at the Junction Between Two Schedules A and B for Fractionated Radiation

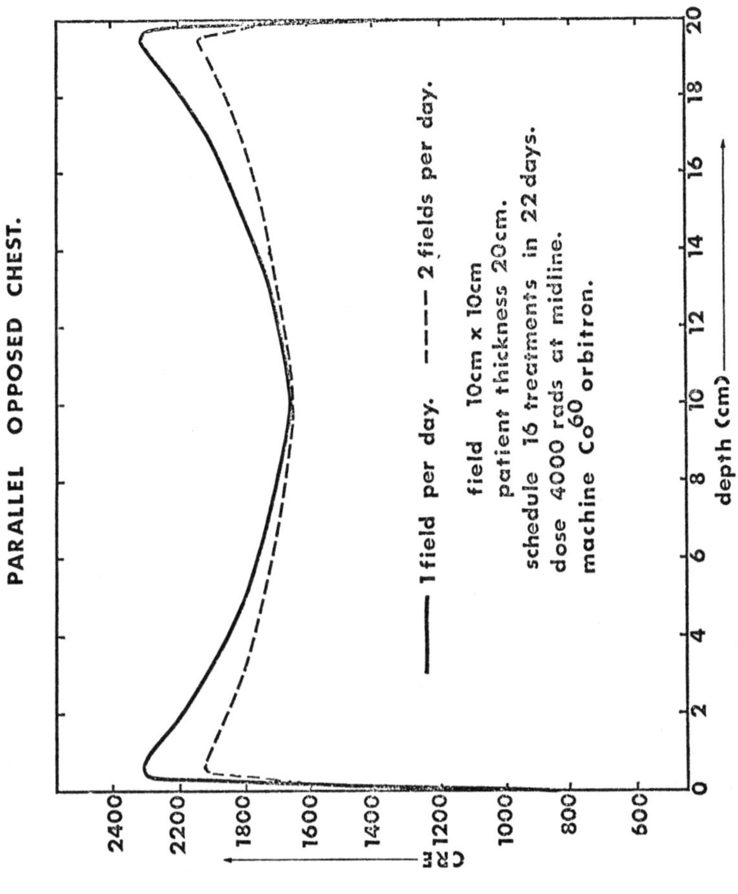

Figure 3. Diagram Showing the Enhancement Effect Resulting When Doses of Different Magnitudes from Two Schedules in a Parallel-opposed Treatment are Given on Alternate Days Instead of Both Fields Being Given Daily

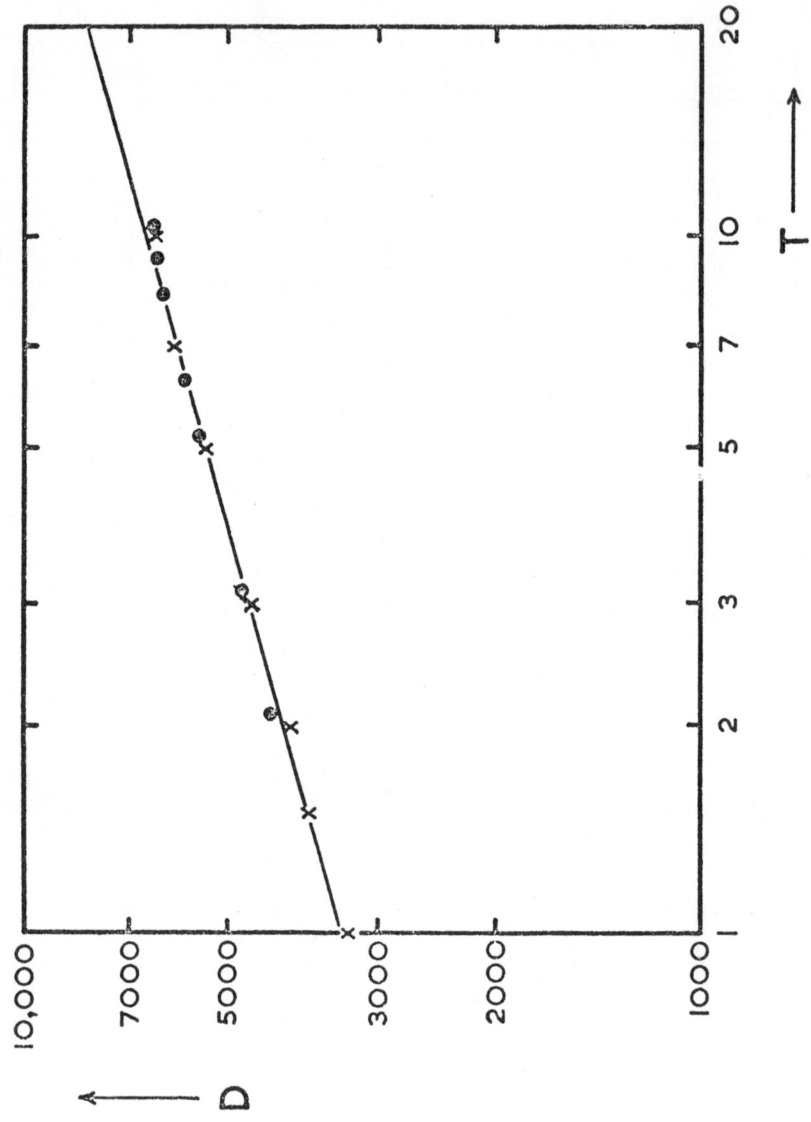

Figure 4. Graph of Total Dose, D (in rads), of Radium γ-radiation Against Total Time, T (in Days), for Various Treatment Schedules of Constant Dose Rate Which Achieve Normal Connective Tissue Tolerance (Logarithmic Scales)

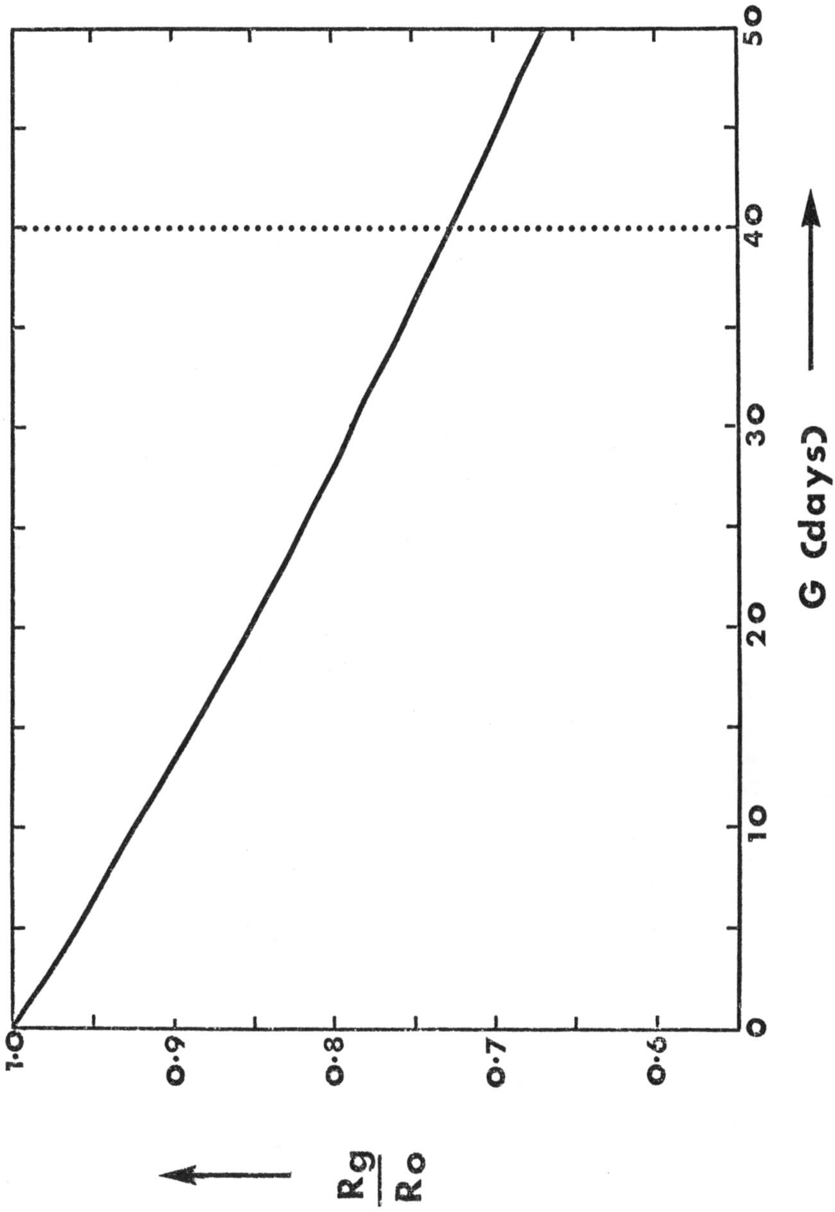

Figure 5. Relationship of the Fractional Decay in CRE, R_g/R_o, Which Equals $\gamma(G)$, to the Gap in Treatment, G (Days)

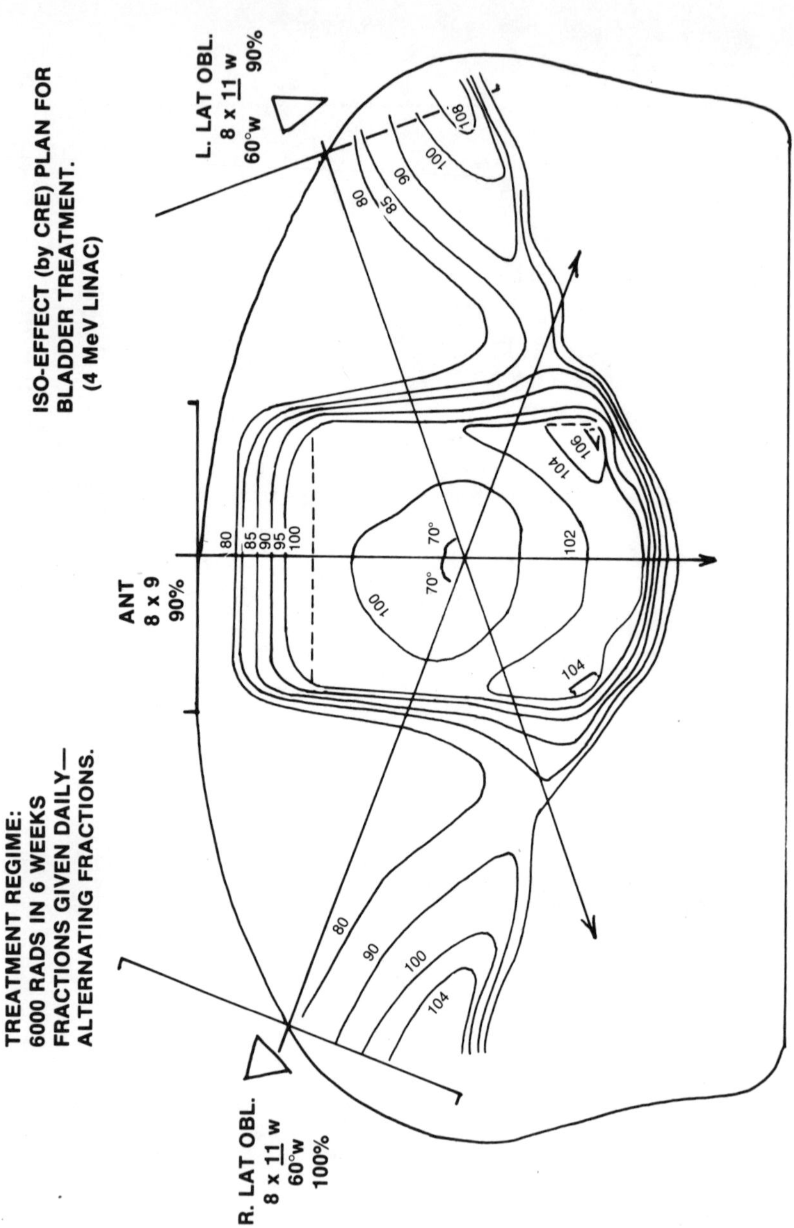

Figure 6. Iso-effect (iso-CRE) Computer Plan for Treatment of Carcinoma of the Bladder (4 MeV Linear Accelerator). Possible High Dose Effect Regions Visible in Latero-posterior Margins of Treated Volume)

4. Dose-Volume Relationships

M. Busch
U. Rosenow

Clinical observations, theoretical models, and radiobiological experiments demonstrate that the dependence of local tumor control, or of normal tissue radiation damage on absorbed radiation dose may be represented by a sigmoid-like curve. In addition, Herring and Compton (6) found a dependence of local tumor control on tumor volume, or number of cells: the larger the number of cells, the more dose necessary for the same control rate. Dessauer had stated in 1925 (2) that the larger a tumor is, the more difficult it is to cure.

On the other hand, the larger the irradiated tissue volume, the smaller the dose required to yield a given tissue damage rate. Local tumor control and tissue damage are dependent on volume in different ways, and both effects cannot be represented by the same radiobiological model.

Local Tumor Control

There are some marginal conditions influencing the formulation of a radiobiological model for local tumor control by irradiation which are applicable to clinical observations:

1. We can assume that small—but not too small—parts of a tumor react independently from one another when irradiated. Evidence for this assumption is found in data like that of Fletcher and Stovall (4), who reported in a retrospective study in carcinoma of the floor of the mouth, that the rate of local necrosis increases with too large a locally absorbed dose, and that the rate of local tumor recurrence increases with too small a locally absorbed dose.

2. It is assumed that smaller tumors (or smaller parts of a large tumor) show reactions to radiation similar to the reactions of larger tumors. The dose D needed for a defined local control rate h of a

small tumor must be multiplied by a factor f to get the same control rate H for a larger tumor:

$$h(D) = H(f \cdot D), f > 1. \quad (1)$$

3. From assumption 2 and the statistical multiplication law, it follows that the local control rate of a tumor H (D) is the product of the control rates h (D) of its (not too small) parts. In the case of a homogeneous dose-distribution and N equal volume parts V_o of the total tumor volume V we get:

$$H(D) = h^N(D) = h^{V/V_o}(D) \quad (2)$$

and

$$h(D) = h^N(f \cdot D) = h^{V/V_o}(f \cdot D) \quad (3)$$

4. Further conditions are:
h (D) = 0 for D = 0
h (D) = 1 for D = ∞, and
$0 \leqslant h(D) \leqslant 1$.

The following function for the local tumor control rate fulfills all the conditions mentioned above:

$$H(V,D) = e^{-(V/V_o) \cdot (D_o/D)^Q} \quad (4)$$

where D_o is the absorbed dose for local control of $1/e \approx 0.37$ of a tumor volume $V = V_o$, and as such is dependent on radiation sensitivity of the tissue. Q governs the gradient of the curve and may be considered as a "multitarget component."

Function (4) may be transformed into a power function with base 2 as follows:

$$H(V,D) = 2^{-(V/V_o) \cdot (D_{50}/D)^Q} = 0{,}5^{(V/V_o) \cdot (D_{50}/D)^Q} \quad (5)$$

where D_{50} is the dose for a 50 percent control rate of a tumor volume $V = V_o$.

With Q = 19.7, function (4) can be fitted nearly identically to one of the curves published by Herring and Compton (6)(Fig. 1). Our deviances from the curves of Herring and Compton for smaller volumes are because the exponent of function 4 can be considered a logarithmic transformation of the exponent in the model of those authors.

The exponent Q may also be estimated from clinical data. From the data of Shukovsky (12), Q is 12.6; from that of Stewart and Jackson (13), Q is 11.9. It seems that a value of 12 should be a good approximation to start with.

Figure 2 shows the fit of the tumor control model, i.e. function 4, to clinical data of Stewart and Jackson as given in Table 1. The effect of doubling the tumor volume is also represented. To achieve the same control rate, the dose has to be increased by approximately 300 rads, or 5 percent.

The extension of the model to inhomogeneous dose-distributions results in the following function:

$$H(V_u,D) = 0.5^{(D_{50}^Q / V_0) \cdot \int_0^{V_{Tu}} dV/D^Q(V)} \tag{6}$$

where V_{Tu} is the total tumor volume.

By using equation 6 the effect of inhomogeneous dose distributions on local tumor control rate can be estimated. This effect cannot, of course, be investigated without considering tissue damage as well, as tissue tolerance is the main limiting factor to radiation cure of tumors, and maximum cure rates are derived by optimal radiation doses.

Also, there are other factors influencing local tumor control or tissue damage, which may be taken into account by further extending the model. Some of these are the homeostatic control of the tumor growth (3), or the influence of radiation on tumor specific immunity, as discussed recently by Gallmeier (5) (can radiation increase the frequency of metastases?). Therefore, the model is a first step in the effort to describe the rather complicated subject of radiation sensitivity of tumors and normal tissue.

Tissue Damage

The radiobiological model for tissue damage is based on assumptions similar to the one for local tumor control. The probability for a larger volume of tissue to stay free of damage from a certain radiation dose is considered to be the product of the respective probabilities of its not-too-small parts. Using further marginal conditions as above, an expression of the probability W to remain free of tissue damage is derived as follows:

$$W\,(V,D) = e^{-(V_T/V_{To}) \cdot (D/D_{Wo})^P} \tag{7}$$

or

$$W\,(V,D) = 0{,}5^{(V_T/V_{To}) \cdot (D/D_{W50})^P} \tag{8}$$

where P is used to describe what can be considered as a multitarget component. D_{W50} is the dose at which 50 percent of the tissue volume $V_T = V_{To}$ remains free of damage. P again may be derived from clinical data. The available data (7, 8, 10, 12) lead to values for P from 6 to 39, the differences possibly due to large statistical uncertainties. From the radiobiological experiments of Phillips and Margolis (11) a P equal to 16 can be derived (see Fig. 3). The larger the P, the more homogeneous is the biological material.

Equation 8 may be extended for a more general application, i.e. for inhomogeneous dose distributions, and different radiosensitivity of different tissues to

$$W(V_{Ti},D) = 0.5^{\frac{1}{Vo} \sum_{i=1}^{n} \frac{1}{(D_{W50i})^P} \cdot \int_o^{V_{Ti}} D^P(V_i)dV_i} \tag{9}$$

where V_{Ti} = volume of tissue i

$D(V_i)$ = Radiation dose in tissue volume dV_i, dV_i being a volume element of V_{Ti}

n = number of different tissues

The probability of tissue damage S may be defined as

$$S\,(V,D) = 1 - W\,(V,D). \tag{10}$$

Figure 4 shows a best fit of the expected probability for tissue damage to the data of Stewart and Jackson (13) on necrosis of the larynx in irradiated larynx carcinoma, stage 3 using a P of 16 as in Fig. 3. There is also good agreement of equation 8 with older data of Holthusen (7) on the occurrence of telangiectasis of the skin after irradiation.

Cure Probability

The cure of a tumor patient who does not yet have metastases depends on the cure probability of the tumor as well as the probability of his remaining free of tissue damage caused by irradiation. This means that the cure probability is a product of the probability H of local control of the tumor and the probability W to remain free of tissue damage:

$$U = H\,(V_H, D_H) \cdot W\,(V_W, D_W) \qquad (11)$$

The curve derived by this equation reaches a maximum at the dose optimum.

By using equations 5, 8, and 11 the influence of volume on the overall cure probability can be calculated. In Figure 5 the volume effect is shown, using values of $Q = 12$ and $P = 16$, as before. In agreement with clinical experience, it follows that the optimal dose must be higher for larger tumor volumes. Also, the cure probability is reduced for larger tumor volumes, and further reduced if a layer of healthy tissue around the tumor is included in the target volume to ensure that all tumor cells get the intended dose.

Discussion and Conclusions

The assumption of an independent radiation reaction of smaller parts of tumor or healthy tissue, respectively, may not be valid in practice. However, several conclusions can be drawn which correspond well to clinical observations, or have a high degree of plausibility, in spite of the simplicity of the formulation. In particular, this model allows the following inferences:

1. A larger tumor has a smaller prospect of being cured than does a smaller tumor with the same dose and a given radiation sensitivity.
2. Whenever a greater volume of tissue (target volume) is irradiated with a certain dose, the frequency of radiation damage is also greater.
3. Radiation damage can be described by the product of irradiated volume and a high power of the dose absorbed by this volume (the volume integral of a high power of the individual doses which compose the total dose).
4. The prospect of cure can be improved if the primary tumor is included in the smallest possible volume given a relatively high

dose, plus the additional application of a suitably adjusted low-dose irradiation technique to areas of regional lymphatic spread.

5. In the case of localized small area irradiation (9) with suitable adjustment of the target volume to the tumor volume, the optimum dose is independent of volume. By comparison, when a standard irradiation method with constant target volume is applied, without regarding the actual tumor volume, then a somewhat smaller dose must be given to the smaller-sized tumor than to the larger tumor, in order to obtain the maximum prospect for survival.
6. The prospect of cure depends not only on the clinical stage classification, but also on the size of the primary tumor in the early stage.
7. The radiation sensitivity of a tumor should be defined according to inclusion of a standard volume, for example, by the 50 percent probability of cure for 1 ml of the tumor in question.
8. Homogenization of the dose distribution in the tumor area markedly improves the local tumor control rate. The improvement of the tumor control probability is especially significant if the inhomogeneity of the dose distribution in the tumor is improved from ± 10 percent to ± 5 percent, while further improvement produces no considerable advantage. Inhomogeneity of the dose distribution at a level of ± 5 percent in the tumor volume cannot be obtained by Telecobalt radiation. It may be obtained by megavolt X-ray irradiation. Therefore, the use of accelerators in radiation therapy may be preferred over cobalt units. The extent of expected improvement in the prospect of control of a tumor through homogenization of the dose distribution in the tumor area is shown in Figure 6.
9. Deviations in the applied dose from patient to patient produce, as expected, a flattening of the curve of the tumor control rate as well as that of the radiation damage rate. Likewise, too great a biological inhomogeneity of the material (individual variations in the radiation sensitivity of tumors and tissues) has the same effect. In the case where these deviations remain under 5 percent, the effect on the steepness of the curves is minimal. With wider deviations the probability of survival of the patient is decreased.

REFERENCES

1. Buchelt, L., *Ablauf und Ausmass der Lungenfibrose in Abhangigkeit von der Strahlentherapie des Bronchuskarzinoms*, dissertation, Marburg (Lahn) (1966).
2. Dessauer, F., in H. Meyer, *Lehrbuch der Strahlentherapie*, Berlin/Wien (1925).
3. Ellis, F., "Relationships of Biological Effect to Dose-Time-Fractionation Factors in Radiotherapy," in *Current Topics in Radiation Research*, Amsterdam (1968), *4*, 357.
4. Fletcher, G. H., Stovall, M., *Radiology, 78*, 766 (1962).

5. Gallmeier, W. M., "Tumorimmunologische Phänomene: Theoretische Grundlagen, klinische Bedeutung," *Gemeinsamer Kongress der Deutschen und der Osterreichischen Röntgengesellschaft*, 298 (1973).
6. Herring, D. F., Compton, D. M. J., "The Degree of Precision Required in the Radiation Dose Delivered in Cancer Radiotherapy," *Computers in Radiotherapy: Proceedings*, Brit. Inst. of Radiology (1971).
7. Holthusen, H., *Strahlentherapie*, *57*, 254 (1936).
8. Lindgren, M., "On the Tolerance of Brain Tissue and Sensitivity of Brain Tumors to Irradiation," *Acta Radiol. Suppl.* 170 (1958).
9. Martius, H., *Strahlentherapie*, *100*, 329 (1956).
10. Phillips, T. L., Buschke, F., *Amer. J. Roentgenol.*, *105*, 659 (1969).
11. Phillips, T. L., Margolis, L., *Front. Radiat. Ther. Onc.*, *6*, 254 (1972).
12. Shkovsky, L. J., *Am. J. Roentg.* *108*, 27 (1970).
13. Stewart, J. G., Jackson, A. W., in Easson, E. C., "A Clinical Approach to Neutron Therapy," *Current Topics in Radiation Research*, Amsterdam (1968), *3*, 175.

Table 1

Local Tumor Control in Carcinoma of the Larynx, Stage 3, for Fractionated Radiation

Control rate	03	05	07
Absorbed dose (rads)	5250	5500	5750.

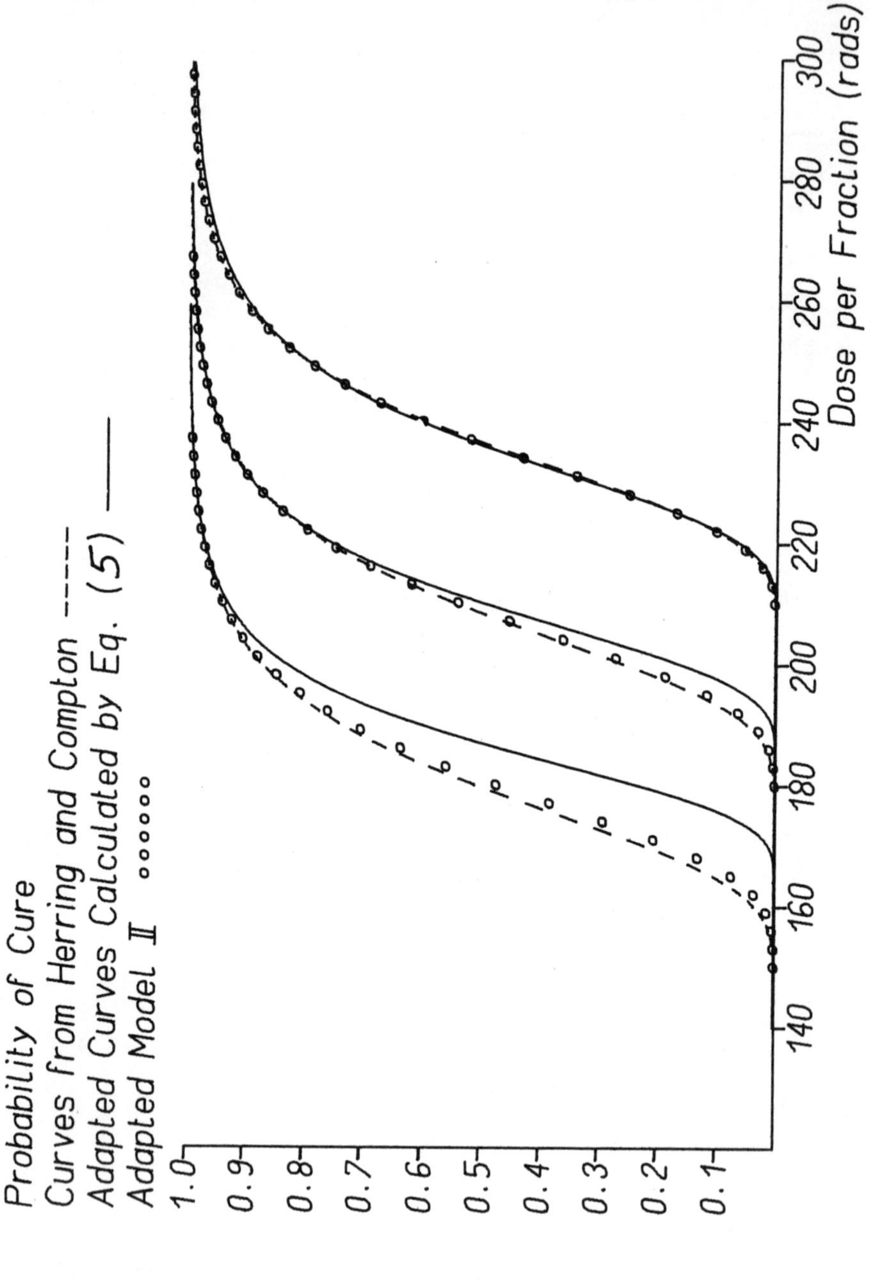

Probability of Cure
Curves from Herring and Compton ----
Adapted Curves Calculated by Eq. (5) ——
Adapted Model II oooooo
1.0
0.9
0.8
0.7
0.6
0.5
0.4
0.3
0.2
0.1
140
160
180
200
220
240
260
280
300
Dose per Fraction (rads)

Figure 1

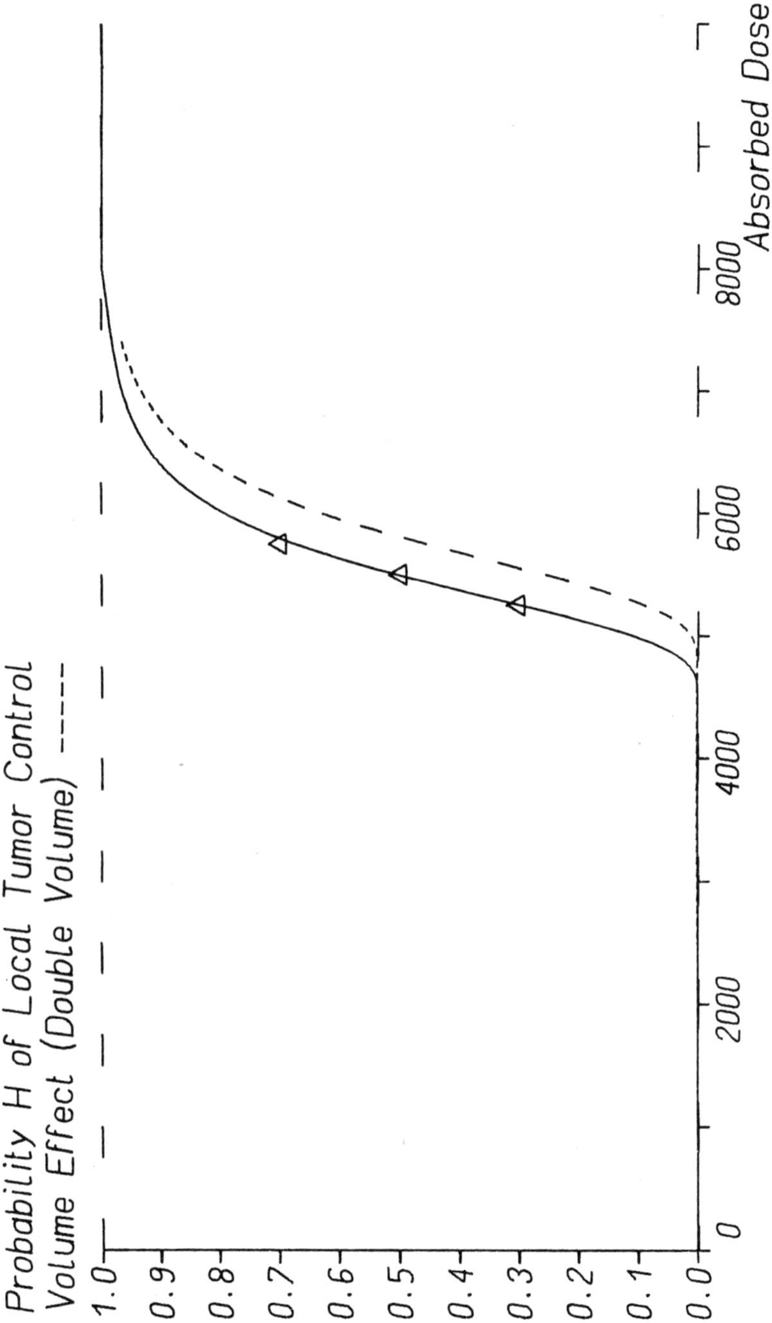
Probability H of Local Tumor Control
Volume Effect (Double Volume) -----
1.0
0.9
0.8
0.7
0.6
0.5
0.4
0.3
0.2
0.1
0.0
0
2000
4000
6000
8000
Absorbed Dose

Figure 2

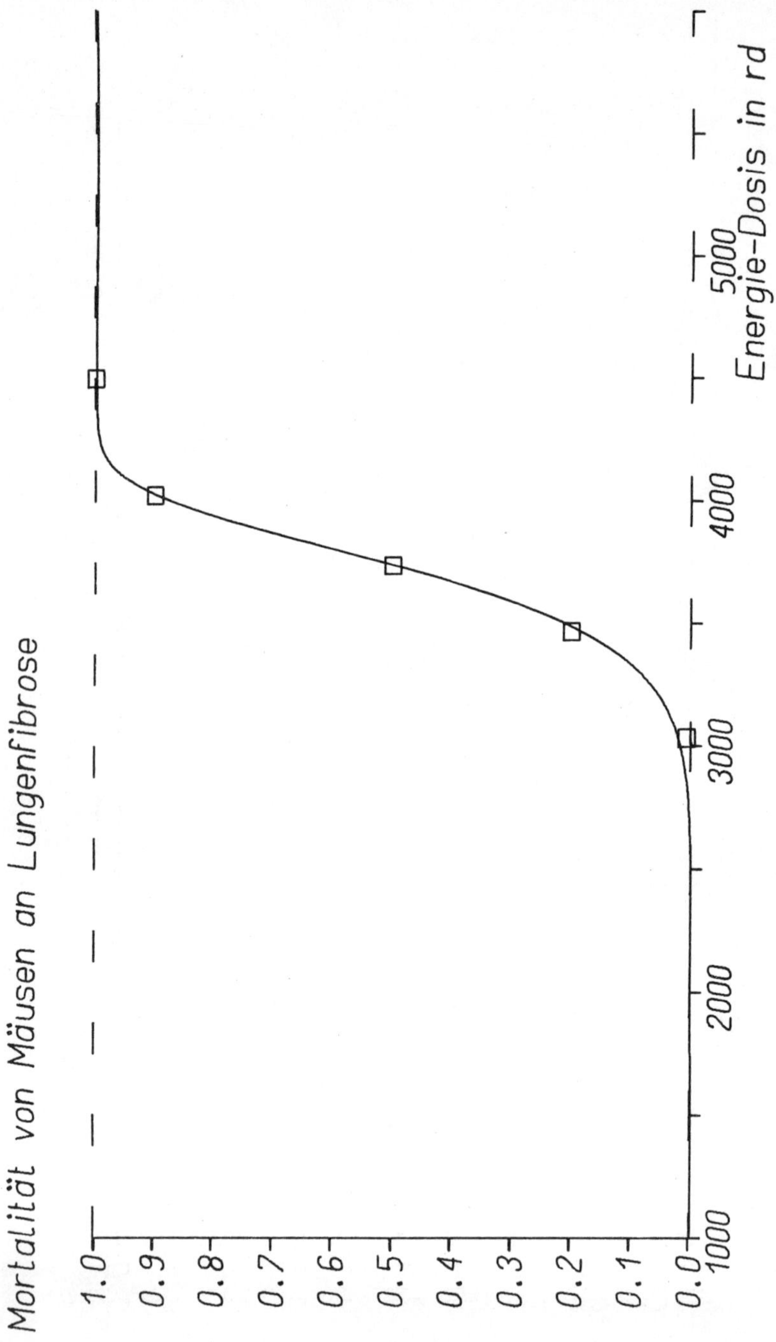
Mortalität von Mäusen an Lungenfibrose
1.0
0.9
0.8
0.7
0.6
0.5
0.4
0.3
0.2
0.1
0.0
1000
2000
3000
4000
5000
Energie-Dosis in rd

Figure 3

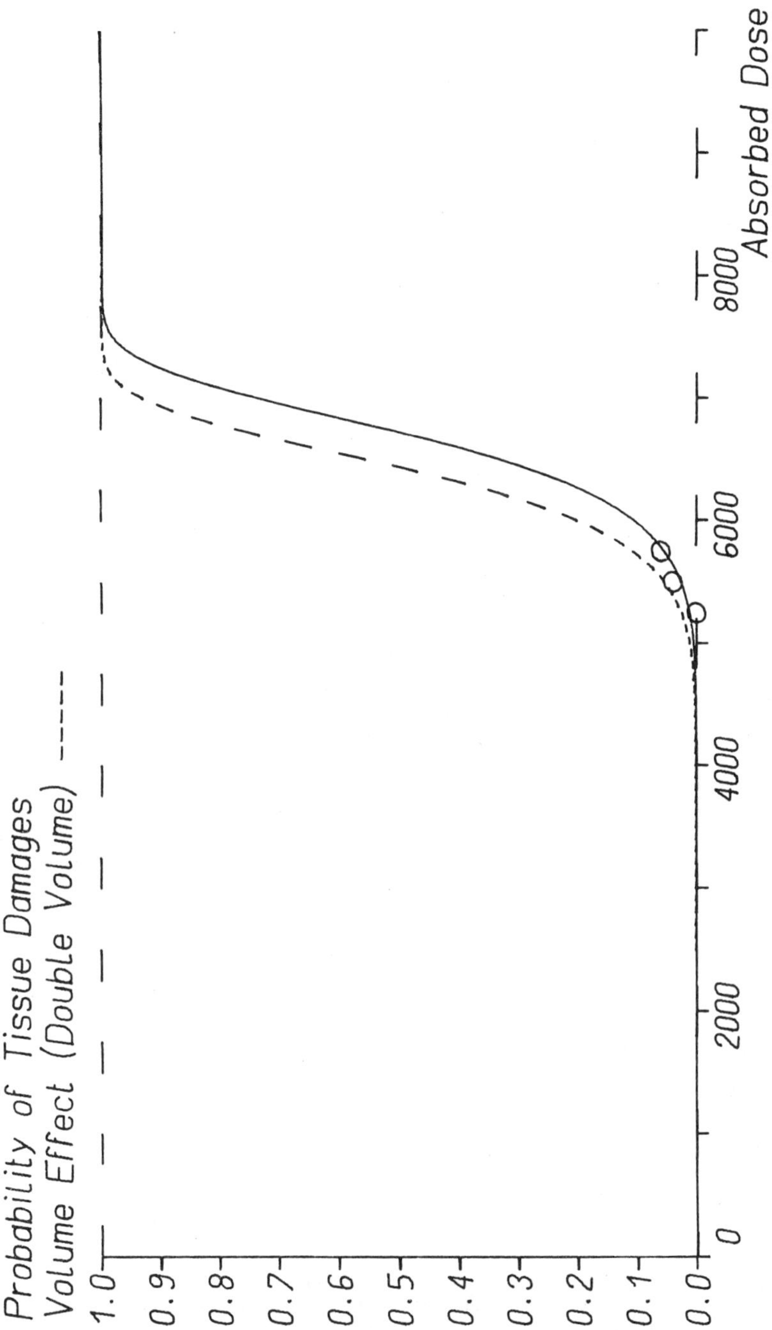
Probability of Tissue Damages
Volume Effect (Double Volume)
Absorbed Dose
0.0
0.1
0.2
0.3
0.4
0.5
0.6
0.7
0.8
0.9
1.0
0
2000
4000
6000
8000

Figure 4

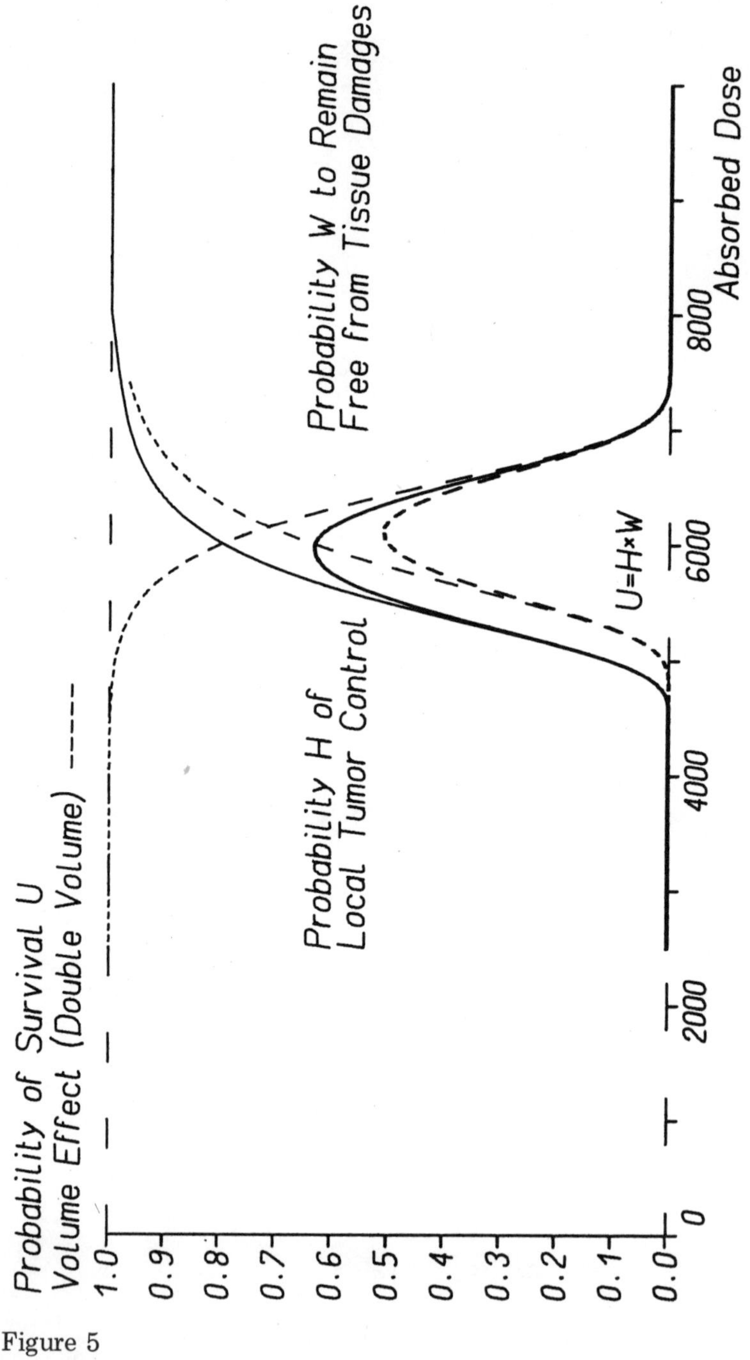
Probability of Survival U
Volume Effect (Double Volume) ----
Probability H of
Local Tumor Control
Probability W to Remain
Free from Tissue Damages
U=H×W
Absorbed Dose
0
2000
4000
6000
8000
0.0
0.1
0.2
0.3
0.4
0.5
0.6
0.7
0.8
0.9
1.0

Figure 5

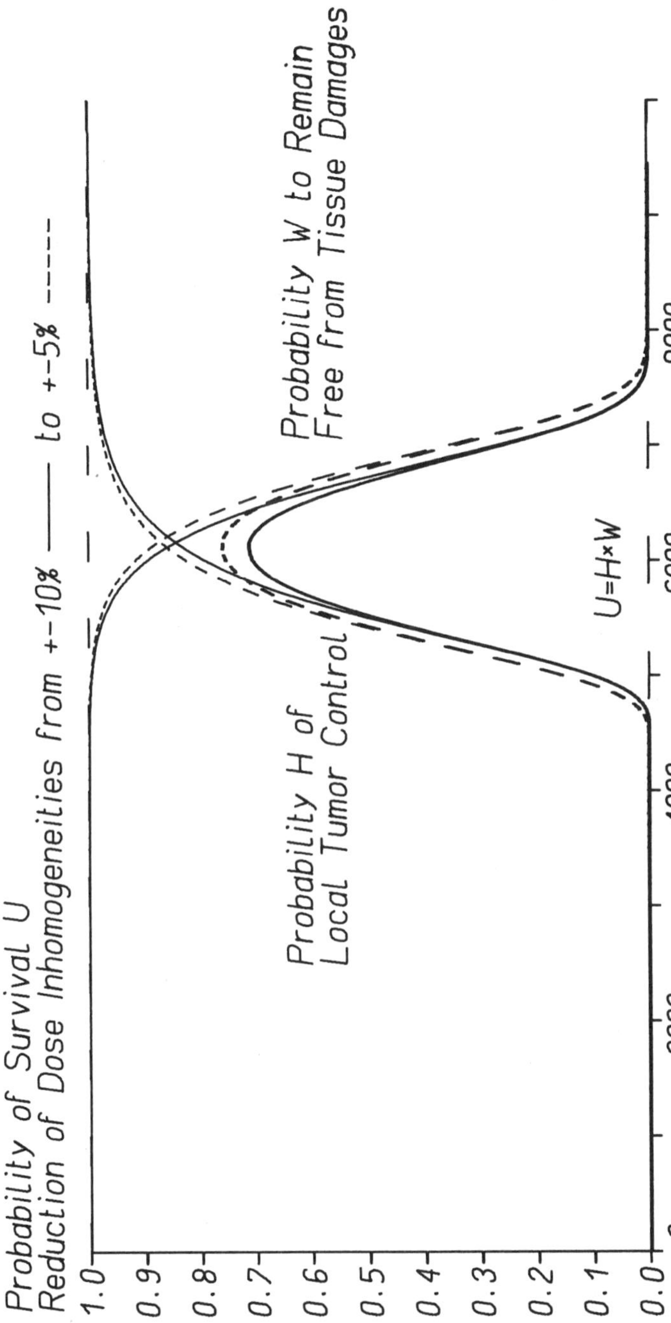
Probability of Survival U
Reduction of Dose Inhomogeneities from +-10% —— to +-5% -----
Probability W to Remain
Free from Tissue Damages
Probability H of
Local Tumor Control
U=H×W
0.0
0.1
0.2
0.3
0.4
0.5
0.6
0.7
0.8
0.9
1.0
0
2000
4000
6000
8000

Figure 6

5. The Application of the Computer in Radiation Therapy Decision Making: Cell Kinetic Considerations

M. L. Griem

In 1959, Quastler and Sherman described a method of studying the cell proliferation kinetics in the intestinal epithelium of the mouse (1). This classic paper described the use of tritiated thymidine as a method of marking or labeling cells undergoing DNA synthesis. By using tissue sections cut very thinly, it was possible to identify various compartments of the cell proliferation cycle (Fig. 1), in the tissue section to identify cells undergoing mitosis, and in the overlying photographic emulsion identify cells containing radioactivity in the nuclei by counting the labeled nuclei. This classic paper led to the important symposium on cell proliferation held in Dublin in 1962 (2). In that symposium a number of methods of measuring cell turnover were reviewed and in the same proceedings both tumor and normal tissue kinetics were discussed. Mendelsohn, in that year, pointed out the importance of the concept of growth fraction and a method of measuring this factor (3). In 1961 Terasima and Tolmach pointed out the variations in the radiation sensitivity of cells in different phases of the cell cycle (4). Subsequently, Sinclair and Morton analyzed another tissue culture and showed similar findings. Later Sinclair pointed out the cyclic X-ray responses in mammalian cells in vitro and that cells in late stages of DNA synthesis were 2.5 times as resistant to radiation as cells that were in the process of mitosis (5).

In 1966 Mendelsohn set forth some of the problems facing the radiation therapist in attempting to use some of the new concepts of cell proliferation kinetics and cycling radiosensitivity to improve the patient with cancer (6). In that discussion Mendelsohn pointed out that a number of parameters were not available to provide the needed information to help in decision-making. Little was known about the cell turnover rates in human tumors. Subsequently, Steel outlined some of the knowledge concerning the cellular proliferation in tumors and pointed out the importance of the knowledge of the growth fraction and of the cell loss in the analysis of the way a tumor behaves (7).

In 1968 Fry organized a symposium on normal and malignant cell growth (8). In that monograph of the proceedings of the symposium, Dethlefson pointed out a method of measuring the proliferative rate in tumor using radioactive iodinated precursors of DNA (9). Also in that symposium Mauer pointed out that the nondividing leukemic cell population in children presented a particular problem and that careful analysis of this nonproliferating population could lead to improved treatment methods with drugs and irradiation (10). Also in that monograph human epithelial tumor growth curves were discussed in some detail by Tubiana (11). Since then the biologist has used many of the techniques developed by the radiobiologists to understand the interaction of cancer chemotherapeutic agents on proliferating cells. The site of block in the cycle has been analyzed in detail. A thorough analysis has recently been published by Madoc-Jones and Mauro in a review article (12). A number of drugs enter the cell at one phase of the cell cycle and create a block at another phase. Steward and Hahn have used some of these facts to develop computer models for suggested methods of using cancer chemotherapeutic agents (13). Recently, Mendelsohn has again focused our attention on the nonproliferating cells in an analysis of the cell kinetics in breast cancer (Fig. 2). In this analysis of Mendelsohn and Dethlefson, two breast cancer lesions in the same mouse were analyzed—one a slowly proliferating and one a fast proliferating tumor. In a detailed analysis based on the figure, the flux of cells moving into the nonproliferating compartment represents one of the major considerations in the rate of growth of the tumor. It is important that as one considers this type of problem, the computer lends itself to analyzing some of these newer concepts in tumor growth.

Mendelsohn points out, "All aspects of cancer therapy have a kinetic involvement. In radiotherapy the growth kinetics effect, the rate of tumor shrinkage, the design of optimum fractionation, and an estimation of the number of tumor or normal cells at risk and the use of the combination or other treatment modifications to increase the therapeutic ratio of tumor to normal response. In chemotherapy the same problems repeat themselves and also in addition the use of cycle-linked agents demands a keen insight into cell cycle behavior and the non-cycling cell. Finally, in surgery as well as radiotherapy and chemotherapy, a knowledge of the growth rate provides the framework within which one predicts and interprets the likely times of recurrence, the response to therapy and the probability of cure" (14). Yet with all these limitations, multiple-drug combinations have been developed and drug irradiation interaction has been used to improve the response of tumors in the clinical management of a number of patients with cancer.

A second use of the computer has been to analyze the role of oxygen in the modification of the radiosensitivity of self-renewing cell systems. Lerch (15) has used some of the models developed by Sacher (16) and the data of Revesz to do computer modeling of rates of reoxygenation (17).

Recently, Mendelsohn pointed out that the computer might be used in decision-making and that families of therapeutic operating characteristic curves (TOC) could be generated from known data concerning the probability of tumor ablation and from data concerning complications of treatment (18). To this analysis, he and his colleagues have added the cost analysis of a medical decision-making from the standpoint of outcome of such treatment. This whole concept has been beautifully discussed in a recent paper by Moore (19), which is recommended for reading.

Summary

In radiotherapeutic decision-making, a number of pieces of information have been made available in the past fifteen years to improve our knowledge of tumor and normal tissue growth. We have learned much more about the action of radiation during the cell cycle. A host of cancer chemotherapeutic agents have been analyzed in a similar fashion. With this knowledge, some models have been developed using the computer to improve our ability to study tumors. We should see further progress in this field as we gain greater understanding of tumor and normal tissue behavior.

REFERENCES

1. Quastler, H., and Sherman, F. S., *Exp. Cell Res.*, *17*, 420 (1959).
2. Lamerton, L. F., and Fry, R. J. M., *Cell Proliferation*, A Guinness Symposium held at University of Dublin, Trinity College. Philadelphia, F. A. Davis Company (1963).
3. Mendelsohn, M. L., *J. Nat. Cancer Inst.*, *28*, 1015 (1962).
4. Terasima, T., and Tolmach, L. F., *Nature*, *190*, 1210 (1961).
5. Sinclair, W. K., and Morton, R. A., *Rad. Res.*, *29*, 450 (1966).
6. Mendelsohn, M. L., "Radiation Effects in Tumors," in *Radiation Research*, ed. G. Silini, Amsterdam, North Holland Publishing Co. (1967), 659.
7. Steel, G. G., *Cell and Tissue Kinetics*, *1*, 193 (1968).
8. Fry, R. J. M., Griem, M. L., Kirsten, W. H., Eds., *Normal and Malignant Cell Growth*, New York, Springer-Verlag (1969).
9. Dethlefsen, L. A., "Incorporation of ^{125} Iodine-Labeled 5-Iodo-2'-Deoxyuridine into the DNA of Mouse Mammary Tumors," in *Normal and Malignant Cell Growth*, ed. Fry, R. J. M., Griem, M. L., and Kirsten, W. H., New York, Springer-Verlag (1969), 186.

10. Mauer, A. M., Saunders, E. F., and Lampkin, B. C., "Importance of the Non-Dividing Leukemic Cell," in *Normal and Malignant Cell Growth*, ed. Fry, R. J. M., Griem, M. L., and Kirsten, W. H., New York, Springer-Verlag (1969), 168.
11. Tubiana, M., Frindel, E., and Malaise, E., "*In Vivo* Cell Kinetics of Human Cancers," in *Normal and Malignant Cell Growth*, ed. Fry, R. J. M., Griem, M. L., and Kirsten, W. H., New York, Springer-Verlag (1969), 202.
12. Madoc-Jones, H., and Mauro, F., "Site of Action of Cytotoxic Agents in the Cell Life Cycle," in *Handbook of Experimental Pharmacology*, new series *38/1*, ed. Sartorelli, A. C. and Johns, D. G., Berlin-Heidelberg-New York, Springer-Verlag (1974), 205.
13. Steward, P. G., and Hahn, G. M., *Cell and Tissue Kinetics*, *4*, 279 (1971).
14. Mendelsohn, M. L., and Dethlefsen, L. A., "Cell Kinetics of Breast Cancer: The Turnover of Nonproliferating Cells," in *Breast Cancer: A Challenging Problem*, ed. Griem, M. L., Jensen, E. V., Ultmann, J. E., and Wissler, R. W., New York-Heidelberg-Berlin, Springer-Verlag (1973), 73.
15. Lerch, I. A., *Radiology*, *101*, 683 (1971).
16. Sacher, G. A., and Trucco, E., *Radiat. Res.*, *29*, 236 (1966).
17. Littbrank, B., and Revesz, L., *Brit. J. Radiol.*, *42*, 914 (1969).
18. Mendelsohn, M. L., "Radiotherapy and Tolerance," in *Frontiers of Radiation Therapy and Oncology*, ed. Vaeth, J. M., Baltimore-London-Tokyo, University Park Press (1972), *6*, 512.
19. Moore, D. H., II, and Mendelsohn, M. L., *Cancer*, *30*, 97 (1972).

This investigation was supported in part by USPHS grant CA-14599, the Department of Radiology, University of Chicago, and the Franklin McLean Memorial Research Institute (operated by the University of Chicago for the Energy Research and Development Administration).

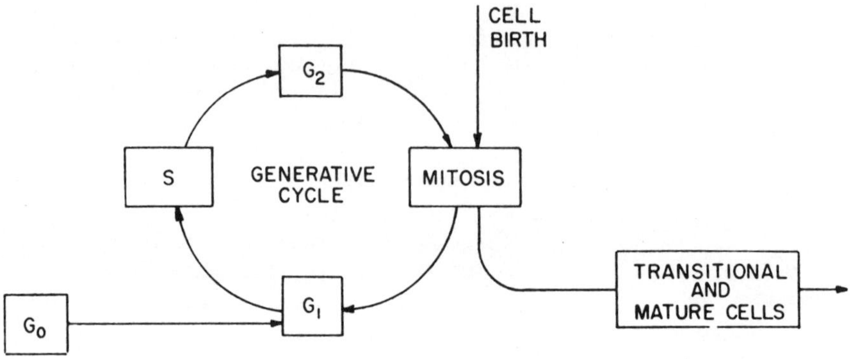

Figure 1. Compartments of the Cell Proliferation Cycle

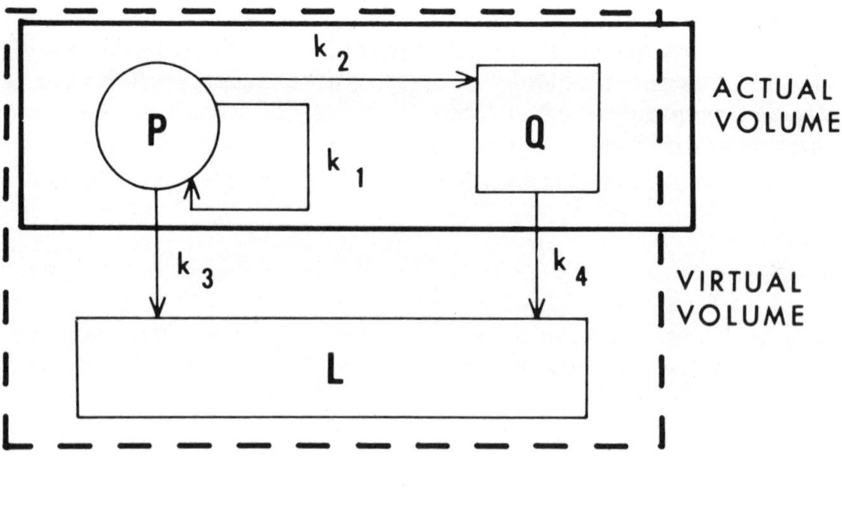

Figure 2. Cell Kinetics in Breast Cancer

6. Cell Kinetic Systems: In Vitro

E. B. Douple

I. Introduction

Today's radiation biologist, striving to contribute to the understanding of the basic interactions of ionizing radiations with living systems and to a rationalization and further improvement of radiation therapy as treatment modality for malignant disease, may find encouragement in the following observations. First, it would be fortuitous if the radiation therapy treatment regimes of today, even though they were developed over many years of practical experience, represented an optimum time-dose relationship. Second, changes in time-dose relationships could be expected to alter significantly the effectiveness of a treatment regime. Third, cell-kinetic studies performed by exposing mammalian cells *in vitro* to different irradiation conditions may have considerable application to clinical procedures and provide valuable insight into the essential features of radiation therapy as a consequence of the myriad combinations of biological and physical parameters.

Since the development nearly two decades ago of an *in vitro* technique by Puck et al. (1), which yields fairly accurate quantitative data on the proliferative capacity of mammalian cells, dose-response curves have been produced for many types of cells irradiated under many different conditions. Today the techniques for obtaining relatively precise quantitative data on the survival of mammalian cells after exposure to radiation are sufficiently advanced to warrant the construction of mathematical models to aid in the elucidation of the phenomena involved. Numerous techniques, including computer-based methods, have been applied by Cohen (2, 3, 4), Cohen and Scott (5), Steward and Hahn (6), Fischer (7, 8), Hethcote and Waltman (9), Brown et al. (10), and many others to predict the surviving fraction of irradiated cells. Reports such as these have demonstrated that, given sufficient information about certain critical parameters, one can proceed to evaluate hypotheses, account for the time course of radiation-induced changes in the survival properties of different cell populations in several cell-kinetic systems, and extend this information to the evaluation of such differences in treatment as continuous irradiation versus several multi-fraction irradiation regimes.

The pertinence of mammalian cell studies *in vitro* to radiation therapy is illustrated, for example, by the isosurvival curves for the 10^{-10} survival level constructed by Elkind et al. (11). The curves predicted a range of required total dose consistent with those used in clinical practice, and the calculations for generating the curves used single-cell survival parameters very similar to those observed in *in vitro* experiments.

It became very apparent from the first *in vitro* studies on cell kinetics that radiotherapy could be made more rational and more efficacious if it were based on the kinetics of the cell cycle. To this date, however, the details of the kinetics of cells in tumors have remained elusive and complex. The *in vivo* studies are complicated by parameters that may change because of variations in tumor size or variations in patterns of anoxia. The survival properties of several groups of constituent cells may remain unknown, and systemic effects may produce serious complications. Since the characteristics and responses to ionizing radiation of tumors over the whole period of their development are far from being known, it has become essential that we understand basic kinetic changes in rather simplified, controllable systems. Although no single system will serve as an adequate kinetic or biological response model for all tumors or for all normal tissues, some *in vitro* systems have been developed as better models from which kinetic information can be gained and extended to predict improved clinical therapeutic designs.

II. Exponential Growth Phase Systems

When mammalian cells are plated in media in culture dishes, the cells settle to the bottom, attach, and under the appropriate conditions begin dividing. After an initial lag period, the population will eventually enter an exponential or log phase of growth, as illustrated in Figure 1.

These exponentially growing cell populations have been used most frequently by radiobiologists as a kinetic system to study the radiation response of human cells. The use of nucleic acid precursors and autoradiography in these studies has elucidated such cell-cycle parameters as the generation times and lengths of the pre- and post-DNA synthetic phases. Much important information has been obtained, including many of the basic parameters of mammalian cell survival, such as estimates of D_o, D_q, and extrapolation number, n. As a result of numerous fractionation studies, like the classic split-dose experiments of Elkind and Sutton (12), valuable information regarding repair and recovery phenomena has been obtained under conditions of active growth.

Using various synchronizing agents, many workers have studied radiation response characteristics of cells in different parts of the cell cycle. Several reviews of methods and criteria of mammalian cell synchrony have been reported, including the reviews by Sinclair (13) and by Nias and Fox (14). Terasima and Tolmach (15), Sinclair and Morton (16), and many other authors have reported marked differences in radiosensitivity for cells in various parts of the cell cycle, and cell-cycle radiosensitivity differences have also been reported between cell lines.

The radiobiology of cultured mammalian cells has been reviewed in a text by Elkind and Whitmore (17). Some authors have extended results of these *in vitro* exponential growth-phase systems to models for the optimization of treatment schedules, suggesting that it may be possible to plan differential killing by radiation of one cell line over another on the basis of the differences in their age responses. Differences in initial slopes of survival curves might contribute to clinically observed variations between the radiosensitivity of tumors (the 1974 L. H. Gray Memorial Conference focuses attention on the clinical significance of the low-dose region of the mammalian cell survival curve). Survival curves obtained with different types of cultured cells have not been determined with sufficient accuracy at low doses with fractionated exposures to conclude whether their shapes are significantly different. Important differences might well be found which may account for the variety of responses of various tumors, and between tumors and normal tissue after fractionated irradiation using doses in the clinical range.

When cell kinetic characteristics are considered, however, exponential growth-phase systems might not represent the best cell kinetic systems for measurable solid tumors in animals or man. For one thing, too high a fraction of clonogenic log-phase cells might be cycling per unit time. This is not to say that all that has been observed in studies of log-phase cells is irrevelant to solid tumors. Indeed, dilute log-phase cultures of solid tumor cells with minimal intercellular competition or contact may be good counterparts of very highly proliferative solid tumor cells in the proximity of a blood vessel. But it must also be recognized that large differences in growth rates, changing growth rates, and changing proliferative stages within the clonogenic tumor cells can be expected to influence significantly the response of a tumor to radiation.

III. Plateau Growth Phase Systems

If the culture of cells illustrated in Figure 1 continues growing *in vitro*, the cells will eventually reach a plateau phase of growth and they will eventually form a confluent monolayer and a fairly constant cell number per dish. This plateau phase may persist for a period of several days, and in our laboratory V-79 Chinese hamster cells have been held as unfed cultures for a total of fourteen days. Plateau-phase cell cultures have been characterized in some detail, particularly in the laboratories of Hahn at Stanford and Little at Harvard. Hahn and Little (18) have reviewed in considerable detail the characteristics of plateau-phase cultures as an *in vitro* model for human cancer.

If the medium is not renewed throughout the period of growth, the plateau is reached, probably because of exhaustion of one or more substances in the serum. The addition of serum to these unfed cultures causes the cell number to increase and reach a higher final cell density. The final cell density is influenced by many factors, including the serum concentration used at the beginning of the experiment, the number of cells initially plated, and occasional shaking of the dishes during incubation.

If the media of the cells in exponential phase of growth is renewed daily, beginning around day 5, the plateau phase is reached at a higher cell density, as a result of crowded conditions. These crowded populations are called "fed" cultures, and they may be maintained almost indefinitely with regular medium changes.

Hahn and Little (18) have shown that both plateau cultures, fed and unfed, are dynamic cell systems in which cell loss into the culture medium is balanced quantitatively by a limited amount of cell proliferation, and consequently these cultures represent *in vitro* cell-renewal systems.

In unfed cultures of Chinese hamster HA cells, Hahn has shown that cell viability remains high for several days, cell death remains low (1-3 percent per day), less than one percent of the cells are in cycle at any one time, and perhaps 20 to 30 percent of the cells are arrested in the G_2 stage of the cell cycle.

The cell viability was shown to drop with time in fed plateau-phase cultures and after 4 to 5 days in plateau phase, only 30 to 40 percent of the cells being clonogenic. Cell death was estimated to be about 10 to 15 percent per day, and the S phase of the fed cells was greatly extended compared to the S phase of exponentially growing cells (18 hours compared to 6 hours, respectively). Much more mitotic activity was reported in fed cultures than in unfed cultures. Differences were reported by Little between the Chinese hamster HA cells and Chang human liver cells (LICH) for both fed and unfed plateau-phase cultures.

Important differences have been reported between fed and unfed cultures with respect to their response to ionizing radiation. Hahn has reported no repair of sublethal damage in fed cultures, but the ability to repair sublethal damage is present in unfed cultures. Furthermore, the fed cultures did not reflect the ability to repair potentially lethal damage, whereas unfed cultures may possibly repair such damage. However, Little has reported no reduction in extrapolation number or in repair capacity in dense cultures of Chang liver cells. In the future it may be of importance to compare the cell kinetics of the unfed plateau-phase cells with the cell kinetics of cells in solid or ascites tumors that have a poor nutritional status.

A radiation-induced depression in the rate of flow of G_1 cells into S has been reported to occur in some mammalian cells after exposure to several hundred rads, but has not generally been observed in established lines of human cells. Little demonstrated this using a line of human liver cells (LICH) having a doubling time of approximately twenty-four hours and a pulse-labeling index of 35 percent during exponential growth. When plateau phase cells were used, however, the initiation of DNA synthesis was significantly delayed by irradiation—an effect that may be a general occurrence in many slowly proliferating cell systems. For these cells the D_0 dose was consistently lower and the extrapolation number somewhat higher in plateau-phase cells.

There is evidence that some *in vivo* tumors may have regions with labeled mitoses curves similar to fed plateau-phase cultures with an elongated S period, while in other tumor systems the durations of cell-cycle phases appear to be independent of the location of the cells in the tumor. This may offer a partial explanation for the tremendous variation in responses of tumors to fractionated courses of radiotherapy.

Since plateau-phase cultures may be maintained for several days, these cell kinetic systems can be used to evaluate the effects of fractionated irradiations regimes. Cell survival data will become more meaningful, however, when more detailed kinetics information is obtained for the older plateau-phase populations.

IV. Spheroid Tumor Models

Although plateau-phase cultures may be the best *in vitro* representation of solid tumors that can be obtained with conventional cell-culturing techniques, they lack at least two important features of the *in vivo* tumor: (1) extensive, three-dimensional intercellular contact; and (2) differing metabolic environments due to diffusion limitations. Systems have recently been developed for growing three-dimensional clones in a semi-solid medium (19, 20). In addition, multicellular "spheroids" of Chinese hamster V-79 cells have been grown in suspension culture, and this system may uniquely simulate many characteristics of solid tumors, since they are morphologically similar to the tumor cords of some animal and human tumors. Spheroid culture methods were first reported by Sutherland and his associates in 1970 (21, 22, 23), and they have been applied to a variety of radiobiology experiments, particularly by Sutherland and Durand.

The spheroid culture system is intermediate in complexity between standard culture systems and tumors *in vivo*. The cells are stirred at low speeds and allowed to form spherical aggregates. The cells then continue to divide, and the spheroids have a growth curve similar to that of many solid tumors: they may eventually contain as many as 10^5 cells. A radiosensitive G_1-like noncycling population of cells develops slowly and is maintained in the presence of neighboring, highly radio-resistant, hypoxic, internal noncycling cells and normally cycling cells which are relatively resistant and asynchronous. Metabolites, including oxygen, do not reach central areas of large spheroids, and central necrosis is observed in spheroids greater than 300 microns in diameter.

Very large spheroids contain approximately 20 percent hypoxic cells, a percentage similar to that of many tumors *in vivo* (24). Cells in this system can also be maintained for very long periods of time, and the spheroids may represent a superior *in vitro* system for the investigation of therapeutic techniques, both chemotherapeutic and radiotherapeutic, applicable to solid tumors. The investigations of Sutherland and Durand have demonstrated an increase in radio-resistance for cells irradiated in contact as small spheroids rather than as single cells, an increase that was not observed when colonies of comparable size were irradiated on plates (25). Their investigations have also indicated a capacity of enhanced repair of sublethal radiation damage when V-79 cells are grown and irradiated as spheroids.

In a recent report by Durand (26), the response of spheroids was assayed by placing entire spheroids in petri dishes and observing cellular outgrowth. Spheroids were also reduced to single cells by trypsinization at various times post-irradiation, and viability of the cells was determined by conventional colony-formation methods. In addition, spheroid volume and cell content were monitored as a function of time after irradiation. "Cure" of spheroids, as indicated by lack of cellular outgrowth but not spheroid volume change, correlated well with single-cell survival. Cures were achieved only when every cell was killed. Repopulation was reported when spheroid volume was decreasing and volume was not indicative of cell density or total cell number.

The spheroid kinetic system offers several advantages over *in vivo* systems. Like most *in vitro* systems, indirect host-tumor interactions are removed. With 10^4 to 10^5 cells in each spheroid, cures for the tumor models can be assayed at survival levels comparable to those which can be studied by conventional colony-forming techniques. The endpoints, such as cure, regression, cell density, and cell survival can be intercompared, since other indirect factors should be minimal. Large numbers of "tumors" can be studied with the convenience of *in vitro* manipulation methods without the added expense of maintaining host animals. Kinetic parameters like cell loss, cellular repair and recovery, and repopulation can be studied as the net survival changes. A disadvantage of this system is that rigorous statistical analysis is hampered by changing spheroid characteristics dependent upon spheroid density, the feeding schedule, and the history of the population (25, 27).

V. Conclusion

Since interpretation of experiments with animal tumors is complicated by immunological and other host-tumor factors, *in vitro* kinetic systems have an important role to play in the study of response of cell populations to radiation, including fractionated irradiation regimes. Many important radiobiological concepts have been obtained from studies using exponential kinetic systems. Noncycling cells, however, may constitute a majority of the cell population of many solid tumors, and therefore their radiation response is of considerable importance, particularly if these noncycling cells may be responsible for tumor recurrence. Plateau-phase kinetic systems and spheroid tumor models may represent very important kinetic systems, which may be used to test computer-based methods of predicting the surviving fraction of cell populations exposed to fractionated irradiation regimes.

The spheroid tumor model system simulated morphologically certain solid tumors and may have a similar growth pattern. This model offers the ease of manipulation typical of an *in vitro* system. However, this is a mixed population of cells with respect to nutritional status, oxygenation, and proliferative activity. Spheroids have proved very useful for studying certain aspects of the dynamics of oxygenation and reoxygenation of hypoxic cells after irradiation, and for studying the effects of radiosensitizers (28). The system is particularly amenable to the study of common radiobiological endpoints, such as cure, regression, and cell survival.

Most *in vitro* systems lack complexity, notably the absence of vascularity. Also, few tumors in patients are known to have generation times as short as those of cells cultured *in vitro*. Many *in vitro* cell cultures have different parameter values, such as lower D_q values, than cells assayed *in vivo*. The plateau-phase kinetic system and the spheroid-tumor system offer great potential for fractionation experiments, and information can be gained from them which cannot be obtained from exponential growth systems or only with great difficulty from *in vivo* systems. If descriptions of tissue-culture measurements are to be extended to tissues and tumors, and if computer-based models that are currently available are to be applied to cell kinetic systems *in vitro*, the stochastic properties of the proliferation processes in the kinetic systems will have to be defined more adequately, particularly in older plateau-phase cultures and in older spheroids. Dynamic models must be developed to account for the major shifts in survival parameters during fractionated treatment regimes.

ACKNOWLEDGMENT

This work was supported by NIH Contract 71-2087, DHEW.

REFERENCES

1. Puck, T. T., Marcus, P. I., and Cieciura, S. J., *J. of Experimental Medicine, 103*, 273 (1956).
2. Cohen, L., *Computer Programs in Biomedicine, 3*, 27 (1973).
3. Cohen, L., *Brit. J. Radiol., 41*, 522 (1968).
4. Cohen, L., *Radiology, 101*, 419 (1971).
5. Cohen, L. and Scott, M. J., *Brit. J. Radiol., 41*, 529 (1968).
6. Steward, P. G. and Hahn, G. M., *Cell Tissue Kinet., 4*, 279 (1971).
7. Fischer, J. J., *Acta Radiol. Ther. Phys. Biol., 10*, 73 (1971).
8. Fischer, J. J., *Acta Radiol. Ther. Phys. Biol., 10*, 267 (1971).
9. Hethcote, H. W. and Waltman, P., *Radiation Research, 56*, 150 (1973).
10. Brown, B. W., Thompson, J. J., Barkley, T., Suit, H., and Withers, H. R., *Radiology, 110*, 197 (1974).
11. Elkind, M. M., Swain, R. W., Alescio, T., Sutton, H., and Moses, W. B., in *Cellular Radiation Biology*, Williams and Wilkins, Baltimore (1965), 422.
12. Elkind, M. M. and Sutton, H., *Nature, 184*, 1293 (1959).
13. Sinclair, W. K., in *Normal and Malignant Cell Growth*, Springer-Verlag, New York (1969), 90.
14. Nias, A. H. W. and Fox, M., *Cell Tissue Kinet., 4*, 375 (1971).
15. Terasima, T. and Tolmach, L. J., *Biophys. J., 3*, 11 (1963).
16. Sinclair, W. K. and Morton, R. A., *Nature, 199*, 1158 (1963).
17. Elkind, M. M. and Whitmore, G. F., *The Radiobiology of Cultured Mammalian Cells*, Gordon and Breach, New York (1967).
18. Hahn, G. M. and Little, J. B., *Current Topics in Radiation Research Quarterly, 8*, 39 (1972).
19. Dalen, H. and Burki, H. J., *Exptl. Cell Res., 65*, 433 (1971).
20. Shinohara, K. and Okada, S., *J. Radiat. Res.* (Japan), *13*, 109 (1972).
21. Inch, W. R., McCredie, J. A., and Sutherland, R. M., *Growth, 34*, 271 (1970).
22. Sutherland, R. M., Inch, W. R., McCredie, J. A., and Kruuv, J., *Int. J. Radiat. Biol., 18*, 491 (1970).
23. Sutherland, R. M., McCredie, J. A., and Inch, W. R., *J. Nat. Cancer Inst., 46*, 113 (1971).
24. Van Patten, L. M. and Kallman, R. F., *J. Nat. Cancer Inst., 40*, 441 (1968).
25. Durand, R. E. and Sutherland, R.M., *Experimental Cell Res., 71*, 75 (1972).

25. Durand, R. E. and Sutherland, R. M., *Experimental Cell Res.*, *71*, 75 (1972).
26. Durand, R. E., *Brit. J. Radiol.*, *48*, 556 (1975).
27. Durand, R. E. and Sutherland, R. M., *Cancer Res.*, *33*, 213 (1973).
28. Sutherland, R. M. and Durand, R.E., *Int. J. Radiat. Biol.*, *22*, 613 (1972).

QUESTIONS

NEURATH: This may be a naive question, but how, if you have a monolayer of confluent cells in an equal-size dish, can you have ten times as many cells if they are fed than when they are unfed?

DOUPLE: The size of cell may be one particular difference, but it's cell density that's more important. The cells are packed more tightly, and the observed difference here has to do with the tightness of the grouping of these cells.

ELLIS: Did I understand you to say that this spheroid method had only been used successfully on one type of cell?

DOUPLE: It's only being used with the V-79, a nononcogenic, Chinese hamster lung-cell culture.

ELLIS: And yet, with a bigger number of cells you need a bigger dose to get rid of them?

DOUPLE: That's right: as with larger tumors, larger doses are needed. This has been studied particularly by Dr. Durand. But the interesting observation is that there isn't a good correlation between the volume of the tumors and the ultimate cure of the "tumor."

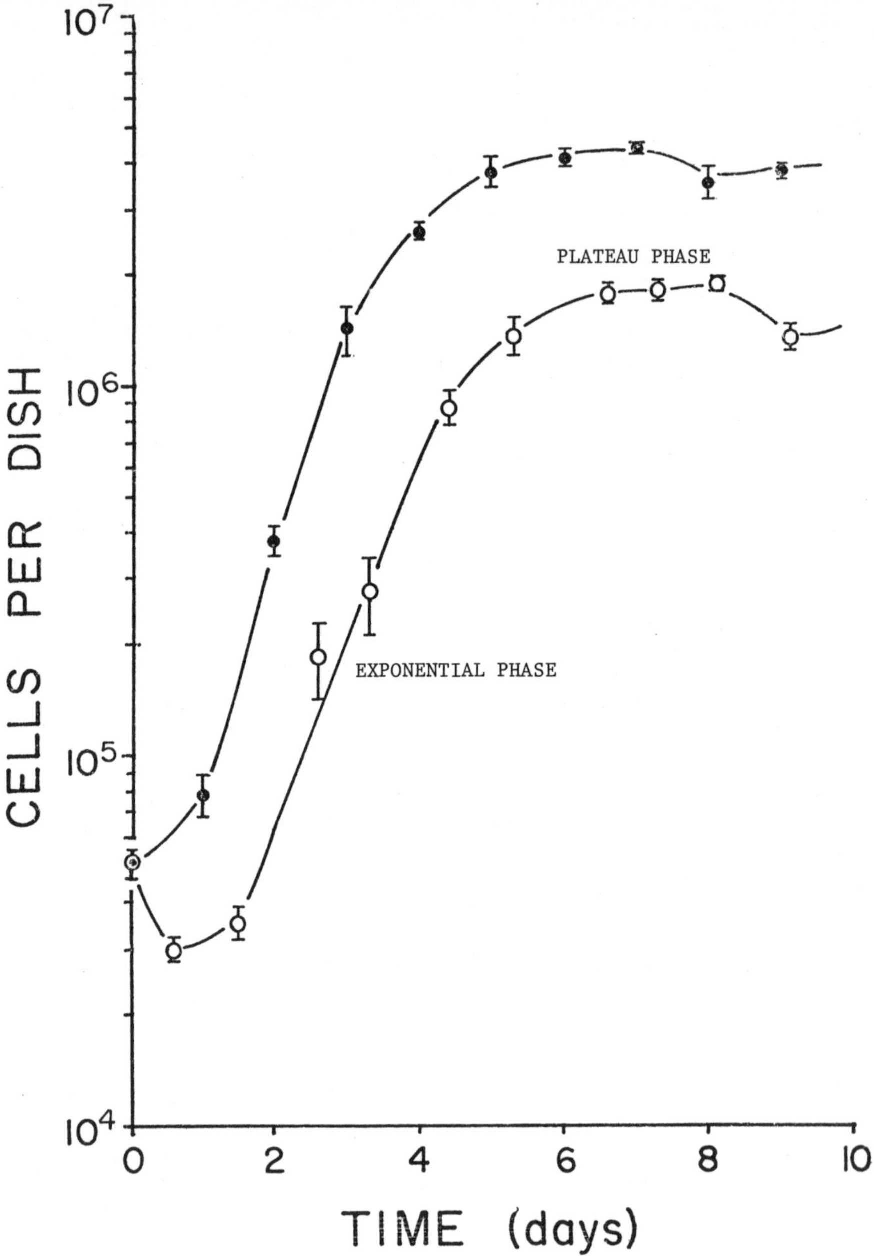

Figure 1. Growth Curves for V-79 Chinese Hamster Cells (Closed Circles) and MTG-B Mouse Mammary Adenocarcinoma Cells (Open Circles) as a Function of Days After Subculture

Session VIII: Panel Discussion. "Data Base and Parameters for Cell Population Models"

Chairperson	*Panelists*
L. Cohen	E. B. Douple
	F. Ellis
	M. L. Griem
	J. Kirk
	U. Rosenow

L. COHEN: All contributors to today's session are invited to discuss an important corollary to our topic—namely, what kind of data do we need in order to decide which if any of these models are applicable.

Dr. Ellis, do you think there are any kinds of clinical data or any specific clinical experiments that would help to define the validity of NSD or other similar systems? What would you like clinical experimenters to do?

ELLIS: I feel that there's good reason to experiment with relatively resistant tumors such as melanoma, fibrosarcoma, rhabdomyosarcoma, and osteogenic sarcoma. Very often these patients have hopeless conditions, so there's good justification, I think, for carrying out randomized clinical trials—finding out, for instance, if large doses given once weekly or with similar long intervals would yield different results from daily treatment with the usual 200 rads per day fraction.

L. COHEN: Do you anticipate getting a different response?

ELLIS: I anticipate curing some of the cancers which you wouldn't cure with the ordinary fractionation system.

DOUPLE: May I comment along those lines? I think more needs to be done in evaluating quantitatively the morbidity following treatment with ionizing radiation. I suggest that we look at the hyperbaric studies, for example, where morbidity is apparently a real problem.

ELLIS: We've got morbidity studies. In carcinoma of the cervix, for instance, we plotted response against dose in rets and have shown the increase in rectal complications with dosage. The effect on the tumor depends on the cell survival parameters for these tumors, and they're probably all different. But the two responses are parallel—you get an increase in the freedom from carcinoma cells in specimens excised, with a curve going up with dose and the incidence of complication going up with a curve that's almost exactly parallel to it.

L. COHEN: I think we could emphasize this question in relation to the tumor registries, or whatever data system is going to be kept, particularly how we should record dosage in every tissue and organ traversed by the beam, because these are the data required to analyze such questions in the future. Dr. Kirk, do you feel there's any special type of clinical experiment that would help to resolve some of the problems in developing your system for application?

KIRK: I should think one of the obvious ones is the matter of gaps in treatment. That is one of the areas where there is the least information.

L. COHEN: Do you want us to do split-course experiments?

KIRK: I think split course experiments would be a help, but in the present literature, experiments with split doses are reported in terms of cure rates, with no comments, or at least none that is practical enough for use about the effect on normal tissue. Another point is that information is scant on the relationship of dose and volume.

L. COHEN: Dr. Rosenow should comment on that. I'm sure he would like every clinician to record as much data as possible on field sizes and volumes.

ROSENOW: There is very little clinical data to which we could apply our formula—especially, data on the reaction of healthy tissue. I don't know if you can do any experiments on that.

L. COHEN: Every day healthy tissue is being irradiated, and every radiotherapy center has been doing so for many years. The problem is to get at the information. Even data on the absence of a reaction is important.

ELLIS: It's not enough just to record the volume. You should record the actual site, and I don't mean by that just whether it's a larynx or an abdomen. I mean which part of the larynx. My belief is, for instance, that the important structure in the irradiated larynx is probably the arytenoid cartilage. If irradiated to a high dose, that cartilage will necrose. Whereas, if you treat the thyroid cartilage—which has a bigger area of perichondrium—it won't necrose because it still has got some nutrition. I feel, therefore, that it's not just a matter of volume in cubic centimeters, but probably—and this is just a suggestion—that it's the proportion of the organ concerned. In the instance I've just mentioned, it's the proportion of the perichondrium of the thyroid cartilage to the whole of that perichondrium that might be important. Clinically, Dr. Wang of Massachusetts General Hospital has said that he finds that if he can keep his radiation rather anterior to the arytenoid cartilage he has much better clinical results. Similarly, we know that if you treat the whole of the lungs you get a very different effect from when you treat just a portion of the volume of the lung.

L. COHEN: You wish to record the fraction of every organ treated?

ELLIS: You may be able to record it by taking radiographs in some instances, and filing copies of the radiographs. That might be important as a way of deciding whether it's volume in cubic centimeters or the proportion of the organ that matters. I think the same thing applies to the bowel. We know it applies to the kidneys.

GRIEM: We've been analyzing the complication of treatment of cancer of the cervix, and we find that the bowel injury is also related to the previous history of inflammatory disease, and previous surgery in the pelvis. I think we have to record not just the treatment parameters but a whole host of factors related to the condition of the patient—whether the patient has hypertension, anemia, and other medical factors.

DOUPLE: Along the lines of what Dr. Ellis has proposed, it seems to me that some type of staging system, an anatomical staging system, perhaps analogous to that used in identifying carcinomas, might be something that might be of value in terms of recording this information.

L. COHEN: Staging the normal tissue volume?

ELLIS: The normal tissue volume related to the dose.

ROSENOW: Could I add just one more remark? In reference to our model in which we consider a certain critical volume of tumor with which the body can cope by the way of immunity. Let's say that the number is 1,000 cells or 10,000 cells below which a tumor would not yet be considered as malignant. So we need some knowledge, too, about which stage, or which number of cells, a tumor could be considered as a critical mass.

RAGAN: There are so many things that could influence the reaction and complicate the design of tumor registry systems. The problem is not to include less in our tumor registry systems, but more—including the diet of the patient during the schedule and a thousand and one other things that may be important.

GHILEZAN: I should like to speak as a clinical radiotherapist about the volume factor. It can be very well correlated with the TMN systems. There is a great difference between the tumorcidal dose necessary for eradicating a tumor which is in the first two stages, compared with a T-3 volume. For a T-3 tumor you need generally 1800 or 1900 rets for eradicating, and only 1700 rets for a T-1 or T-2 lesion.

In regard to reoxygenation and redistribution, there are interesting data about twice-a-day radiation which permits a better redistribution of the cells in the tumor, giving better results obtained in T-3 and T-4 lesions. This kind of approach is useful radiobiologically but also affects the clinical point of view.

With more advanced lesions we have better results with a longer fractionation and a longer protraction. With longer treatment times we have fewer complications. This is true for the larynx and also for abdominal tumors.

SMITH: One difference between the NSD and CRE concepts, as I understand it, is in respect to the variation with number of fractions in the NSD concepts using partial tolerances. If one gives, let's say, one third of the total number of fractions, one gets one third of the total effect; whereas this is not true with CRE. I would like to ask what the other models predict and what the experimental evidence says.

ELLIS: With the NSD concept it's assumed that tolerance is related to cell killing, whereas the CRE is related to a kind of observable clinical effect. That seems to me the essential difference. In the NSD concept you stick to one level of tolerance; in the CRE it tends to cross those levels of tolerance.

KIRK: The difference is really more of a mathematical point of view of your definition of scale. You're trying to reach one endpoint, normal tissue tolerance, and there are many ways you can reach it. You can take different functions that will reach that same point. We've chosen one that is compatible with a concept of scale in which each different level is proportional to dose, which in addition leads to a simplification when you're going to continue radiation. I don't think there's anything more fundamental here than a change of scale.

ELLIS: The things we hear about are what happens in animals or *in vitro* cultures, which tell us the kind of way to think about things. But I believe, if we really want to optimize treatment, we've got to have some way of taking a piece of the tumor and finding out what the cell parameters are. If we can do that, then I think we should be able to make a real advance. This demands a change in technique. It's not enough to show with one or two epithelial tumors, or one or two sarcomas, that they behave in a certain way, because there is a big spread in the behavior of tumors. Every radiotherapist knows of cancers that have got worse during the treatment, while another melts away. We can't assume that what applies to one tumor will apply to another. We can assume that while there are variations in a normal tissue, there is going to be more uniformity in the behavior of normal tissues.

L. COHEN: Dr. Ellis is asking biophysicists and engineers to devise some system whereby we can get feedback of information during treatment so we know what the cell population is in every tissue we irradiate.

V. Workshops

Session IX: Workshop on Computer Program Validation and Documentation

Chairperson
D. J. Wright

Panelists
J. S. Clifton
J. R. Cunningham
J. G. Holt
U. Rosenow

WRIGHT:

The theme of this 5th International Conference includes "Aid to Developing Centers." In this context I define a developing center as one starting to make use of computers for radiation therapy treatment-planning, even though as a therapy department it may have been in existence for many years and has an excellent reputation.

Earlier in this conference the phrase "computer credibility" was used. Originally, computer output was suspect and often laboriously checked by hand calculations, and if a difference was discovered, it was assumed that the latter was correct. I do not recall doing a manual dose distribution for 4096 points, which is what the computer program I use does, so that it seems to have been a somewhat irrelevant evaluation process. Nowadays, computer output is almost considered as divinely inspired and as such cannot err. This approach is probably as bad and certainly inaccurate. Also, earlier this week, it was said that the human is an excellent computer, but a poor hard-copy unit. This is really what we should discuss as validation-documentation.

The American Association of Physicists in Medicine (AAPM) Computer Committee recently discussed a protocol that addresses itself to these problems. The protocol is listed to serve as a starting point for discussion, and after giving some background for this document, I shall ask the panel in turn for their comments before opening the meeting for general discussion.

I am particularly concerned, because of the wide circulation and continued modification of computer programs, that their original validity may be lost. In the United States there are many groups using similar programs—for example, Garrett Holt has a group serviced by a central department at Memorial, New York; there are over 50 PC users; commercial services of computer planning are increasing—and still there are many using their own programs. Even the United Kingdom, with its National Health Service running a computer service, is not immune to the proliferation of programs, since, apparently, there are funds available to develop new programs but no funds available to install equipment to use existing, proven programs. Program proliferation is expensive and just possibly hazardous.

Validation-testing can turn up some odd, unexpected results. Recently, I was testing a program for radium needles and found that it gave dose rates at 2 cm from the perpendicular bisector of a 3 mg needle that were 100 percent in error! Repeating the test for a 30 mg needle gave correct results. This discrepancy lay in a round-off problem due to fixed point calculations. The importance here, however, is that the documentation accompanying the program had not warned me of this problem. A second problem turned up in an external beam program when it was used to calculate a "box" technique for four-field irradiation of the pelvis of a patient who was 45 cm from here to there (laterally). In such a plan the dose to the femoral heads may be of interest and these lay more than 30 cm deep to the contralateral field. The basic TAR data used in the computer program only went to 30 cm and was not extrapolated. Dose values calculated there were garbage. Now this can be lived with if it is known beforehand; otherwise one must be quite astute to recognize invalid output. Yet another, similar problem came to my notice this morning. A friend at another hospital uncovered a program bug when he tried using it for 6 MV planning. Previous testing for Cobalt and 4 MV had not revealed this particular limitation.

So, this is the point—if you ask someone (in the United States) whose program they use, they will probably say "Cunningham's"—but Jack probably doesn't know the individual user who got the program from someone else—probably with many modifications enroute to make it more user-oriented or to fit different computer configurations. The validity of the original program cannot be assumed to hold for its mutated offsprings.

This is why the AAPM Computer Committee feels that some protocol, as listed here, is desirable. Although some details might not be applicable everywhere, we listed those we felt important, and I'll briefly run over the various points.

Responsibility for use of computer-generated data must be accepted by the user and cannot be laid to the original author. I think everyone accepts that. The user must satisfy himself on the suitability and validity of any program he employs. This will entail at least the comparison of results with those obtained by the original author, and comparison with actual measurements which may, in fact, be necessary and are usually desirable. This check becomes more essential if the computer system, the language, or the basic input data for therapy equipment differs from that of the original author. Such a comparison must be made by a radiation physicist or similar expert in radiation.

An author—and this is where we're going to put some work back on a few people—an author who is willing to provide a program for others to use must also provide the following information: flow chart; basic method of calculation with equations; lists of approximations; assumptions and limitations; list or source of basic data used; extent of applicability of the program; some test examples; and the date of the particular version of the program. No user should attempt to use a program for patient care if this information is not available. I gather that there might be some problem to get this sort of information; programs that are supplied by commercial companies, but this probably can be circumvented either by a nondisclosure agreement with the company or by writing your specifications before you hook up with this company, saying precisely what it is that you want.

The AAPM Computer Committee would be willing to serve as a repository of copies of this documentary information, with the idea that the AAPM would contact the authors every so often to find out if there have been any major bugs or updating, we would then arrange to publish this in *Medical Physics.*

For the purposes of this policy statement, the term "author" would be interpreted to cover not only the original individual or institution that supplied the program, but also those who have subsequently modified such a program and have documented their version under the guidelines listed. Currently, the AAPM is planning a series of specific cases of treatment-plan computations as a starting point for validity testing.

CUNNINGHAM:

I agree with you, documentation is of the greatest importance. I might use your list as an agenda and comment on each item in turn.

By "flow chart" I assume you refer to the way the operator interacts with this system, what he does, what he needs, where the information comes in, and where the output goes. This sort of flow chart is more important than a flow-charting of the program calculation, which can be very difficult to read by the nonsophisticated user. In this context advertisements often state that certain programs and computers can be used by people who don't know anything about computers—which, in my estimation, implies very unsophisticated users. In a sense I feel they may be the wrong users, but I may be a little far out on that.

The basic method of calculation is absolutely essential and must be included in the documentation. By this I mean a statement of the physics of the calculations, the physical assumptions, what approximations are made, and what limitations exist (e.g. does the data go beyond 30 cm). My earlier programs had that limit, previously referred to, but now they include extrapolation, which naturally is less good the farther you go; so the results are perhaps just new garbage. This really also concerns the applicability of the program.

A list or source of basic data that are used is absolutely essential to the documentation, as is the date of the particular version of the program. It's almost incredible, to my mind, that programs and calculations are made without references, or a statement of where the basic data came from and where it was tested—but this happens often.

Much of this is housekeeping, essential but not very rewarding. I recall getting a phone call from someone who wanted to know why they got a particular answer, using "my" program. I did not know the caller or where he got the program but when he sent me his problem (well documented) it appeared he had used a program listing dated differently from the documentation he had. Luckily the housekeeping had been done and his problem could be sorted out.

HOLT:

I basically agree with the points that have been raised. Documentation will not clear up all the problems of misuse, or the problem of programs obtained "through the back door," since these may have been changed in innumerable ways unknown to the original authors.

If we are to produce a document (similar to that we are discussing), it should include guidance as to how one can test the program. This is perhaps an even more important aspect of our concern. For instance, turnkey systems like the PC 12 or RAD 8 are initially made to be a black box to the user, and one should, in a sense, protect oneself by receiving guidance as to how this black box may be tested. Manufacturers, to some extent, were not quite aware of all the limitations of their programs, and for other reasons they may be somewhat reluctant to disclose all the contents of the black box. This is just like a dangerous drug—its inherent danger and usefulness should be known and should be *made* known. It is even more necessary when equipment is distributed to people relatively unknowledgeable in computer applications.

There are, I'm sure, tests one can devise to check the validity of a program systematically. However, all programs probably have hidden features that their authors are unaware of. One of our programs occasionally gave strange answers. Their strangeness was evident to an experienced treatment-planner but could be overlooked by a less experienced individual. The wrong answers could be prevented by fudging the input by a millimeter but it was some years before the reason for the program fault was found. This is no protection, and no tests can be devised against such a problem, since one doesn't know where the error is going to occur. It is necessary to devise a test that is most likely to cause trouble if the software has some unforeseen strange features to it.

There are several points to be considered in any kind of system. First would be the inherent accuracy of the computation model, from the physics aspect. Unless calculations of the Monte Carlo type are used, one is bound to use a simplified model that imposes conceptual or physical limitations. Even a simple model is not calculated to its fullest capability of accuracy in most computer programs, if only because of limitations imposed by the economics of storage. These limits, as Jack Cunningham pointed out, should be known.

Some statement is needed about the accuracy of peripheral hardware and its limitations. For example, digitizers may have inherent inaccuracy in this transfer, and although the stored data may be accurate, a simple copy of the display (for instance by Polaroid camera) may have a good chance of transferring a significant error. Again, the user should be made aware explicitly of this possibility of error.

A third point is the interpretability of output. Now that's a terrible word, but I couldn't find a better word. I mean, by it, what does the printout we get really mean? How have the results been normalized? Frequently, a program based on TARs is normalized to the dose ("in air") to a miniphantom without the patient present, and this result would be altogether different from a "skin dose" normalization. A more complex normalization interpretation would apply to a noniso-centric, non coplanar, multiple-field plan. It is necessary, then, that the output of a program be clearly stated, with all its implications. In our time-sharing network we have some seventy-five users, and daily we get calls—from physicists—for aid in interpreting output. One should have a very clear explanation of what comes from the black box of a standalone system.

If the suggested protocol is adopted, it should be more than just a document consisting of tests and illustrations. It should give guidance to the user as to what he should expect in a good treatment-planning system. Many potential users have heard arguments about big versus small machines and don't know which system to choose. In the suggested document it would be possible to list what could be reasonably expected and what is possible so far as the state of the art is concerned. What can the system do? Versatility is, of course, a matter of choice. Another important point is convenience. How are data acquired and displayed? Is the system interactive? Much of this is actually related to cost, and cost is important, but cost is also related to accuracy, because all these features are interrelated. Our panel should give the prospective user some idea of the interplay between these various aspects; accuracy of computation model, accuracy of peripherals, interpretation of results, versatility, convenience, and cost.

CLIFTON:

I will start with your protocol as an initial document, in an attempt to be provocative and, I trust, neither rude nor insulting.

It strikes me as a document written by physicists, for physicists, and as far as a computer program is concerned, it looks entirely at symptoms, not cause. One could easily translate this into a second-hand car salesman's spiel.

Responsibility: You buy a second-hand car, you're the driver. You are responsible if you run somebody over with it.

Validity: If you buy a second-hand car, you must satisfy yourself it has a steering wheel and a wheel on each corner.

Documentation: This is precisely what a second-hand car salesman would use. He would say, "Look, the body work is first class; it's got jolly good chrome fenders, new mufflers; two radios"—and what have you. What he doesn't tell you is the state of the motor, and has the car any brakes?

This is, I think, the hub of the problem. The fact is, it does not matter what program you are trying to transfer from place to place unless you document what goes on within the computer.

We have been talking about the periphery of the problem. I'm going to be a bit heretical, but most of our dosimetry programs have been written by physicists to solve dosimetry problems without regard to how the compiler in the computer goes about its business. We heard Garrett Holt refer to unexplained glitches in his program, and the only way to lick this problem is to bury FORTRAN. Any time you have *GO TO* statements and programs with multiple ports of entry, you can never guarantee what will happen when you run them on another machine. We have to go over to a compiler like ALGOL or PL/1, where you can use a modular structure and define specifically what each module does, with one way into it and one way out.

There is where I come back to documentation. It is necessary to document specifically the interface between modules and how it operates. Only then can you transfer programs between computer systems with a reasonable hope that they will run without getting some strange bugs. Common statements are a frequent source of such bugs—particularly if matrix calculations are done.

Somewhere right at the start of this documentation one must include information about how the programming is done. I do not see how you will ever satisfactorily document the straggly dosimetry programs we have now. They may be good physics dosimetry, but they are awful computer techniques.

ROSENOW:

It seems that not much has been left for me. I would like to consider the first point on your list—responsibility—because I think we must keep the various responsibilities in mind before thinking of documentation. I don't quite agree that responsibility rests with the user. Consider not the second-hand car but the first-hand treatment machine. Although the main responsibility for the application of radiation lies with the physician, the radiotherapist, a good deal of responsibility rests with the manufacturer and also with the physicist.

I think the same applies to a program, at least to one distributed not only commercially but also, somehow, officially. Part of the responsibility lies with the author (the manufacturer), and another part with the user, split up into the responsibility of the physician and maybe the physicist or computernik. In the future this situation may become more frequent, with departments without physicists or computer specialists available but using a computer program. There may be many users with no local persons familiar with the program details.

Documentation has two aspects. One is the documentation of the program itself—but that ranks second in my list of priorities. Most important, I think, is the User Handbook, giving sufficient detail to allow the physician, especially, to take over responsibility for applying this program. So I see documentation for application as a separate problem from documentation of what is in the black box.

Again, by analogy to the use of the treatment machine, there should be regulations—possibly legal—containing minimal requirements that must be fulfilled to use a program for radiation treatment-planning. Other working parties, including one in Germany, have tried setting up standards in this area, but their results are only recommendations without a legal base. I think it is very important to make such standards, with respect to the use, the application of a program, rather than with respect to the documentation of the program itself. These standards should cover such questions as how the output of the program is used, and what assurance is there that the output is regularly checked by the user?

One final point. The suggested protocol mentions a test example to be supplied with the program. I think it is very important that test examples covering the whole range of applications in a department (and this may vary from department to department) be provided. These examples should be run regularly every month or so to be sure, as far as we can, that the program is running consistently.

WRIGHT:

We had envisaged two types of test examples. The first one would be supplied to me by the person that I got the program from so that I can check if my equipment reproduces his result—a check really on any adaptive changes required by my configuration. The second type is more of the kind you mentioned: a test of applicability of the particular programs to my particular needs.

Garrett, how do you handle this question of responsibility among the members of the Memorial Network?

HOLT:

The legal responsibilities are a nebulous question that will not be resolved unless a decision—some court judgment—is made. We assume responsibility for the maintenance of software and the development of programs. To this end we insist that potential users spend time at our institution in training before they become operative. It is a joint responsibility, though we assume the moral responsibility for program integrity. The legality has not been challenged in almost ten years of operation.

CUNNINGHAM:

I represent, in a sense, the opposite end of a Gaussian distribution of opinion regarding responsibility. I've taken a different approach, because of different conditions but probably both mine and Garrett Holt's are equally reasonable. I have no idea of who now has my programs or how they may have been modified. I have assumed they are in the public domain and now the property of whoever uses them. As far as I know this has never been tested legally.

HOLT:

There are innumerable versions of our programs circulating, some of them obtained through the back door. Some may be very old, and for them we obviously have no responsibility.

CUNNINGHAM:

The two situations may not be very different. I've done one thing which generally may or may not be useful. I have dispensed pieces of paper—program listings. Partly, it was on purpose as the only operational way to do it, but partly it was so that the receiver could do what he liked with it, except that he had to process it—to type it in—to make it a program. He was now the possessor, the owner of that program. I think the responsibility might change if the user received a tape or disc or deck of cards and did not process it himself. I operate this way also for the selfish reason that when a person is interactive with the program to the extent of getting it running, he has then solved a lot of problems and got rid of some bugs. He'll need to ask me fewer questions. This is a self-protecting thing.

I wanted to raise a point about the user of a program. There are two concepts here—the actual user and the responsible user. The former may be a technician operating the console under the direction of someone else who may be a physicist or radiotherapist. One should clarify and distinguish between these two users and the two different situations they pose.

WRIGHT:

I think this is comparable to the relation between a technologist setting up a therapy patient (the actual user) and a radiotherapist (the responsible user). In the context of the suggested protocol, the "user" would have to be the responsible user—the therapist possibly, because other people in his department are blanketed by his coverage.

CUNNINGHAM:

I raise this point particularly in the context of documentation because the documentation required for these two different people is quite different.

CLIFTON:

I think there is a third class of user here. Our discussion has concerned itself with documentation for a user who wants to use the program as it stands. In my experience, most physicists are ornery enough to want to change it. This will require a different degree of documentation and a different degree of validation to that which would satisfy a user who is using the unaltered program.

Test examples have been mentioned. They are fine but have certain limitations, the basic one being that the correct operation of the program for one or two test examples can immediately create a false sense of security. If someone else runs the test, and it works, he says "O.K., the system flies." Many years ago our first treatment-planning program ran on an old Elliot-80 machine and was the only program that used all the core. After a month the manufacturer started using it to test the core, since it would throw up parity bugs undetectable by their own tests.

ROSENOW:

Wouldn't you agree that regular checks on a therapy machine don't give a false feeling of security? I think that is a comparable situation and in the same way you have to make regular checks on the program —not just an initial check once and for all.

PROGRAM LANGUAGES

RENNER:

I think that the suggested protocol should state that the program language be specified precisely—not just as FORTRAN or PL/1 but as the particular extended form of that language. Frequently, people are unaware that they are using an extended language that is not a universal extension. This raises a further question. If you have a program written in a standardized language (whatever that means), can you assume that when it is transferred to another computer, of another manufacturer, with different compilation, it will run if both manufacturers have guaranteed that their machines use the same standard language?

PRASAD:

I do not agree that FORTRAN is not a useful and convenient language. Many institutions (certainly in this country) have physicists whose programming capabilities are limited to FORTRAN. If one dispenses with it, then programs will be limited to a few highly sophisticated institutions with large computer capabilities.

LIDOFSKY:

I am involved in teaching elementary programming courses. They are given in ALGOL or PL/1 or FORTRAN or BASIC—it doesn't make a bit of difference, each can be learned easily. The big problem is that all of these languages are not available on all machines. In the United States currently you are almost sure to settle on FORTRAN 4. People should be urged to use PL/1 or ALGOL as they become more generally available.

HAHN:

The computer-science community is beginning to make inroads on the problems of a specific language with what is called structured programming. With it we are talking of modular programs, each module having a very specific input function and output, and we try to avoid *GO TO*'s which make programs perform in a crazy way. FORTRAN is not an ideal language for structured programs, but it is one we have to use and one we'll be with for a long, long time.

DREW:

I'm sorry Clifton hasn't defended himself on the use of FORTRAN or ALGOL. I believe the question is not how easy it is to use or transfer a language but how easy it is to validate the program. A program of 200-300 lines is virtually impossible to validate. Test cases only prove it works for those test situations. As long as there are *GO TO's* and common statements the program may flip out. We have to make sure that is impossible, and a structured modular program is needed. FORTRAN really cannot handle this. Surely if we learn FORTRAN, we can learn ALGOL or PL/1.

JAMESON:

If you set your mind to it, programs can be written that are transferable from machine to machine. We set out with this objective and have run programs on five different manufacturers' equipment, and they've run easily. The first time we transferred, there was a certain amount of work, but after that the subsequent transfers were very easy.

ROTHMEIER:

The topic of computer languages is always a fun one and ought to be worth a couple of days' sessions. It is possible that FORTRAN is not optimum. ALGOL and PL/1 are neat but not often used. The reason that some FORTRAN programs may have unpredicted outcomes is that the programmer himself has not been educated in a good style of programming.

CLIFTON:

I thought that when I said we should bury FORTRAN I would get this reaction. Many of us use FORTRAN. However, the basic construction of the language is such that if we continue using it, validation of programs is a nonstarter—simply because of the re-entry type of statement that you have in FORTRAN. You can never, ever be certain what the computer does when it compiles such a program. Many people use FORTRAN, and we will go on using it, but we ought to start looking at things like PL/1—they are a lot better.

PROGRAM TESTING

HOLT:

Although documentation of programs is necessary, this is going to be difficult to obtain. I know in our institution we have no funding for it. We have one man furiously writing programs but hardly any of them are really thoroughly documented in the way the protocol suggests. However, most of us that use these programs know some of their weaknesses and could devise a series of tests designed to bring out errors. To start simply, one can test that the program reproduces a certain beam distribution and then proceed to devise tests of difficult mathematical points, such as boundaries between contours—in other words how does the program handle critical situations? All of us know many of these situations, and it should be possible to give the user such a set of problems for his computer to solve. The proper execution of these problems, or the satisfactory explanation of what happens in these cases, will help the user understand how the program performs, what its limitations are, and how to interpret the output.

WRIGHT:

May I pose a question to the rest of the panel? Do you think an international working group could be set up to follow Holt's suggestion and devise a series of test programs? Naturally, the needs of different users vary and a test set may not be all-inclusive, but for very specific problems (for instance, that of adjacent contours) would this be feasible?

ROSENOW:

This is similar to checking one program against another, and it is not possible to provide test examples for all different programs since they need differently structured input data. If you don't provide this input data in the appropriate form for each program this would not work.

CLIFTON:

On the face of it, it's worth while, but can one do it quickly enough? One is trying to evaluate a basically dynamic area. By the time a test procedure is established and tried on a program, the programmer already has advanced to a newer version of the program which invalidates the test.

CUNNINGHAM:

I don't know whether the idea is possible and I'm not sure I feel it's desirable. Devising a state of mind for testing is possibly desirable. The operation of a program in a computer is the use of a tool—and the tool itself is irrelevant—but the operation of the program is to make a statement of physical fact. In this context, the fact is an absorbed dose at a point in a patient, or something analogous. The test is, then, is the prediction correct? So the test method is the same as for any other physical fact, i.e. an experiment to confirm it. So I'm not sure one can devise test examples; one can devise models, but I think a state of mind has to be engendered so that if you make a statement you must check it.

WRIGHT:

Certainly the final test has to be against actual measurements. A subcommittee of the AAPM Computer Committee has been toying with the problem. I found that six years ago a similar group was doing the same—trying to get an all-inclusive list—and getting nowhere. We decided recently on a new approach. First let us run a few very simple, even trivial, tests as a pilot scheme to get our hands wet and learn the problems of running tests per se. We chose a single needle, a plane implant and a Fletcher-Suit after-loading radium applicator—with no external beams—they would be harder. We are expecting data on these from ten groups (so far we have three). We are just looking at the mechanics of getting various groups to run similar problems. When we've got that under control, then we can consider how to evaluate the results that have been supplied. When we've got all the data, we expect to publish our experiences in *Medical Physics*.

RESPONSIBILITY AND DOCUMENTATION

SUNTHARALINGAM:

Having heard the discussion so far, I feel we have only muddied the water. There are two aspects to the whole problem: the turnkey system and the institution with programming expertise.

A turnkey system has a commercial aspect and there are different motivations and competition between the manufacturers. The term "turnkey" implies a black box that the user will not be interfering with. He will follow the instruction manual and try to get an answer. Now it is left to the responsibility of the purchaser. Am I satisfied with just this or can I get additional information about the black box from the manufacturer? As with other items in radiation therapy, the purchaser can write his strict specifications and requirements and if the manufacturer of the black box is willing to give this documentation, then he may have a sale.

The institution that has developed its own program represents the other aspect. They may have sufficient documentation—for their own use—and are happy with it. If, now, I as an interested party want to use their program, it is *my* responsibility—not that of the author—to try to find out what assumptions were used, what information is available, and whether the program will be suitable for my application. I should take the responsibility to evaluate this.

The examples given by the chairman were not proper simply because they do not represent the case of the actual user. If you do not use the programs routinely, you may not be aware of limitations,, whereas if the problem is posed to routine users, they will probably be aware of its restrictions already. We should commend institutions that have developed programs for their use. They are not trying to be the number one car salesman, they have generated programs for themselves, and we who may be interested in going to these individuals must assume responsibility for what we get.

I am disturbed that the suggested protocol is placing additional responsibility and work on an author, just because he is willing to help another institution. Perhaps this could be reworded. If I want to use his program I should try to get what I need—the basic assumptions, list of basic tables—we should not require the author to supply this.

JAMESON:

When we went to a time-share company, initially the contract said that the company would not be responsible if anything went wrong with our work. We protested, and since we had the backing of a government agency, this was changed and responsibilities are to be shared. This does show that responsibilities can be shared within the whole system.

KIJEWSKI:

A great many programs are developed under government grants and I think they should be distributed as widely as possible, but it is with the documentation that many of these programs fall down. No one can use them because the author has not bothered to write down what he has done. I think the protocol should be very strongly worded that we demand from the author that this documentation exist.

KARZMARK:

Documentation is important. As to the debate whether the author or the user should supply it, I think the author, as defined in the suggested protocol is uniquely capable of providing it. However, if you impose too many requirements on him, his good will may become exhausted. There has to be some mechanism of support for this documentation. Certainly you want it in hard copy, and if you ask the author to provide it, he will make some special effort to ensure the validity of his documentation and exclusion of dubious statements. This is essential and costly. Prospectively you could require authors to document programs as they are developed. Retrospectively, for programs developed five or ten years ago by public money, I doubt if this can be done, though conceptually it is desirable.

CUNNINGHAM:

The references to public money are absolute red herrings in an international situation. No money that is going into a program developed in Sweden has relevance to public money in Canada . . .

KARZMARK:

But if documentation is to be supplied widely, there will be costs involved, and imposing specific requirements may incur costs for which additional funds have to be sought.

I believe the protocol should also include a point Wright alluded to. One does develop an awareness of bugs in existing programs, and there should be a mechanism to investigate them (preferably with some degree of confidentiality) and to correct them, as this is an important part of overall responsibility.

DREW:

One thing has disturbed me all week, and I think it has been forgotten this morning as well, and that is the patient. Nearly everything we have been dealing with is geared toward treating some poor blighter on the stretcher—and we gaily talk about bugs, gaily talk about the program that may or may not work, forgetting the shattering effect it will have when this bug crops up. We are dealing with human life and have to be far more careful in approaching the use of computers. We are developing somewhat of a cavalier attitude, but we are not producing programs for credit-card billing, where mistakes can be corrected. Documentation is part of this. We can't force an author to provide documentation, but we should strongly recommend to any user that he not get or use a program that has not been thoroughly documented.

LIDOFSKY:

What is in it for an author to take the trouble to document a program? Somehow he has to gain some advantage from this effort. A well documented program in a repository constitutes a worth-while publication, and this may be, in a sense, the author's reward. If the program was grant-aided and such a publication results, then it may be easier to get another grant.

RENNER:

If the author of an undocumented program should die, you may as well bury the program with him. I find it very necessary to document my own programs, so that a colleague can take it over when I am on vacation, or just because five years from now I may not remember what I did in a program I wrote.

JAMESON:

Frequently, a lot of time can be wasted working on some one else's program, because one thing is missing. You may have what the author has written, his scientific ideas and his approximations, but what you do not have is why he had done it this particular way.

HAHN:

What we're talking about here is, obviously, a continuum. At one end is the ideal document, which I think has never been generated and probably never will be. At the other end is the program with absolutely no documentation. Obviously we're all interested in transferability—nobody wants to do over and over again what has been done before—and obviously we all want ideal documentation. However, if the program is going to be worth while for you to replicate, you will ask for it even with no documentation; and as Cunningham says, you might do a better job through being forced to learn it the hard way.

This does point up the fact that undoubtedly the responsibility must rest with the user. Since we cannot predict the performance of any program under all circumstances, we must have a responsible person who reviews the output and evaluates if it is right or obviously wrong. The suggested protocol looks pretty good, I think. It is a realizable, workable set of program descriptions and is something to aim at.

We have been talking about a marriage between physicists in medicine and computer scientists. What Clifton calls a limitation of certain programming languages is really a limitation of computer science. What we need is good computer science practice and a good programmer who will do thorough meaningful documentation because he needs it for himself and he needs it for his institution, and hopefully he would like others to use his program.

ROTHMEIER:

I'd like to come back to the question of who does the documentation, and that is always a problem. Some people argue that the author is the best one to do it because he knows it best, and other people argue that the receiver is the best one to do it because there is no better way to learn the program. The question of incentive here is definitely important. There's got to be some mechanism to provide incentive, and there's nothing like paying someone for documentation because it just takes a lot of time.

Now the second point is that your proposed documentation does not include computer-programming documentation. That's probably something that shouldn't be left out, depending upon the purpose of the documentation. If the purpose is for some other programmer to maintain it, then you have to have more detailed documentation, and that's a bigger job. Some of this can be handled by forms with checklists, or lexicons of all the variables in a program, and that alone may be enough to get a new program started. A definition of the data base used is another essential part of this documentation. I would guess that an author of a program could provide that documentation in a day or two, if he knows the program. Programmer-oriented documentation probably takes weeks, though it really depends on the size of the program. Our discussion on documentation of approximations and assumptions has focused on the dosimetry problem, but I wonder if it could be broadened to include things that may be more specifically relevant to information systems as well.

A PROTOCOL FOR COMPUTER PROGRAMS

HENDERSON:

At the last meeting at Uppsala, there was considerable discussion on standardization of terms used in radiotherapy, particularly with regard to radiotherapy equipment, and there was a proposal to sort of set up a working group to continue this. In the meantime, the IEC [International Electrotechnical Commission] has started producing draft recommendations and, in particular, Technical Committee 62 deals with electrical equipment in medical practice.

Just one aspect of it, the safety aspect, covers 285 pages of fine print. A subcommittee of TC 62 deals with high energy equipment and equipment for nuclear medicine, and a particular subset of that has produced information on beam teletherapy and particle accelerators which does cover movements used and is relevant to the computer programs.

I feel that the standardization aspects of programs would come under the IEC. It is hoped that their recommendations are incorporated into the standards of individual countries. Their documents have sections on safety and documentation which could well apply to much of what we have been discussing, the documentation of the equipment and use of equipment.

The point that I would like to make is that, as far as I can see, there is no subcommittee of the TC 62 which is specifically dealing with computers. It might well be that some working group from this Conference could produce—or make the nucleus of—some protocol document that could be taken over and incorporated in the IEC.

CLIFTON:

We are concerned, in the end, with the treating of patients, and we have spent most of this morning's discussion concerned with documentation. I'd like, therefore, to make just two comments, in summary, on those two points, First, we *are* treating patients. If you treat patients with any form of drugs, the drug house that provides you with a drug is required by law to tell you of the known side effects of that drug. I see no reason at all why, if you use turnkey systems or similar systems are put on the market for radiation treatment-planning, the known side effects of those programs should not be equally specified.

The second point is this: any documentation you receive on any program you should view in exactly the same way that you would view the reference for a would-be employee. Namely, you read it, and you consider not only what is there but what it does not say, because that's what you need to know.

CHU:

I should like to ask how the AAPM would implement such a protocol as we have discussed? A computer program repository is a voluntary group of users. If I wish to use a particular program, it's because I know of its source—not because it is registered at a repository. If the repository receives a program, they are merely a committee who can only review the write-ups but are without ways of testing the program and verifying the documentation. The protocol is a guideline for the author, but the validation of a program still rests with the author. If someone uses an undocumented program, how are you going to reprimand him?

WRIGHT:

The intent of the protocol was to serve as a guideline for users. The items listed are those we felt should be documented. The validity tests were purely a starting point for the users. There is no suggestion that the repository (AAPM committee or other groups) will pass judgment on whether a program is good. The suggestion is rather that there would be available a suggested series of test examples against which the prospective user could test a program. We are not providing a Good Housekeeping Seal of Approval.

GOITEIN:

The only thing certain in life is program failure. We seem to be seeking a comforting certainty, a safety guarantee that can never be given. No program can be uniquely defined, and the possibilities, allowing for microsecond cycle time and the permutation and combinations of work, are infinite. What we are trying to do is not set up a formula with exactitude but instead improve reliability of what we are doing by setting benchmarks and guidelines.

A protocol must reflect the great difference between a purchased turnkey system and somebody's program that is given to you. There are two things this committee should offer regarding turnkey systems. First are the guidelines to physicists, as to how they exercise the responsibility that they will be saddled with. What is an adequate set of tests? How should they establish the validity of the turnkey system? Something specific—for example, what a complete check might involve—would be helpful. It is very vexing if the manufacturer has not provided the basic source of data, the method of computation, and the fundamental physics involved. The actual physics may be very different from what was intended. One particular area of concern would be the interpolation procedures, which are very important and can produce errors of factors of two in certain regions with unsophisticated methods.

It is also helpful to have guidelines for what one might reasonably ask for with a borrowed program. Of course, our in-house programs may have a different level of documentation; they may have known bugs and unworkable options. I know it and can handle it, but I would not let these out in this form.

KARZMARK:

The problem of protocol and whether people will follow it, I think, is an important question. I think I would agree with Dr. Rosenow that, initially, such protocols are exemplary, and I think you'll find that even manufacturers, to the extent feasible, will tend to follow them. In fact, in many areas manufacturers are looking to larger organizations to set standards and specifications, because otherwise they find themselves in the unenviable position of having every single customer set individual specifications, and that is chaotic for them.

CUNNINGHAM:

I think probably many aren't aware that, on the international scale, the IAEA convened a panel on this subject last fall. One of the panel recommendations was that the IAEA ought to act in some form as a repository of programs. The real context there was aid to developing nations or developing centers. But there is, in that sense, a mechanism for an international repository of programs.

SUNTHARALINGAM:

Mr. Chairman, I was wondering if we can formally, at this international conference, make a request to the international body, the IAEA, asking if they could undertake the setting up of a committee to look into this matter of protocol, rather than have each individual country, through their physics organizations, doing it. Committees in individual organizations often lack financial support. If the financial support comes from an international organization, and an international committee is set up, some action may be forthcoming with benefits similar to those received by radiation therapy over the last ten years through other international committees.

ROSENOW:

We have some very incisive regulations in different fields of radiation application—for example, radiation protection, use of isotopes, and use of treatment machines; also in the field of electrical safety, and so on. But there are no such regulations in the field of radiation treatment-planning, and especially in the field of computer applications. I think it is very necessary that we have some sort of legal base for doing this kind of job, especially in the situation where a program is developed in a department, or taken over from another department using this program. I think in view of the patient and in view of the doctors using this program, it is very important to supply the radiotherapist with any means to accept these responsibilities. He should have the possibility of knowing as much about the program or the system used as is necessary to apply it safely and correctly to the patient. In the case of an in-house program, maybe only the physicist or the computer specialist knows all the details. We have to somehow protect the doctor, the applying physician, against any probable errors or mistakes which can be made with this program. So I think it would be very good if someone, maybe some international committee, would set up a list of minimal requirements, especially in respect to the handling, or application of programs for radiation treatment.

HOLT:

I also feel that there is a strong need to provide the documents that will give some guidance to a responsible user, somewhat along the lines that have been discussed. I feel that, desirable though it might be, it would take longer working through an international committee than it would if it were handled by a local committee.

WRIGHT:

In conclusion, may I say I feel that the sense of the group here today, both on the floor and on the platform, is in favor of motherhood and the protocol, and I would suggest, unless there's any strong disagreement, that I will contact the members of this panel, and that in the

Proceedings of this conference, a document similar to this AAPM proposal, with perhaps some of the additions that were referred to from the floor and from the panel, will be incorporated.

A PROTOCOL FOR COMPUTER PROGRAMS IN RADIATION THERAPY

being a document derived from discussion by the AAPM Computer Committee, with modifications from discussions at the Fifth International Conference

(1) *Responsibility*: Resides with the user, not the original author.
Comment: Author in this context means *any* supplier of a program. If a turnkey system is used, it is possible that the responsibility may be shared with the supplier.

(2) *Validity*: The user must satisfy himself that a program is valid for his purposes. This will probably involve running a series of tests; making comparisons with radiation measurements made by a radiation physicist; and running some tests of constancy of program operation.

(3) *Documentation*: The following items require documentation before any attempt to use the results for patient care is undertaken.
- (a) Flow chart (showing inputs and outputs of system).
- (b) Basic method of calcuation.
- (c) Lists of approximations, assumptions, and limitations (both of soft and hard ware).
- (d) Listing (or source) of basic data used.
- (e) Extent of program applicability (e.g. types of therapy equipment for which the program has been used).
- (f) Test examples so user can decide that program changes have not distorted the operation.
  (Comment: These tests are conceptually different from those recommended as validity tests.)
- (g) Date of version of program.
- (h) Description of program language (and extension) of the original version.

Comment: Good computer-programming science methodology should result in such documentation being routinely produced for each new program. This is to be strongly recommended. Retrospective documentation becomes extremely difficult. Modular programming is to be preferred as leading to more easily defined program operation and reliability.

(4) *Program repository*: A repository with the capability to publish updated information should be set up. AAPM has offered to do this, but IAEA might be more logical.
Comment: The main reason for this stems from the way programs

have been disseminated widely from their original sources. Original authors do not know who may be using their older programs. Those users may need documentation which the original authors now do not utilize. A central repository could serve as a resource in these cases. The repository would not carry any responsibility for program validation.

(5) *Protocol Implementation*: This protocol could be promulgated by an international body. It could be agreed to by national groups. Subsequently it would then be the preferred approach, and usage by turnkey system designers and others could lead to rapid implementation.

Session X: Reports of Workshop Directors on the Establishment of an International Radiotherapy Data Bank

Chairperson	*Panelists*	
F. W. Lane	J. M. S. Prewitt	M. L. Griem
	J. A. Henry	M. Stovall
	L. Cohen	L. Davis
	D. P. Ragan	B. Olsen
	S. Clampitt	

LANE:

The session this morning is devoted to the concept of an international radiotherapy data bank. For many years, radiotherapists have collected statistics as a means of analyzing past performance. With the advent of computers, the temptation to collect has been difficult to resist, and computerized radiation therapy registries have proliferated at an amazing rate. The time has now arrived to combine efforts to develop a more efficient method of collecting statistics. Through national or international cooperation, the possibility exists to develop a large data bank which could be used for a number of purposes:

(1) to determine radiation effect on normal and malignant tissue
(2) to define end results of treatment with some statistical validity (and)
(3) to act as a substitute for randomized clinical trials as a basis for the evaluation of radiation therapy techniques.

This concept was raised initially at the Second International Conference on the Use of Computers in Radiation Therapy at Chicago. At that time the opinion was expressed that "given proper cooperation, it should be possible to arrange uniform collection and analysis of data throughout the world." It was considered necessary first to agree on the desirability of this concept, and, secondly, to decide on the ways of accomplishing it. The principle gained some support, but the mechanism for accomplishing the desired end was never vigorously pursued. At the Third International Conference in 1970, the concept again surfaced. Frank Ellis proposed that data should be "collected if possible on an international scale, since the more cases embraced by the scheme, the greater would be the significance of analyzed results." Various facts of the problem were considered, and a vigorous exchange of ideas took place, but again there was little dialogue after the adjournment of the conference.

At Uppsala, two years ago, the working group in radiobiology again took up the torch. Under the chairmanship of Dr. Moller of Gottenburg, and with the aid of such present congress members as Judith Prewitt, Lionel Cohen, James Kirk, and Stig Stenson, a statement was made that "the group considered it would be of great value to collect statistics on an international basis as a data bank for radiation effect on normal and tumor tissue. From this data bank, any topic of interest could be studied and cure rates could be assessed with sufficient statistical significance." In the immediate post-congress period, Judith Prewitt traveled to Geneva to present to the I.U.C.C. a proposal sponsored by the National Cancer Institute regarding such a radiotherapy data bank. This was enthusiastically received, but no further commitment was made.

In short, after six years relatively little progress has been made. The desirability of a data bank seems reasonably established, but the actual mechanics of accomplishing it are still unsettled. It has been frequently stressed that the aim of this particular conference is to point the way toward a determination of future efforts in the radiation therapy computer fields, rather than to describe the current state of the art. Under this directive, it was decided to use the occasion of this Fifth International Conference to promote the long overdue radiation therapy data bank. To this end workshops were held which were directed toward the following topics: goals of a data bank; information requirements; mechanisms of handling data, quality control, and mechanics of informational security. Subchairmen were assigned to summarize the consensus of these workshops for the session this morning.

Before these papers are presented, however, I should like to make one further comment. In addition to considering the format of a registry, I think this conference should take the giant second step of determining the mechanisms of actually establishing such an entity. This would entail establishment of an on-going international committee with responsibility to lay the foundation for such a cooperative venture; to determine the location and repository for the data bank; and to report back to the next international conference the feasibility of such a venture. I doubt that an international registry will ever be established if we talk about it only on a biennial basis at these conferences. We need interconference work, and a committee to do it.

REPORTS OF WORKSHOP DIRECTORS

PREWITT: *Goals for an International Radiotherapy Data Bank*

The working group on registry goals started with the assumption that there was interest in exchanging information about oncologic radiation therapy on an international level, and went on to consider the functions which such an effort might fulfill. The primary purpose, of course, is the improvement of health care delivery through critical evaluation of past experience and careful planning of prospective clinical trials.

Computer usage in radiotherapy is well accepted for compiling archives, scheduling patients, and constructing empirically reasonable treatment plans. During the conference at Dartmouth we have seen excellent examples of such endeavors. Attention should now turn toward mechanisms for improving the end results of therapy by utilizing computer-based radiobiologically motivated, and clinically validated treatment models of optimum therapy regimes. Pilot studies by several radiotherapists and biomathematicians indicate that this is both feasible and worth while. A radiotherapy data base representing a large collective clinical experience associated with a companion radiobiological research data base is of utmost importance for this endeavor.

First, the establishment of such a data base would lead to acceptable standardization of the medical record, which could facilitate an exchange of ideas not only in radiotherapy but also in other fields of medical practice.

Secondly, with a broad-base coverage, a retrospective data base could partially substitute for prospective clinical trials designed to assess protocols and optimization criteria.

Thirdly, retrospective data could give us information on extreme dosages—data that are unattainable now because of moral and legal restraints.

Fourthly, it could help determine whether present differences in techniques are major or inconsequential, and whether meaningful gain can be expected from applying the fine details of cell and tissue kinetics.

Lastly, these data bases could form the basis of a valuable teaching aid for future practitioners of radiotherapy.

In our group we considered rather briefly an example of what a record might contain. A detailed analysis of records must correlate effects on tumors and on normal tissue with the original conditions and treatment. The records should be complete and based on experience. The facts that are known to be important should be included; this, of course, is a very difficult job. Also, facts that are suspected to be significant should be recorded, but one must not go overboard and record everything. Records should be accurate and complete; they should be the responsibility mainly of the physician. The data should be language independent in deference to our international tongues; this is now a possibility with the state of the art of computational linguistics, particularly in medicine. The items to be covered should include details of identification, of relevant etiological factors, of conditions bearing on the relationship of treatment to end result, of treatment factors, and of follow-up.

On the more detailed level, we reviewed a proposal that Dr. Lionel Cohen and myself worked on at the last meeting. It included what we then called the minimal information requirements for a statistical evaluation of therapy; this, later, we revised simply to informational requirements, the minimal being redundant. This included a general clinical record, a radiation therapy record, and surgical, medical, and chemotherapy records. Most attention was paid to the general clinical and radiation therapy records, in the belief that the others would fall into line following similar formats.

The general clinical record included items of identification; social data; diagnostic data, including histologic, cytologic, radiologic, and other criteria; information on staging and grading; management policy, whether this is curative or palliative; and information on follow-up, including contingencies and survival times.

Linked to these would be the radiation therapy record, containing information on identification (not only of the patient but of the therapy center), the management policy, radiation modality, treatment pattern, detailed dose plan, treatment factors, local reaction, systemic reactions, tumor response, and final disposition of the case. Many of us hope an encoded form of the actual treatment plan will be included.

Needless to say, central to the success of such an effort is the spirit of international cooperation in studying informational requirements, standardization of nomenclature, validation procedures for data, and methods for maintaining integrity. Feasibility must first be demonstrated on a small scale with careful and intensive monitoring before a large commitment is made. The use of free medical text versus constrained data structures and formats is now possible, with the aid of computational linguistics. Perhaps this could be encouraged and would be a good mode for the physician data entry on fixed forms.

Attention must also be paid to the null record—the case where you simply don't write anything down. This doesn't mean that nothing happened. We hope that this type of effort will lead to greater physician acceptability and fewer errors.

In summary, the working group believes (1) that it is now time for a five-year plan, (2) that a select group can initiate the data base, and (3) that mechanisms for support for the sessions of this working group will be forthcoming.

LANE:

The type and amount of information required for a radiation therapy data bank varies according to one's concepts. There's the comprehensive approach, which entails the collection of large amounts of data in the hope that its analysis will lead to important conclusions. With modern computers this is relatively easy to carry out. The obvious problem with this approach is the physical collection of such massive amounts of data, which is difficult to accomplish. On the other extreme is the type of data collection which is devised for a specific investigation, with specific questions in mind. These two concepts have been brought up at previous conferences, and have been discussed at length. We shall now hear from Professor Henry from Brussels, to see what the consensus of yesterday's workshop was with regard to information requirements for the proposed Radiation Therapy Data Bank.

J. HENRY: *Informational Requirements*

Mr. Chairman, it is amusing that you should select somebody whose native language is French to summarize a discussion in English. Not only is there a possibility that he has not entirely understood what was said, but there is also a possibility that the congress will not understand what he has to report. Fortunately, Dr. Prewitt has already told us much of what was discussed regarding informational requirements.

If you wish to have a useful data bank, it should not be just a simple tumor registry, like that which exists in most countries today, nor should it be a registry of unused data. It should be useful, and it should be used.

If you wish to have a large number of people participating, you must begin in a pragmatic way with minimal requirements for information. This does not prejudice against the registry with more extensive information. These would also include, of course, the minimal requirements, and I think would give some incentive to the others to extend their registers.

To use our report as an example, at the beginning we have the usual administrative data. Then we include general information on the patient, not forgetting to state whether the patient has had treatment for cancer previously elsewhere. A means is available to avoid duplication of patients who have been treated in more than one institution.

Also, information is included regarding starting date of treatment, whether it's the initial treatment or recurrence. Another important point is the location and extent of the tumor. This data raises the question of how to classify extent of disease; whether T.N.M. or some other classification should be used. I feel that we must accept the international classification; if it is not a good one, we have to change it. When many centers use their own classification, it's not possible to compare results. If we institute an international data bank, we should stick to one international classification, and accept it.

The system must be open. It must be arranged in such a way that later surgical, chemotherapeutic, or pathologic data can be added to the radiotherapy information.

As it is intended to be a radiotherapy data bank, the type of treatment must be recorded; the tumor dose; the number of individual fractions; and the length of protraction. This is the minimal requirement. We should know whether it's preoperative or postoperative treatment, palliative or curative, and whether it has been radiotherapy alone or combined with other modalities.

The most difficult part of the record is the follow-up. In this should be included the reactions that you can see both early and late. It is not too difficult to determine the sequelae of treatment, with a computer to keep track of patients.

These are the minimal requirements. To develop them further, we felt that it would be useful to gather a working group to see what is being done now and what we would need for a clinical trial. But if we wish to have something to present within two years, I think that those minimal requirements should be considered in the next few months.

LANE:

To ensure consistency in any registry system an acceptable basic vocabulary must be developed. This pertains to all sorts of things—disease sites, histology, staging, and certainly the factors involved in radiation treatment. Agreement on these variables is essential if we are going to collect data that are free of confusion. Dr. Cohen has been given the task of summarizing suggestions for standardization of data.

L. COHEN: *Standardization of Data*

Standardization of Data, as outlined by Professor Henry, will need to systemize information on the site of the disease, the pathology, the therapy applied, and the results. Now exactly half of our task has been done for us by the American College of Pathology, which has made available various systematized nomenclatures. I think we have all agreed that we will adopt this specification in toto; to attempt to redo this system would be merely wasting time.

The World Health Organization is involved in producing international specifications of disease. That section relating to oncology is to be updated in 1976 and will be in a form compatible with NCI's systematized nomenclature. The systematized nomenclature of Berenson, SNOMED, will be made available to all users in the form of a field trial addition very soon.

Basically, it has been proposed that the clinical record will cover five fields—topography, which refers to anatomical site; morphology, which includes all pathological information, both gross and microscopic; functional changes, both biochemical and clinical; etiological factors; and treatment procedures—surgical, radiotherapeutic, and chemotherapeutic.

Our task is the last part of the operation. Among the procedures will be the radiotherapy record. Here it would be relatively simple to standardize the data because radiotherapeutic data in this are largely numeric.

Dr. Prewitt mentioned the type of variates that we would need to record. There are some complicated or sticky areas, and one of the most difficult to resolve is probably staging. For the radiotherapist, staging information is used for treatment-planning purposes as a means of so locating the target volume to include the disease in its known extent; for the statistician, staging is used to compare results. Staging information could be empirical and in the traditional format it is dangerous to modify or to try to improve acceptable staging procedures, for reasons which Professor Henry has pointed out. Staging information could be obtained, however, in a general form by using the SNOMED classification, which is really a combination of topography and morphology. If we know the pathological changes in all organs and situations of interest, we have specified the primary site of the tumor, and where the regional metastatic extensions are to be found.

I am not quite sure how this can be handled computer-wise, but these subdivisions can be broken down with any desired degree of refinement. The extent of the disease can be then entered as a data set, which could be analyzed on the basis of this kind of topographic and morphologic information.

The rest of our task is not difficult. To specify dosage, we merely have to decide whether we want to specify Roentgens, rads, minimum tumor dose, maximum dose in the target volume, etc. There are many ways of presenting doses, but these are things which can be specified. The fractionation scheme is a matter of numbers of fractions and sizes, and their distribution in time and sequences. The time of treatment is a matter of recording the dates on which these various procedures were done, and assuring that the sequences can be extracted from the computerized record.

Size of tumor is a rather more complicated situation. Entering length and breadth and penetration, so as to give an estimate of volume, is possibly adequate, but possibly not.

Recording of tumor response is a matter of observing the site, extent, and volume of the tumor at initial treatment and observing it at follow-up intervals thereafter. The reactions in normal tissues is a matter of defining the pathological and functional state of every organ of interest traversed by the beam before, at the time of, and at follow-up periods after the radiation.

LANE:

The ideal data entry system for a computerized registry has yet to be designed. The major problem with any registry system is the human effort required to collate data. Information has been proven much more accurate if collected by physicians as part of their ordinary work. Consequently, every effort must be made to devise some sort of data-entry system which would entail a minimum amount of work from the professional staff, and which could be completed by the physician himself.

Another recurring problem with registries is the lack of pertinent data when charts are reviewed retrospectively. This might be avoided by a system that would use a checklist to keep track of data.

Lastly, an ideal system might allow for direct data entry into the computer, avoiding some of the clerical errors that might arise with key-punchers and other middlemen. Don Ragan of the Mallenkrodt Institute of Radiology in St. Louis will now report the Workshop on Data Entry Systems, which was held yesterday morning.

D. RAGAN: *Data Entry Systems*

In the introduction I was asked to summarize the consensus of the group on data entry systems. This is hard to do. If I had only one thing to say about our discussion, it would be that there was no consensus.

If I were given the task of designing a widget, it's imperative that I know what a widget is supposed to do. In this sense it's hard to design a data entry system without having some feel for what kind of useful purposes these data will be put to. Drawing on what previous speakers have said, I would conclude that the uses to which these data are to be put are reasonably standard: end results, survival, etc.

The initial feeling of the group was that the mode of data collection will have, by and large, a great effect on the success or failure of the system. It has implications on validity of the data; implications on physician acceptance; and, of course, implications regarding the cost of a patient information system, either locally or internationally.

The group discussed a number of possibilities for data collection. Multiple choice forms were viewed by some as the only economically feasible solution to the problems. Free form dictation is unbeatable for simplicity and physician acceptance. Touch-screen entry, again, is really great for physicians. Some people believe that the data base must be the primary record, for reasons of validity or efficiency. For each of these areas you'll find people who are religiously in favor of a particular approach; and I think for good reasons. Each of us, in our own institutions, has seen a data base that has failed for one reason or another, and we're very sure we don't want our international data-collection system to fail in the same way.

With an international approach to a registry system there is a need to accommodate the diverse predispositions of contributing individuals. In previous efforts to get community cooperation, frequently, people have been alienated when their system was excluded because of some quirk in the way data were collected or utilized.

This implies a need for establishing a common denominator in terms of data—or, as the previous speaker has said, "the minimum that's needed." This could be used as a start which we can all agree on. I'd like to suggest that we're not going to get very much from an approach that leads to an accommodation of a diversity of data, or the union of all data sets that are participants.

What is needed is a well-defined interface. If I design a piece of electronic gear to fit my computer, the best thing I can do to ensure success is to define the interface well. With a well-defined interface, I can put it on other machines and understand what it is doing. The same is true of an information system: if the interface is simple and straightforward, I've simplified my task.

Unfortunately, the problems that were brought up in our planning session are not simple ones; they're not the kind that any of us can resolve in a meeting like this. Therefore I think there is a need to establish an ongoing working group to work on these problems.

I suggest that the technical or computer details have by and large been the stumbling blocks to previous systems. More is needed than a supersophisticated computer system in order to get the registry off the ground.

Let me toss out a couple of things for discussion: No one in the meeting so far has addressed the point of what can be done differently in an international data base as compared with existing regional data bases—which are organized almost identically with the suggestions made here. And these bases have failed 100 percent. What's going to be different about *our* effort? Why should I, as an individual, recommend to my physicians that they invest their time in this international effort?

Secondly, a tacit assumption has been made that the international registry should be an end-result kind of operation. I suggest that from the point of view of data entry, in-putting all data on everyone is almost a prescription for failure. In the initial stages perhaps we should be considering a radically different approach, perhaps a protocol approach. In fact, I would point out that the only kinds of registry efforts that have succeeded in this country are ones that have been directed. In Mel Griem's case, for instance, this was a Hodgkin's Disease study, where the subset of data is reasonably small compared to everybody's data.

LANE:

To be simplistic, the purpose of any data bank obviously is the analysis of the final data. Hopefully, by systematic analysis of multiple records we can find better ways of treating our patients. Stuart Clampitt, of the University of California Medical Center, San Francisco, will now summarize the workshop of Output and Data Analysis.

S. CLAMPITT: *Output and Data Analysis*

I'd like to preface my remarks with some comments I made when we first began the workshop. In my observation there are three ways in which these data bases tend to fail. Usually they do not get established in the first place unless there is an agreement on the information to be put into them. This tends to be the overriding consideration in establishing a data base. Do you like the information that is in it? Has information been left out which you feel is necessary? That sort of thing. The next problem is the survival of the system, or its use by people in the field. This has quite a bit to do with the data-input procedures. If you can satisfy those two prerequisites, you can usually ensure survival for at least several years, or until you have enough information to start doing some sort of analysis of the data. At *that* point, however, if you have not provided some sort of assurance that the information you've put in can be retrieved, your system fails.

Almost all systems that fail have done so at one of those three levels. As the system is optimized to satisfy the first two conditions, I hope people will not forget the last condition: retrieval.

I'd like to start with the group's conclusions on retrieval which seem to have met with general agreement. A number of participants stressed the importance of fast retrieval. The speed estimates varied somewhat according to tasks and according to participants but generally fell in the time range between a fraction of a second and five seconds.

The types of tasks mentioned for this kind of high-speed response were CRT displays of any portion of an active patient's medical record, and hard-copy generation of the same location of any reasonably well defined subset of either active or inactive archival data.

I'd like to add a few additional retrieval tasks that were not brought up and that I believe the state of the art supports. They would include survival-rate analyses, both fixed interval and actuarial; distribution histograms for continuous and discrete variables; correlation analyses for two variables; simple descriptive statistics for single variables, such as mean and standard deviation; staging frequencies; and percentages and survival analyses by stage. The participants generally agreed that there were some statistical analyses that did not have high-time priorities.

Acceptable performance times were tossed around and ranged from minutes to days. Generation of hard copy would tend to fall into this latter category. I would suggest that poorly defined retrievals—such as finding patients treated with radiotherapy in 1974, or those receiving postoperative radiotherapy on the department's Cobalt unit—would be the sort of appropriate slow retrieval problems you might define. Nonclinical retrievals for the purposes of billing, scheduling, and evaluation of departmental performance are the type that do not need to be done in seconds.

I should mention that some of my earlier statements reflect a personal bias—for example, that the total medical records should be computerized. The main criticism regarding this concerns the loss of such graphic data as photographs of the lesions, the anatomical drawings that some doctors like to use to record disease, dose plots from dosimetry, etc. With the exception of photographs, all of the other graphics are sparse enough to be included in the computerized record, and are retrievable for subsequent hard copy. I should like to suggest that putting the record in the computer should mean a gain in information, rather than a loss. I won't try to define "gain," but it involves a number of different categories, the least of which may be completeness.

The last area that I want to mention concerns the need expressed in our workshop to resolve the conflicts between the two basic retrieval tasks in medicine—patient health care, where you're working mainly with one record; and clinical research, where you're working with a large number of records. Many of you are aware that currently the largest effort to computerize the medical record is in Burlington, Vermont, under the direction of Larry Weed. This PROMIS system handles the first retrieval task—patient health care—very well. At the moment no attempt is being made to handle the second retrieval task: clinical research. It's illustrative of the need to bring these two tasks together that this failure of PROMIS is probably the major reason why Weed's system includes a number of hospital departments but does not include Radiation Therapy.

Several speakers in our workshop suggested ways to resolve this conflict. All suggestions were basically the same: create two data bases. The clinical research data base would be a proper subset of a medical record generated by the computer rather than through duplicate recording and would include only data that could be meaningfully retrieved across a significant number of patients. This secondary, smaller data base would be used as an archival system as well for studying large groups of patients, perhaps eventually from many different countries, as we are discussing in our International Data Base.

Not everyone expressed total agreement with such a dual data base, however. I'd like to suggest that this problem is not a unique one for us or for Larry Weed or even for medical information; it's been with us for as long as people have tried to use a variable format in an inverted tree structure for their records. The problem was solved many years ago; I'd like to mention briefly the solution and how it might be applied to the radiation therapy data base. Each record in the data base is prefaced by a fixed format header, including 10-20 percent of the data in the variable records. I suggest that this header can be identical to our earlier mentioned clinical research data base. It would then allow rapid retrieval across the active medical record data base. By "active" I mean patients who are about to be treated, patients who are being treated, or patients who are close enough to treatment to need very close follow-up. The header can be modified, every time the medical record is updated. It's a relatively trivial task to construct an archival data base consisting of these headers, or arrange for routine copying of the headers of the medical records into the archives whenever the archives are mounted on the system. This can guarantee that archival retrieval is always as current as the medical records themselves.

LANE:

Stuart's report leads us directly into the next topic on the list for this morning: the Computerized Radiation Therapy Record. Mel Griem, of the University of Chicago, has had a great deal of experience in this, and I'll turn it over to him.

M. GRIEM: *Medical Record Replacement*

Stuart is a tough act to follow, because he already has said everything I'd like to say.

The question is whether one should computerize the radiation therapy record. At the Chicago meeting I presented the IBM approach —that is "It's Better Manually." I think we've come a long way since then.

About two or three years ago in our own group, we looked around to see whether it might be possible to computerize the patient record. We visited a number of places and we came to certain conclusions. This morning we've discussed the concept of the data base. We need initial identification; the general information, which Stuart just mentioned; treatment plans as carefully defined by Dr. Henry and Dr. Cohen; follow-up information as well as tumor-specific data related to specific protocols. Then somehow this computerized record must be handled so that the data are retrievable.

In the process of developing our system, we looked around at various tumor-registry approaches. We found that for everyone that was working there were six that were not working. The reason for their failure was the poor quality of the data, which were degraded by secretaries, by punch cards, by forms, and by total system failure.

If one were to do a systems analysis of the radiation therapy record and of a radiation therapy department and then check the interaction between it and their resultant data, one might get some ideas.

Initially the patient is seen in the radiotherapy department. Information must be gathered about his identification. There is the initial interview, and certain hard copy must be generated immediately. Then the decision is made as to whether the patient should be treated or not, data are entered, and an active file is created.

Let's say the decision is that the patient should be treated. There are various possible interactions while the patient is being treated, and the computer or the medical record or the radiotherapy chart must interact with the patient and the physician. Again hard copy or some sort of display must be readily available.

Finally, after the completion of treatment, the computer might interact in the follow-up procedure in a number of ways. The patient must be scheduled for follow-up. This entails a computerized letter suggesting that he come for examination. When the patient arrives, the computer might make sure that the physician examines the right areas, measures the proper nodes, and gathers the correct information.

I think that there is a role for a computerized radiation therapy record. There may not be a simple solution for producing it; in fact there may be half a dozen methods of approach. It seems essential, though, that at least as we design systems, (1) we consider the physician input as being essential; (2) that verification, a very important thing which we will hear about shortly, be possible; (3) that we have certain abilities to standardize the quality of this record; and (4) that ultimately analysis of what we have done can be readily generated to create our international radiation therapy data bank.

GENERAL PANEL DISCUSSION

LANE:

I would appreciate it if the panelists could come to the podium so that we can start a general discussion on the papers so far presented. I'll take the Chairman's prerogative and ask the first question, or, really, reraise the point that Don Ragan has already raised. What are we going to accomplish by establishing an international radiotherapy data bank, and how is this different from some of the data banks that we've already set up?

PREWITT:

I think we hope to gain by the international data base a broader exchange of information than is possible on a local or national level. We want to share innovations and experiences that transcend what goes on in any one radiotherapy department or in any one region of the country. This is the impetus; by pooling experience, we can gain much new information regarding epidemiological factors, treatment techniques, and such.

SHRIVASTAVA:

I wonder if we are aware of any other international data banks, whether in medicine or science or technology? Maybe a look at these would give some insight into our problem.

PREWITT:

There's at least one data bank somewhat similar to the one we are proposing, namely the International Immunotherapy Data Base, started at the National Cancer Institute. The data base for this differs from ours in that it deals largely with experimental rather than clinical data. However, I think it is important for us to realize that such a data base has been started and is beginning to be of value.

SILER:

I should like to call attention to a system in which K. C. Tsien and I played a part, since it might be directly applicable to the problem at hand.

The system I refer to has been operational for some years. It was presented at the RSNA Meeting a couple of years ago, and later at the Toulouse Conference. This particular system carries along two different items. It is a recursive structure, with one portion serving as a description in text terms of the particular data. The cells that correspond to this can be stored in a variety of formats: binary codes, multiple punches, text, fixed-floating point numbers, etc. Consequently, it is quite flexible. The data themselves are stored somewhere else.

If we were to utilize a structure similar to this, I think we could begin to employ the computational linguistics that Judy Prewitt mentioned, not just on the data but on the description of the data. Perhaps in this way we could open the possibility of mapping the staging system—granted, not with the greatest confidence in the world; but what is Stage IV in one place is highly unlikely to be Stage I in another. Perhaps this system could be useful in serving as a basic mechanism for the implementation of an international data bank.

The system does permit one to set up any data structure desired. We have had stored something like 2,000 cases of breast cancer. I can give an idea of the complexity of the data when I say that a printout of the data description—not the data itself—on a particular patient runs about 6 feet on lined, printed paper.

Just one more comment on the ability of the Group to get things started. As you remember, the automation got its approval at the 1968 Conference of this body. Subsequent to that meeting, the Committee on Radiation Therapy Studies of the National Cancer Institute set up a subcommittee on automation to determine tentative specs. The project was advertised and eventually funded. Perhaps some such course might serve to get this thing on the road. We do have the precedent that this body has a good feel for the way things should be going.

LANE:

Thank you. Don, I think you've got some comments?

RAGAN:

Yes, I'd like to address myself to this system because it exemplifies the problem that we are always running headlong into. Tsien's system puts a heavy burden on the analysis end of things. For input it works well: It's flexible, and it accommodates most sources of output. When you get to the analysis, however, it becomes a real problem to determine the definition of the data. What they cover and how they cover it. Statistically speaking, it is not well defined. I think you know that personally I do not like the PROMIS system as much as my colleagues do. However, I'll have to concede one point: it was developed to be not so much a computer system as a problem-oriented way of looking at medicine. It is the specification of the problem that allows for a systematic and careful delivery of health care. Tsien's system is the opposite of that. That is, don't look at the problem, just collect the data.

HENRY:

One can ask whether, in such an international data bank, consistent analysis will improve the physician's input. Sometimes the opposite is true: the secretaries who take care of the data should improve the physician's input.

GRIEM:

I would like to disagree with that. I don't see how the secretary can improve medical information.

HENRY:

They don't make the data better. However, sometimes the physicians don't record the right information, and if you have people who check them, you can frequently remind them that the forms are incorrectly filled out. That's what I mean, mainly that you'll improve the work if there is some system to control the situation.

CLAMPITT:

I agree with Dr. Henry. The problem here, though, is that in the system he is describing, what the doctor does is fed back to him. Thereafter he can evaluate whether a good job had been done. If you put the information into a system that has no structure, you have no way of evaluating whether you're doing a good job. There is no feedback.

NEURATH:

I'd like to turn some of the things around a little bit. As Don Ragan and others have pointed out, what you want to get out of this system really determines what you put in and how you arrange it. One quick way to approach the problem before creating a bigger international bank is to utilize data banks already in existence. Suppose this group could direct questions to existing data banks, which can give answers from their existing data.

In our own experience we have found that we can't answer a lot of the questions that are being put to us. Almost every new question sets up a new problem. We can answer it partially, but not entirely. The second problem we find is that even though we can theoretically answer the question, there are faults in the data that come up: the answers don't look right, and then you find things that are wrong. This is the kind of experimental approach to the creation of a system making use of existing ones that might be worth while at least to explore.

CLAMPITT:

I've found that at the present state of the art in radiotherapy, we're having a great deal of difficulty answering a few general questions. I agree with what you say, Peter (Neurath). But perhaps, it would be profitable to have some specific goals. There are questions that you must ask of any data base, either an existing one or a proposed one. I would just like to mention a few of these questions. At the moment I think there are only a few we're even prepared to ask, let alone answer. One of them is whether you can stage all recurrences of cancer, based on information for the sample that you're collecting. And what do you do if staging criteria change? Can *you* change? Can you split your base population into all subsets of interest? Maybe we can ask that question in such a way as to set up some sort of performance criterion. Those are the types of questions we must answer. Others have to do with end results—but, there are a relatively small number of questions on end results that can be asked.

GARY-BOBO:

The system we talked about yesterday has been running routinely at our cancer center in Montpelier since 1965, and we have data on almost 30,000 patients.

I would make just two comments regarding this. First, there are two types of data banks. One is a skeleton of the clinical facts; the other goes into greater details about one sort of tumor, say Hodgkin's or breast disease. They are both useful, but in a different way. From a practical point of view the questions asked are about epidemiology and the final-result survivals. To have full details on radiotherapy treatments would seem useful in a restricted area but useless at the international level.

GRIEM:

We have the same data in the United States, from the National End-Results Group, where selected hospitals and selected tumor registries in certain parts of the country put in such data. As one of the participants, I feel that that data bank is totally inadequate. The quality of the data is excellent, but the amount of data is inadequate to do the type of studies that Dr. Cohen and a number of other people have requested. I feel that we should not repeat the same mistake.

CEDERLUND:

I would like to know who would be able to use these data and for what purposes? Only the participating radiation therapy centers, or any center? Just a physicist who wants to find out what centers use ultrasound, or a journalist who wants to write a paper on radiation therapy, or a manufacturer who wants to do some promotion? And how much could you get out of it for what cost? Could you simply write a letter and say "Please send me by return mail, free of charge, a copy of everything you've got"?

LANE:

I'm not sure we can answer those questions, but maybe. I'll let Lionel Cohen have a try.

COHEN:

I think I'd like to give an example of what might be asked of this system. A radiotherapist might ask the question whether recurrence in breast cancer is different when the patient is treated five days a week as compared to two days a week. With any local group of patients, if you start breaking the data down according to stage, dose, number of fractions, total treatment-time, and such, you've fragmented your rather limited data into very small groups. With the international data bank, a radiotherapist could get the world's supply of breast cancer dosimetric information and end results and do a statistical analysis. In other words to answer the question would require a variety of different treatment schemes to look at, which you won't find in any one city or any hospital; you may find the answers if you can tap the resources of all the centers in the world or all cooperating institutions.

PREWITT:

Let me reemphasize Lionel's (Cohen) remark from the point of view of one involved in planning. It's valuable to know what is being done, and what the level of the success is, so that limited resources for research may be distributed in the best possible way.

NEWTON:

I am far from being a data-base expert, but as I've been listening here, some things have been going through my mind. The problems you're addressing with respect to what information should be gathered and what questions should be asked are very deep medical, epidemiological, and statistical questions. I suspect that you all know better than I that it is going to take a couple of years to really resolve this to the point where you can go ahead with a solid data bank of international/national scope.

I've been wondering what we can ask the people in the computer science field to do technologically to be ready for us when we reach the point of international data banking. Here are some of the things I am hearing, as a person not deeply involved in this area. They are things that may have some feedback to you. (1) There's a tremendous amount of information to store, (2) There are going to be local idiosyncracies in the way people want to gather and store data, and (3) There is a tremendous data-verification problem. I am not too sure that this is going to work as well in a long-loop situation to one single central data bank as it would in tight-looping to regional data banks. When we think in the international domain, there might be data banks in each country or in large countries such as the United States, in certain regions, with correspondence to a major center.

If this is going to be so, maybe we should be doing something analogous to what the network people did when they started planning for ARPA nets, i.e. to define what are going to be the essential elements in the data base. To start, we should do some research on the devices to make it possible for people with different kinds of computer approaches in different countries to communicate with one another;

this, essentially, is a network problem and amenable to computer science. Second, let's look at some of the work on intelligent query-and-answer systems for data bases, so that once we get this horrendously big data base, we can begin to ask meaningful questions of it and get meaningful answers.

LUNDY:

I am not in this business at all, but I would point out that there are specialists in information-retrieval these days. This certainly is not an exclusively radiation-therapy problem, or even an exclusively medical problem. I am wondering whether we are involving some of these people who specialize in information-retrieval to help in planning the kinds of questions that should be answered? Certainly, the physicians are the people that have to define what data goes in and what information comes out, but I think there might be some help from the people who specialize in information-retrieval.

GRIEM:

I think that Carol (Newton) has brought up a very interesting concept. Most radiation therapy departments have some sort of computational facilities on site, and one might assign a fairly high priority to patient and physician interrogation to gather data. This might be in a short, closed loop that would bring out what's been gathered, so that the physician can say, "Yes, that's really what I want to say."

It seems to me that the question of the ultimate quality control of what this local data-gathering might be, the compatibility center-to-center, and how we get at the data are the things you've addressed the question to and also that Dr. Clampitt has mentioned. But how do we get at the information once it is collected?

LANE:

In any data-collecting system there must be built-in mechanisms for maintaining quality control. Errors are inevitably made, and some way must be introduced to find and correct them. What can be done to ensure the validity of medical data in a registry? Marilyn Stovall of the University of Texas System Cancer Center in Houston will report on the consensus of the workshop on quality control.

REPORTS OF WORKSHOP DIRECTORS (continued)

STOVALL: *Physics Standardization*

In a sense, the results of our workshop should have been reported first. After all, if you don't have data worth saving, then you don't have to worry about input or output systems or how to store them.

The group did talk about quality control and the object of quality control, which is to ensure that all data relating to patients are valid and consistent, and satisfy the minimal criteria laid down by the data bank. This implies control of (1) the basic physical data, (2) the application of these data to individual patient dosimetry, (3) the delivery of radiation to the patient, and (4) clinical data and radiotherapy records.

The last item is likely to prove the most difficult to implement; unless a tumor dose-statement is reliable, the information concerning the patient and his disease will become meaningless from the point of view of assessing the results of treatment.

The group proposed that the data bank not take upon itself the task of validating basic physical data. This duty belongs properly to the ICRU and other international bodies. The application of these data and the delivery of radiation, however, certainly fall within the terms of reference of the data bank.

There is abundant evidence that mistakes and misunderstandings are more common in these phases of radiotherapy than most of us would care to admit. This evidence is derived first from the IAEA-WHO Program of dose-intercomparisons using TLD dosimeters. This program has covered a large number of centers in many countries, particularly in developing countries.

Secondly, evidence is derived from the several national schemes of dosimetric assessment which are in operation. The most comprehensive of these schemes is that of the U.S. Radiological Physics Center, based at M. D. Anderson Hospital, Houston. The RPC has so far investigated about 200 institutions by means of direct visits, involving special measurements and detailed review of the local dosimetric and set-up procedures. The results show that for about 20 percent of the treatments studied, the dose delivered to the tumor varies from the stated dose by a margin of more than plus or minus 5 percent. Let me say that again: 20 percent of the treatments deviated by more than plus or minus 5 percent. The actual ranges of errors were minus 48 percent to plus 21 percent. To give meaning to these figures, I might add that in general the 200 institutions surveyed were the larger and more advanced centers.

Such evidence leads to the conclusion that a system of control and assessment carried out by a peer group within each country is essential. The assessment is best carried out by direct visits, involving independent measurements, and if this is not feasible, by dose comparison by mailed dosimeters; a detailed review of the procedures to each institute is essential.

Unfortunately, it is probably impractical to broaden the peer-group control to cover institutes in other countries. But the IAEA-WHO Intercomparison Program provides a basis for ensuring uniformity on an international scale. In addition, these organizations are setting up in various parts of the world a number of regional secondary standardizing laboratories. These laboratories could and should take on the task of ensuring uniformity of dosage in the regions concerned, in terms not merely of the calibration of dosimeters, but of applications and techniques as well.

Finally, we take it for granted that the principal primary calibrating laboratories, such as the NBS, NPL, etc., will continue their policy of intercomparisons so as to ensure the international validity of the rad and other radiation units.

As for the quality control of patient data, the group recognized that this is likely to prove a difficult task. The following guidelines were, however, suggested: (1) it is better to begin with a relatively small number of enthusiastic institutes than a larger number of half-hearted centers. Indeed, enthusiasm and genuine interest on the part of the authorities of the participating institutes and of the individuals actually doing the work are essential. It is also advisable to begin with only a small number of tumors or sites. (2) We assume that the participating institute is supplied with a list of data required by the data bank. It is important that before the data are coded, probably by a relatively low-grade employee, they should be checked over by a physician or by other knowledgeable individuals. (3) The institute should be prepared to supply supplementary information and to clarify data already supplied if so requested by the data bank. (4) Random checking by the data bank of information supplied may prove a useful method, and (5) the problem of specifying tumor dose is particularly difficult. Yet it is central to the success of the project. Ideally, every institute should accept and use a standard definition. The chances of securing universal acceptance of such a definition—and, equally important, the uniform interpretation of that definition—seem too remote to rely upon. We therefore suggest instead that each institute be required to supply sufficient information to enable its own definition of tumor dose to be translated into a standard definition within the data bank. The information supplied must relate to both the spatial and the temporal distribution of the dose within the tumor, the dose to the target volume—if different—and the dose to critical normal tissues.

LANE:

The workshop on validity of data came up with a number of items, as you can see, and there will be a second report on this to be given by Dr. Larry Davis of the Radiation Therapy Dept., University of Pennsylvania.

DAVIS: *Validity of Data*

I only want to spend a few minutes to try to emphasize some of the problems involved with the recording of the clinical data aside from what Marilyn Stovall has emphasized about recording of the physical parameters of radiation dose. The first point is that means must be determined to eliminate mistakes in the data. I think some of these would be obvious and could be checked by the computer programs that are developed. Second, some of these could be eliminated by verification of the data through review by the responsible physician.

I think a larger problem is how to develop consistency in reporting information among participating institutions. Part of this problem results because many of the pieces of information that would be required reflect the judgmental decisions of people who are evaluating patients. Consequently it would be extremely important that all participating institutions have a complete list of definitions of terms required of the information being submitted. This seems one area where quality control would be more difficult, since it borders on judgment rather than obvious mistakes in submitting information.

Some international registries have addressed some of these things in a very limited fashion, such as the International Federation of Gynecology, which has for many years accumulated a limited amount of information about gynecologic malignancies.

My last point is that rather than trying to check exhaustively the validity of the data, it may be more appropriate to have only random samplings of some of the clinical information that might be verified.

LANE:

It would seem that considerable valuable information might be obtained from such an international radiotherapy data bank. In the process of accomplishing this, however, care must be taken not to sacrifice the patients' right for privacy. In Sweden a new Data Inspection Board has been established to register, inspect, and license existing personal registers. This board has the power to determine how a register may be used, what data should be collected, and who can have access to it. It would seem only a matter of time before the United States and other computer-oriented countries would be faced with similar legislation. Thus I think the problem of integrity and confidentiality of data is one that must be considered. Bengt Olsen of Uppsala University will discuss methods of accomplishing this.

OLSEN: *The Problem of Integrity and Confidentiality*

Originally I made an effort to produce a solution to the problem of maintaining confidentiality of data—a solution covering all aspects ranging from application programs to the safety of the computer installation. There are many books dealing with this topic, and there have been numerous conferences on the subject of data integrity.

Since I was quite alone in my working group—I didn't even get the mirror I asked for—I completely changed my presentation. I thought that there could be only two possible explanations for the fact that I was alone: either that everyone knew everything about the subject, or that no one found the subject important.

I am now convinced that the second reason is the true one. Thus I have instead chosen to talk about the importance of the subject and especially its applicability to an International Radiotherapy Data Bank.

Drastically increased possibilities of storing, treating, and combining large person-bound records lead to new risks of abuse of personal integrity. In the hot debate about political, social, and economic goals and ethical aspects regarding individual-based registers, a good balance between the value for the society, the risks to the individual, and the costs of minimizing these risks has to be attained.

The patient's interests are two-fold: (a) to receive adequate treatment, and (b) that data concerning him personally shall not be distributed so that it will have a negative influence on his legal and social status, his chances of getting social benefits or of keeping a job, or, for example, by placing him in a worse position in a court trial.

The hospitals' need for information is well known—they need data banks for aid in administration, treatment, and research.

External interests are also involved.

- Police, judges, etc.
- Insurance companies (for checking claims and evaluating risks)
- Ministry of health (e.g. for checking quality of treatment)
- Tax authorities (e.g. for estimating a doctor's income)
- Pharmaceutical firms (checking and testing drugs)
- Finance investigator (health status)
- Employer (health of new employee)
- Associations for the protection of employees (risks)
- The Military services (ability)
- Relatives
- Research outside hospital
- Private data service bureau
- Domestic as well as foreign political, commercial and military interests, etc.

These potential integrity risks in hospital care emphasized by EDP personal files may affect not only patients but also their relatives. The information can be misused in various ways, for example by organizations associated with the patient.

It might be imagined, for example, that a political party could be interested in having a list of all members of the other parties who suffer from cancer, especially a brain tumor. The information might be used in a pre-election campaign. Now, I hope this will never happen anywhere, but I consider it our duty to build our registers in such a way as to minimize the risks of misuse, and to restrict the access to them.

For regulating open access to the files of public authorities, Sweden has a unique system that dates back to 1766—that is, three years before Dartmouth was founded. The general public has a constitutionally guaranteed right of access to government papers, to all documents received by public authorities or produced by them.

This right of access or "freedom of information" was originally intended as a protection for the citizen, for example to ensure that public authorities treated everybody equally. But in this computer age this openness can be and often is used in the reverse direction.

After years of discussion Sweden got the Data Act in 1973. The purpose of the Data Act is to prevent undue encroachment on privacy from the use of EDP. To prevent misuse of files containing personal information, special permits are required to create such files. A special authority, the Data Inspection Board, examines applications and issues such permits. The main tasks of the Board are:

1. To issue permits to establish and maintain EDP personal registers.
2. To issue directives on the uses to which the register may be put and the items of personal information that may be included.
3. To supervise and control EDP operation.
4. To function as legal adviser and deal with complaints from individual citizens concerning EDP of personal information.
5. To give advice and assistance in matters of EDP, privacy and security.

I will just mention briefly two of the twenty-five sections:

Section 1: *For the purpose of this act:*

Personal information *means information concerning an individual.*

Personal register *means any register or any other notes made by automatic data processing and containing personal information that can be assigned to the individual concerned.*

Individual registered *means an individual in respect of whom personal information occurs in a personal register.*

Responsible keeper of a register *means anyone for whose activity EDP is being carried out, if the register is at his disposal.*

This gives a good basis for discussion. Especially important is the fact that for each register there must be someone who is the responsible keeper of the register.

Section 10: *At the request of a registered individual the responsible keeper of the register shall inform him as soon as possible of the personal information concerning him in the register. When a registered individual has been thus informed, new information need not be given to him until twelve months later.*

Information as defined in the first paragraph of this section shall be given free of charge. If there are special reasons the Data Inspection Board may, concerning a certain kind of personal information, permit a fee.

The provision of the first paragraph does not apply to information which, pursuant to law or statute or the decision of an authority, may not be delivered to the registered individual.

This presupposes that for each register there must be suitable programs for retrieving, updating, or correcting data and for printing out the information. That will given an idea of what is going on in Sweden and what will probably happen in many other countries soon. It has almost led to a new science: "Security and Privacy in Computer Systems." This involves fairly general problems, including: fire, explosion, flood, breakdown, structural collapse, supply failure, theft, espionage, systems faults, data corruption, strike, sickness, civil commotion, and third-party disasters. Here I will talk only about misuse of data. The eleven highest weighted risks at a medium-sized data center are listed in the following:

Threat	*Weighted Annual High Loss US$*
Application Program malfunctions	18 000
Air conditioning malfunctions	12 500
Fire	10 000
Data integrity malfunctions	10 000
Central processor malfunction	9 000
Media damage	9 000
Accidental data erasure	9 000
Supporting software malfunctions	7 500
Computer operators errors	7 500
Programmer errors	7 500
Other equipment malfunctions	6 250

Data integrity malfunctions comes as high as fourth on the list. In order to make your system bullet proof, you have to worry about the following items:

- Recognition of risks and cost/benefit analyses
- Personnel
- Hardware installation

- Localities
- Data preparation and control
- Control of access to data
- File control
- Computer room procedures
- Privacy transformations, coding, and decoding.

Protection of integrity thus consists not only of *technical* but also of *legal* and *functional* components. In the case of an international radiotherapy data bank, the following questions apply:

Who is supposed to use the information and how?
Who is afraid of whom and what?
Who could possibly misuse the system?

The patient is afraid of integrity leakage in general. The researcher is afraid that the whole or parts of his data bank will be destroyed intentionally or unintentionally.

The following four risk categories can be singled out:

1. *Unintentional authorized misuse.* Use of incomplete or erroneous data. Handing over of data to authorities. Cure: Error checks, recommendations, rules, etc.
2. *Intentional authorized misuse.* Certain reports issued by the physician without the patient's knowledge. Cure: Rules, etc.
3. *Unintentional unauthorized access.* When personnel happen to introduce or gain access to personal information without permission. Cure: As in 1, plus identity and authorization control, identity coding, and no lists with names of persons outside the clinic.
4. *Intentional (illegal) unauthorized access (with intention to misuse).* This is the main problem. Someone may get access to data without authorization. He distributes them without any control or they may be used in special illegal ways, commercial or political. Cure: Well balanced information and media protection.

These security problems are generally much easier to solve for batch-type computer systems than for time-sharing systems. In dealing with the problems, special attention must be paid to such areas as:

- Level of authorization, including a discussion on topics such as read only, summarization, selective access, modification, write only, and updating;
- Hardware identification devices, such as keys, badge readers, cards, and individual characteristics;
- Software identification devices, such as passwords (to be used once or permanently), personal questions, and random numbers.

When trying to solve these problems it is easy to agree with F. W. O'Malley that "Life is just one damned thing after another."

Recommendations

1. Analyze the problem of privacy seriously before building the model data banks. Take the necessary steps from the beginning.
2. Strive for uniform security arrangements and standards and international conventions stipulating basic rules on privacy protection. Uniform security standards and international agreement as to minimum privacy protection would be of great practical value and would considerably facilitate international data exchange.
3. Introduce an identification code, so that only the responsible keeper of the register in a particular country could update the international files.
4. No user of the files should get more data than he really needs.
5. Make all employers sign a promise of maintaining secrecy.
6. Make clear rules about sanctions in the event of unauthorized use of data.
7. Do not make big plans for merging large registers. This will perhaps not be allowed. And finally
8. Keep to batch-oriented systems until very safe hardware and software systems are constructed.

With these words I wish the group working on an International Radiotherapy Data Bank all success.

LANE:

I think now we could have the panel come up to the podium and open the session for general discussion.

SHRIVASTAVA:

Most of the policy decisions in radiation treatment are made from whatever data we have at present. Why do we have to make it more valid when we put it in the computer?

STOVALL:

This may partially answer your question. I mentioned a while ago that we found errors exceeding ± 5 percent of the stated dose in 20 percent of the patients treated. Within an individual institution, the physician may have adjusted his dose prescription to compensate for these physics errors. Over long periods of time, perhaps he is treating patients just as well as other institutions, and he is not in trouble as long as he looks at only data for his patients. However, when you start comparing data between institutions, and in particular on an international basis, then we must be sure that we have better data than is now required within an individual institution.

SHRIVASTAVA:

The point that I'd like to make on this matter is not that 20 percent of data is 5 percent off, but that 80 percent of the data is correct! I think that 80 percent confidence at this time in radiation therapy is quite valid.

DAVIS:

I think this depends on what information is required to come from these data and how much research will be done with it. There's a story that's been told several times about the National Surgical Adjuvant Breast Project which is currently evaluating a radiation treatment plan for patients who have had total mastectomies. In the first 100 cases that were accessed to this study, there was a major deviation from the prescribed treatment plan by people who were trying very hard to follow the prescription. Erroneous conclusions will be drawn from such studies where people aren't really doing what they think they're doing, or where they're submitting data that does not describe what was done. I think that if the information in the registry does not describe what happened to the patient, wrong conclusions will be made from research efforts.

GRIEM:

I'd like to second that. With ablation curves and complication curves as close together as they may be in certain treatment decision-making situations, errors like this can lead to complications—such as spinal cord injury, carditis, liver injury, kidney injury—that are unacceptable to society. I think we just can't accept these types of errors in modern radiotherapy departments.

ABEDIN-ZADEH:

As a corollary to what Marilyn (Stovall) has said about standardization of dosimetry, I think there is also a great need for a standardization of definitions. I most appreciate the great efforts of the European Association of Radiology, which has tried to define terminology.

RAGAN:

I'd like to ask if there is anyone on the panel who has in any way developed an estimate for the cost of policing data validity from an international standpoint. Should this burden rest primarily on the local facilities, and, if not, how much does it actually cost to go in and check for accurate information from the actual patient treatment?

STOVALL:

My own impression, and that of the working group, is that there should be national intercomparisons, rather than international ones. Something equivalent to the Radiological Physics Center in the United States could exist in other countries; perhaps it already does and I'm not aware of it. We have to make a plea for physicists to work to certain standards, and there must be on-site peer review of this. As to cost, I can't really say what this is costing us now, but I think it is negligible compared with the overall costs of treating patients.

LANE:

Is the cost being borne by the individual hospitals at the moment?

STOVALL:

No, none of the hospitals involved in any of our reviews has paid for these reviews.

LANE:

May I now ask Dr. Prewitt to summarize the session.

PREWITT: *Summary Remarks on Tumor Registries and An International Cancer Radiotherapy Data Base*

The necessity of establishing local tumor registries in general, and oncologic radiotherapy registries or data bases in particular, is patently obvious to all participants in this, the Fifth International Conference on the Use of Computers in Radiation Treatment. It is necessary to know (1) the signs, symptoms, and history which a patient presents; (2) the most likely etiology and the disease model which constitutes the physician's working hypothesis and *should* provide the rationale for curative or for palliative therapeutic intervention or for refraining from any action; (3) the procedures actually performed by the physician to reduce and/or eliminate discomfort and disfunction; and, finally, (4) the effectiveness of administered therapeutic modalities in terms of end results (i.e., morbidity, recurrence, spread, and mortality/survival). This basic information is germane not merely at the local center of actual patient treatment but regionally and nationally so as to ensure continuity of medical care and efficacy of medical protocols. Moreover, it is also desirable to convert to or to abstract from individual case histories and to create medical archives that are nationally and internationally accessible, so that the collective experience of the medical community can be compared and assessed, and so that health-care delivery can ultimately be cost-effectively optimized without compromising the integrity of the patient. The humanitarian, scientific, economic, and temporal importance of such shared experience is obvious and in harmony with the ethos of medicine.

The decision-making processes in medicine leading to formulation of a working diagnosis and to the selection of a course of patient management are amenable to mathematical, probabilistic, and logical analysis. This approach does not supplant the judgment of the physician, nor does it relieve him from setting goals and assuming responsibility and accountability for outcomes. It formalizes the basis for judgment and casts the relevant factors—or, more accurately, the factors deemed at that time to be medically relevant—into an objective, explicit, and publicly scrutinizable form. To use an analogy, it attempts to dress the medical decision-making process in "the emperor's clothes."

The key to the use of decision analysis in oncologic radiotherapy is the development of a cost/benefit effectiveness function, usually called a figure of merit. This function expresses quantitatively the anticipated merits, risks, and penalties of any therapeutic regime to the patient and to society; the certainty attaching to the outcome; and the cost burdens that must be borne by both the individual patient and family and by the society at large. Obviously, the figure of merit is conditional on a diagnosis or an operational model of disease and cure, and on the state-of-the-art of therapy.

It has become fashionable and customary to call the application of decision theory and utility theory to medicine "rational medical practice." Rational medical practice attempts to optimize the objective function or figure of merit which explicates therapeutic worth quantitatively, so as to select the overall best course of action, according to the criteria that are implicitly or explicitly dealt with formally, and according to the *manner* in which they are dealt with. The mathematics of optimization permits the physician to compute values for parameters appearing in the objective function which indicate the preferred medical behavior; indeed, the same mathematics permits the physician to rank order the therapeutic alternatives.

Far from replacing physician judgment and responsibility, this approach obliges the physician to be articulate and honest about therapy goals, outcomes, benefits, risks, and costs. As a minimum it provides a means for attaching worth to any course of patient management, to make this assessment dynamic as treatment outcome is progressively monitored, and to change the therapeutic regime accordingly as warranted. As a maximum, it provides a means for commensurability—that is, for comparing different strategies and tactics and for selecting the one which is best in some previously agreed-upon sense. Treatment can be tailored to patient-specific characteristics and to the facilities of the local therapy center. In principle, physician capability should not deteriorate; it should thereby be augmented, if not simply vindicated.

In order to apply rational methods to medical practice, a repository of pertinent experience is essential—hence the clinical and research motivations for a radiotherapy data bank, hopefully an international base or bank of structured or organized radiotherapeutic data. The topics bearing on the construction of such data bases have been considered by the various workshops on tumor registries and data bases: (1) goals for an international radiotherapy data bank; (2) informational requirements; (3) standardization of data; (4) data entry systems; (5) data analysis and output; (6) computerized medical records in both fixed and free text formats; (7) validity of data; (8) radiophysics standardization; and (9) methods of maintaining the integrity and the confidentiality of data. The difference between privacy and confidentiality must be acknowledged.

The desire to pursue an international radiotherapy data base has been apparent in our past international conferences on the use of computers in radiation treatment, and still persists at this gathering. Representatives not merely of outstanding therapy centers but of national and world health organizations have expressed enthusiasm and unmistakable willingness to cooperate. It is the hope and the recommendation of the Working Group on Tumor Registries of the Fifth International Conference on the Use of Computers in Radiation Therapy that an interdisciplinary, international nucleus of willing, dedicated, and able volunteers accept a commitment to form a standing working and steering committee for an International Cancer Radiotherapy Data Base (ICRDB). The working committee should include radiotherapists, radiobiologists, biomathematicians, biostatisticians, computer specialists, and information scientists who would convene and correspond over a two- to three-year period, to plan for the next five years. The committee would address itself to the multitudinous problems associated with the ambitious undertaking of establishing an international cancer radiotherapy data base in depth. Note that their task is *not* to work toward the unification and computerization of all radiotherapeutically relevant data and medical records. Rather, their task would include the following: (1) locating existing tumor and radiotherapy registries or data banks and compiling a directory or catalog, including a table of contents and a format description for each; (2) surveying the state-of-the-art of associated and needed hardware and software, especially with respect to data structures and successfully employed management techniques; (3) disseminating this information to colleagues while at the same time soliciting their assistance and comments; (4) anticipating the goals of establishing such a data base—that is, anticipating the questions that are to be answered with the aid of such a data base; (5) ascertaining directions for partial or total revision of terminology, information requirements, data formats, and methods of maintaining data integrity for an international endeavor; (6) selecting perhaps two or at most four organ-sites for which establishment of an international cancer radiotherapy repository is likely to have the greatest payoff or impact in terms of reduced morbidity and improved cure rates; (7) investigating computer and information science techniques, including data-management information systems and networking and satellite communication links, all the while taking cognizance of local idiosyncratic habits and needs; (8) planning for a limited set of demonstration projects to be conducted at qualified centers in order to explore systematically and thoroughly the techniques for the chosen organ-sites; (9) soliciting means to achieve these desires and decisions for an international repository, catalog, or network, and for an on-going international information exchange. The international working and steering committee would have the definite responsibility of continually maintaining contact with colleagues in all interested countries, and would formally report their findings and progress to the entire international radiotherapy community at its next congress, if not before then via newsletters and workshops.

We believe this serious and significant undertaking expresses the consensus of the Data Base and Tumor Registry Working Groups of this Fifth International Conference on the Use of Computers in Radiation Therapy. Furthermore, we believe that such a project is not only now possible but necessary, in order to ascertain the effectiveness of present radiotherapeutic protocols for oncology and to ascertain the potentials for improvement.

GENERAL DISCUSSION

RAGAN:

I'd like to ask if you can identify in slightly more detail what kind of working committees are possible, how people are assigned to them, and what exactly can be expected over the next couple of years?

PREWITT:

Many people have said they would be interested in being involved one way or another with such a steering committee, so that we could get an international exchange of information. In fact, there are more volunteers than would be feasible for such a working group, and, consequently, we need a hierarchical structure for the steering committee, and then perhaps working parties. These latter may be dedicated to a specific project. We may need something done at a certain time, and once that goal is accomplished, the committee will make its report and disband. The main steering committee should be representative, but small enough in size that something can be accomplished at the end of two years. The way those of us who have discussed this committee see it, it would be certainly no more than twelve people, and hopefully closer to six, so that it doesn't get out of hand. This doesn't mean that others will be excluded. This committee is responsible for disseminating information, but it has to be done in a hierarchical fashion in order to make it workable.

We would be able, as I understand it, to get financial support initially for the meetings of the steering committee from the United States sources. Later, I think, other countries would contribute to the project. What happens after that will depend on the recommendations of the committee and the resources (internationally) that are available. The National Science Foundation is planning some key demonstration projects that would demonstrate the feasibility of certain automation techniques in the health field. If these work, maybe other places would duplicate them. At any rate they are being written up, and will be presented for funding.

In this proposal I don't think any of us wants to computerize the world. We just want to see what we can do to establish an international exchange of valuable information through pilot projects under the guidance of a steering committee that is representative of our various technologies and national interests. This steering committee has a very heavy responsibility; they will be few in number, but they have to communicate continually with everybody who is not on the committee. So it's a problem in logistics—we don't want to offend anybody, but we have to get something done.

M. COHEN:

I hate to sound pessimistic, but I've been to more of these international conferences than I care to remember, and I've also worked in an international agency for a number of years. What worries me is this: virtually every international conference I've attended has ended up by making proposals that involve some project or other with promises of steering committees and future collaboration. The success rate of these projects that were so enthusiastically endorsed on the last day of the conference is between 3 and 5 percent. It is a fact of life that the moment we all leave Hanover, we will tend to get engrossed in our day-to-day business, and the resolutions that we made are quietly forgotten. This is a pity, and I'm not advocating it. Quite the contrary. If we have something worth doing, then I think it should be done. We shouldn't just forget about it quietly. It seems to me that the answer is not to go away and set up what amounts to an ad hoc steering committee composed of individuals who happen to be in this conference. I advocate that we work through existing organizations rather than try to set up something completely new.

There *are* existing organizations, in every country. In this country there's the RSNA and many others. In my own country there's the Faculty of Radiologists and the British Institute of Radiology; internationally, there is the World Health Organization.

I would say that the chances of the project continuing and of not fizzling out after three months or less are much greater if, instead of developing an ad hoc steering committee, we try to interest the proper radiological and cancer societies in each country, and work through them. They have already got the machinery to ensure that once a project is going, there are machines for paying people, for obtaining traveling expenses, for ensuring that an item remains on the agenda of the society. Speaking as secretary of the British Institute of Radiology, I would stress that we cannot forget projects, because *they* remain on the agenda, and every time we have a council meeting, someone wants to know what is happening. Whereas, if it is an ad hoc committee, you can forget it as easily as falling off a chair.

PREWITT:

I don't think this time we will end up with an ad hoc committee. The interest that has been expressed here has included that from the National Cancer Institute, the World Health Organization, the Pan-American Health Organization, and various other groups. Consequently, I think that we're starting off on a new tack, with cooperation, sincere interest, and a tremendous number of volunteers—many of whom we'll have to disappoint. We do have the interest of those key organizations you have mentioned. People from all of these groups both here and not here, have expressed this interest. Perhaps for the first time we've got a fighting chance to sustain interest. My sentiments duplicate yours; an ad hoc committee with no backing on a high level will never accomplish much. You have to get backing on governmental level to make anything international work. This time I think we've got it.

CEDERLUND:

Monty (Cohen) almost said the same thing I wanted to say, but in a negative way. All the previous conferences have expressed some interest in this data bank; I'm sure our chairman would like to know what this conference feels. I'd like to suggest that we make some stronger motion this time; that we implore those individuals who either have the authority or know the channels to try to persuade the health organizations in their various countries to give us their moral support; and that those of us who have access to the necessary agency funds see to it that they are made available, and that individuals who have the necessary knowledge and capacity to work this committee dedicate themselves to the project. I don't know the formality of this, but I would like to have some expression from this conference to show that we would like to see it happen.

WILKINSON:

I'm going to take the part of the Devil's Disciple and oppose the International Data Base. It seems to me that as you increase your scope for collecting information from the single institute to a national or international organization, you introduce more and more variables into the system which are bound to confuse the issue. To get useful information, you have to reduce the number of variables, not increase them.

PREWITT:

Just because you have more countries involved doesn't mean that you increase the number of variables. I tried to say very clearly that the steering committee would be responsible for keeping this small until we see that it is reasonable. Thereafter it would grow in response to the desires of the community. It wouldn't get bigger because there were more countries involved. We kept emphasizing minimal information requirements that would help us to do a better job. So more countries doesn't mean more of a mess.

WILKINSON:

I think in most institutes where you have five radiotherapists you've got five variables to start with.

LANE:

I can agree with that, but I think what we are really talking about are demonstration projects to show how or if this will actually work.

Some of the dangers that you are talking about are a little way down the pike.

GRIEM:

It seems that some of the concepts might be tested regionally. Could not some of the things being proposed be tested in a regional group? If they fail there, they are not going to fly any place else.

HANSEN:

I believe that it would be useful to develop concrete proposals with concrete estimates of cost. So far I haven't heard this and I've some misgivings about the possibility of success. So I would think it would be most constructive if this group could prepare a concise statement of the problem, what solutions are available, and what it will cost. Then I think agencies who may be in a position to help could make a better judgment.

MACKINNEY:

In terms of the practice of rational medicine, the proof of the pudding is going to be in demonstrated improvement in survival rates. This in turn will take a matter of ten years, at a minimum. In terms of local studies it seems to me that the problem rests with acceptable standardization. We've all recognized that one place an international body could be helpful is in regard to the criteria under which the international community is willing to accept a study as worth looking at. Certainly there is work to do at the international level, and it has to come first.

LANE:

We are all aware that we have a lot of work to do before we get anywhere. I think we're pushing for the idea that Mel Griem suggested, that we do have some sort of demonstration project that will get the thing off the ground. At a later date we come back and ask that the local project be expanded to a wider base.

SILER:

I would like to support the idea of the international steering committee. I don't think that this is necessarily opposed to the idea of a local demonstration. The problems that we face, especially that of standardization, tend to be global in scope. Unfortunately, the attitude of any single institution tends to be controlled by the person at that institution, like Dr. Griem or, in this case, myself. You know who is pushing the show. I think that we need a broader input of ideas, a scrutinization of the implementation as it progresses, than is possible at any single institution. So while the demonstration projects will be carried out, of necessity, at a few carefully selected places, I would say that we need the global input that a steering committee will develop. This is a terrific job, and I think the consequences of a simple local project, even at the best possible place in the country, is very likely to be a failure.

CLIFTON:

I don't think anybody disputes the desirability of this type of data base. When the chips are down, however, someone has to do the work. Two things stand out for me as far as this discussion is concerned. I would agree entirely with Monty Cohen in that one needs to involve the existing international organizations. On the other hand, there is one serious drawback: by and large such organizations are geared to elect persons to the steering committee who have no knowledge of the subject and no real drive to get things done.

Somehow or other one has to get a mechanism whereby the people on the steering committee are prepared to take off their coats and do some work. In turn, these individuals must have a good working relationship with the international committees, so that they are propagating not their own ideas, but something that is genuinely international.

A second thing comes to mind when we start talking about pilot schemes (which is, after all, the only way we are going to get this to start). One thing we might consider is that we have a number of centers using virtually the same types of hardware. Some of us, hopefully, are using the same terms when it comes to computer science. Therefore we ought to be able to interchange information with a minimum of extra work and heart rending. I suggest that this is where one might look to start, rather than to a large, international system that immediately presupposes a vast computer system and lots of computer time to set up a total new data bank where nobody's initial information will fit. Let's look at those of us who have systems that, in theory at least, ought to be compatible, and start with those.

PREWITT:

I called for a steering committee that consisted of willing, able, and dedicated people—as you suggested, people who would roll up their shirtsleeves and work, and who have connections as well as qualifications. I also tried to suggest that we start with a few demonstration projects where the payoff would be good. We would be very foolish to ignore the good ones already available. To start with those would cut the cost, build on experience, and quickly get us through the first two years. This is the experience I've had in United States projects—pick the qualified ones and build on them and then spread whatever technology you have learned.

CUNNINGHAM:

I wanted to mention that there are probably already in existence a few studies that could be included in the category of pilot studies. At least one of them was carried out at my own institution and is international in scope; it was developed for the Centennial Conference on Laryngeal Cancer that was held in Toronto this spring. It certainly involved multiple countries, and it was for an individual and specific site, a site that was amenable to data handling.

LANE:

I think that what we're trying to do now is to get this idea born. We've had a gestation period of many years, and if we can get it born, it might begin to grow by itself. We have to get it started somewhere.

VI. Implications for Developing Centers

Session XI: Panel Discussion on Obstacles Faced by Developing Countries and Radiation Therapy Centers—the Effect of Computerization

Chairperson	*Panelists*
P. Houdek	R. Abedin-Zadeh
	M. Cohen
	G. Hansen
	H. Perry

HOUDEK:

There has been a great deal of time spent at different conferences and different meetings, organized by different bodies, on the subject of the use of computers in developing centers, but no formula or simple conclusion really has been reached yet. The question is not what the computer can and cannot do; the question should be "What is it feasible to do by a computer in regard to routine radiotherapy?" The majority of procedures involved in routine radiotherapy seek the best possible agreement between the treatment strategy and the treatment actually delivered to the patient. There is more than computer technology involved in this process; there are many other technological activities, as well.

It seems to me that the most important emphasis should be placed on the planning of automation. There are three steps, the first of which is the determination and specification of the center's needs and priorities. The selection of an appropriate technology may be the second point, but I believe it has already been sufficiently discussed here. The final and most difficult step is the establishment of a professional environment at the center which is equal to the proposed degree of automation. This was evident from the discussions on Monday and Tuesday which indicated that this type of dilemma exists in one way or another in the majority of centers.

I would suggest that we reach in our discussion some kind of tentative conclusion as to how international organizations like IAEA or WHO can be more helpful in this respect. This kind of activity seems to me best suited for international organizations, since conferences, like ours, have really no financial possibilities, nor authority to organize needed educational and training programs. I will now ask Dr. Abedin-Zadeh to review the activities of the IAEA in regard to this subject.

ABEDIN-ZADEH:

In the last decade the IAEA has organized three panels in the field of computer applications. The first panel, on computer calculations of dose distribution in radiotherapy, was held in October 1965 and perhaps for the first time brought together radiotherapists, physicists, and computer specialists in a programmed way. The second IAEA meeting, on the role of computers in radiotherapy, was held in July 1967. This panel attempted to identify various radiotherapy activities in which the computer could be used to serve the needs of existing radiotherapy centers. The last panel, held October 1973, was particularly aimed at finding ways in which the Agency and other scientific-medical communities could assist developing radiotherapy centers in establishing and adopting computerized systems. The panel provided the Agency with recommendations which can be summarized as follows:

First, radiotherapy must be regarded as a continuous process, with feedback loops from diagnosis to treatment planning to actual treatment to follow-up. It follows that the full advantage of progress in one sector cannot be realized unless there is some parallel progress in other sectors. It is important for developing centers to understand that the introduction of computer dosimetry does not automatically result in the better treatments of patients. The benefits reaped will depend on the level of preparedness, fitness of the center, and other characteristics. It is therefore greatly in the interest of the patient to ensure that the other aspects of radiotherapy progress have been developed prior to, or simultaneously with, the application of computer methods.

The second was the classification of systems for computerized treatment-planning. Under this discussion it was felt that there are three main categories of systems which operate in radiotherapy centers. Category one consists of batch-computing by transport or telecomputing services. The second category consists of small dedicated computers and medium-sized multipurpose computers, and category three consists of remote-batch terminals plus intelligent remote terminals. Although criteria for each category were formulated, it was not possible to recommend any one of them, generally because the best system for a particular center will depend on many circumstances —for example, the number of patients, the therapy machines available, the proximity of the nearest computer, the efficiency of the telephone system, the utilization of the computer, and the funding available.

Thirdly, for an educational program the panel has made specific proposals for publication. This recommendation was mainly based on technical aids provided by an assisting center to a requesting center. The assisting center might be an existing advanced radiotherapy center or a regional computing center, or perhaps a combination of the two. Within the framework of this project, a research program in computer applications in clinical dosimetry has been initiated by the Agency. The objectives of this coordinated program are to encourage and facilitate the use of computers in developing radiotherapy centers with the cooperation of advanced centers and to test the established computer techniques under local conditions. The program would seek the following studies: (i) development of a computer program for direct, accurate and flexible calculations of the dose at any point in an irradiated volume, adaptable to individual sources and types of machines; (ii) study on the organization of treatment-planning; (iii) study and recommendation on input data and the preparation of manuals; (iv) study on means of long-distance communications for computer input and output exchange, and (v) preparation of local outlets. Up to now, nine institutions from eight countries have participated in the program. The second part is to be devoted to radiation dosimetric data.

Concerning the subject of the present panel discussion, I would like to summarize my comments as follows: the points that should receive most attention are (1) placing emphasis slowly on computerization—having experienced therapists, experienced physicists, and basic equipment—while (2) being aware of the obstacles with which the developing radiotherapy centers are faced in regard to computerization.

PERRY:

My approach is a little different—from the point of view of the physician or therapeutic radiologist. In our country we are faced with this kind of situation: The population is 208 million, and the total of new cases of cancer estimated for 1974 by the American Cancer Society was 655,000. Of that number, 50 percent will require radiation therapy as the primary mode of treatment or in conjunction with a surgical program, a chemotherapeutic program, or some other combination. In the same year there will be 110,000 recurrent cases of cancer, so this gives us a total number of patients requiring care of something like 437,500 cases for 1974. There are fewer than a thousand members of the American Society of Therapeutic Radiologists to care for these patients and a large number of these members are not in the United States but in Canada. The real concern of the radiotherapist is the delivery of patient care. How does that happen?

First, one has to establish a diagnosis of cancer. This does have its problems in many instances. There is the problem with the histologic diagnosis. For those in the audience who have been near the Hodgkin's protocols, we very often have difficulty in making a decision as to the histologic type of Hodgkin's Disease. This is important, of course, in planning treatment regimes, because there are differences in the natural course of the disease according to the histological type—spread, sex, and age incidence. Once we have at least made some attempt at establishing the histologic category, our next goal is to establish (we hope) the extent of the disease. Although there has been great technological development in the first three fourths of the twentieth century, we still have great difficulty in really knowing where all of the tumor is, but we try to make this attempt to the best of our abilities and knowledge. Once this has been established, a plan or treatment policy must be outlined and followed; then one has to determine what the treatment volume should be: the time, the dose, and the other biological parameters discussed previously at this meeting.

The next question is "How do we implement this?" and that is where the computer enters—that is, in the planning, the execution, and the verification of the prescribed treatment. At first blush it may seem easy, but it is not always possible. The radiotherapist is not living in a vacuum, however, and must, of course, cooperate with other professionals, like radiation physicists and technologists. In this area we have, in addition, the computer specialist and, of course, the programmer. The programmer and the computer specialist bring to the setting an impact that the physicist very often does not have in terms of how one can look at systems. We also have to think of the other support personnel, such as the internist, the family physician, the medical oncologist, the pathologist, the surgeon, the anesthesiologist, the administrators, the diagnostic radiologists, the practitioners of nuclear medicine, the nurses, etc. They are all individuals important to the goal of attaining the important thing we are all basically here for, and that is the care of the patient with cancer. The patient's treatment is carried on not in a desert but in some sort of physical facility, be it a hospital or a private office.

The computer is here very important and does assist us in automating some of the functions. While we're treating patients, we require a large quantity of laboratory data, and when the laboratory facility is automated—so that instead of having a hundred little slips, everything is wrapped in a nice, neat format—one can find the weekly or daily hematologic or biochemical status at a glance.

Important for us, though, is how do we get all these individuals, in any setting. Training in a so-called developed or developing country is still one of the most important aspects. In the United States, with fewer than a thousand trained therapeutic radiologists, training of the individual therapist is important; we have made a new thrust, trying to reach young people as early as the secondary school level. In addition, we also must interest the physicists, the programmers, and the technologists in being part of the whole medical scheme for training and in the delivery of patient care.

An important consideration today is the availability of the various kinds of equipment. With airplanes and ships one can easily move equipment to any part of the world, and we all tend to forget the supporting mechanisms. If a piece of equipment is made in Holland, what happens to the person in California who needs parts replacement and technical aid?

What then, in summary, could be the impact of the computer in the delivery from my end as a physician? The impact will depend directly upon the user or users and how they look at things. Many people who "deliver" radiotherapy do not know about the shortcomings of parallel opposed pairs, that the isodose curves are not flat on the outside at the lower energies, that you actually get a kind of bellowing in the middle, and this is important in what happens to your treatment volume and values.

Next on the list would be to standardize and improve dosimetry record-keeping, which has been a large part of the program at the meeting. One factor that was not emphasized, however, was that the records and the registries will be no better than the data you put into the record. If you have no data, no matter how large your bank or how many people you have using it, you cannot get answers.

M. COHEN:

Let me begin by saying how very sorry I am that Ted Sterling was not able to be here. I think many of us who know Ted have missed him very sadly in this Conference. Ted was originally going to chair this discussion, and he wrote to the panel members asking each to prepare a list of ten problems which each member considered to be most difficult, or most germane to the problem of developing countries, and to comment on the possible impact of computers in solving each problem or maybe in making it worse. I, in fact, prepared my list, and I will try to run through it as quickly as I can.

To begin, a cautionary note. I think it links up with what the earlier panel members have already said—namely that it is wrong to regard developing countries as a homogeneous group. I know that the international agencies tend to do so, to refer to the developing countries as if there were some known entity that you could label developing countries. In fact, there are many kinds of developing countries in various stages of development, and each has its own problems. I think we all know that there are even developing radiotherapy centers within so-called developed countries. And so it follows that many of the developing radiotherapy centers will not experience all of the obstacles I'm going to list. The full list will tend to apply only to countries in a very early stage of development.

For convenience I propose to divide my obstacles into four groups. First a general group. Number one is what I call a poorly developed infrastructure. Radiotherapy is a sophisticated activity, which draws upon many other activities both within and outside the hospital.

Within the hospital there are many supporting and associated services —diagnostic, pathologic, hematologic, nursing, maintenance, clerical, administrative, and so on. If any or all of these services function poorly or inefficiently, that will reflect on the working of the radiotherapy department. Outside the hospital there are many firms and organizations which supply the hospital. In developed countries these sources of supply are taken for granted. In developing countries many items have to be imported, and the supply is much more erratic. The external infrastructure also includes organizations that supply services and information, standardizing laboratories, libraries, and so on. In addition, the importance of a reliable, uninterrupted supply of electricity must also be stressed.

The second obstacle is the isolation of radiotherapy. Even in developed countries radiotherapy is a comparatively small specialty within medicine. In a developing country there may be only a few radiotherapy centers, perhaps only one or two, and the total number of professional staff may be very small indeed. Medical physicists, in particular, tend to feel isolated, and even fellow physicists in allied fields outside medicine—for example, atomic energy—may be comparatively few in the country concerned. This isolation from the mainstream of radiotherapy is often aggravated by poor library facilities, a shortage of journals, and insufficient funds to attend meetings and conferences.

The third obstacle is late diagnosis. In many developing areas patients tend to be reluctant to seek medical advice until a late stage. This trend is aggravated by the general shortage of medical facilities for diagnosis. Thus treatment will tend to be palliative or to rely on nonradiation methods. The possibility of radical radiotherapy using complex treatment-planning is vastly diminished.

Now taking those three general comments, what is the likely impact of the computer? My conclusion is that there is little that the computer can do to remedy the situation described. One can only hope that the very existence of computers in a country will encourage the development of the infrastructure I've mentioned. Perhaps one possibility under the heading of the isolation of radiotherapy is to use the computer as a means of producing very rapidly and freely distributing a list of titles of papers, plus addresses of authors, so that the doctors and scientists in developing areas can avail themselves of reprints before the stock is exhausted. Such a scheme was in fact tried by the IAFA some years ago and was successful, but folded because of lack of financial support.

I turn now to some obstacles under the general heading of personnel. First, a shortage of trained personnel at many levels. These include radiation physicists, radiotherapy technicians, physics technicians, workshop and moldroom personnel, and maintenance engineers.

Curiously enough, the one group frequently not in short supply is the medical staff, who have usually been trained abroad.

The next obstacle is the nature of the staff. This situation arises from the way medical care is organized, and from the low salaries paid to scientists and technicians. All too often the medical staff will obtain their main income from private practice, while the scientific and technical staff are obliged to seek a second job elsewhere in order to live. The result tends to be a half-time hospital service in radiotherapy which leaves everyone with insufficient time to devote to any one patient.

The next point is something very rarely mentioned; in fact, it is considered extremely tactless to mention at all, but I'm going to do so nevertheless because I have observed it all too often myself and I think it needs to be said. This is the lack of trust of the physicist by the radiotherapist. This is a disturbing feature of many developing areas. The medical staff tends to be better trained than the physics and technical staffs. They also have a far higher status, both within and outside the hospital. The items that I've already mentioned—that is to say, late diagnosis and the part-time nature of the staff—tend to restrict treatment to comparatively simple procedures such as opposed pairs of fields. This means that the physicist tends to be reduced to the level of a menial who measures the output of the machine, adds up opposed fields, and very little else. He is never given a chance of developing his talents and enlarging his experience. After a time, the therapist assumes that the physicist is incapable of anything of a more demanding nature, and thus a vicious circle is established. As I've said, that isn't usually mentioned, but believe me it happens. I've been in many such centers in the Western Hemisphere.

Now what about the impact of the computer on that little group? The danger here is that the computer will be regarded as a substitute for trained personnel. This it can never be. It is, rather, a tool to be put in the hands of trained people. They have to be properly trained, if only because one day the computer is going to break down and then they will have to know how to work things out by hand. In any case, without proper knowledge and understanding they cannot use the computer intelligently and ensure that the input data are sensible. Provided, however, that this is well understood, there is no reason why the computer should not be a blessing; it will help in the very process of training which is so badly needed. It is probable, indeed, that the pattern will be a computer specialist coming into the medical field from outside and learning radiation physics in order to do the job. I think this is the way it's happened in a number of American radiotherapy centers, rather than radiation physicists learning to do computing, as is the usual pattern in the United Kingdom. One can expect that once the scientist has access to a computer, his status will begin to improve. He will be encouraged to deliver more complex treatment plans, and gradually his standing will change.

The next group is equipment. There's a shortage of dosimetric equipment. All too often, the budget of a developing radiotherapy center has allowed for large radiation machines, often on money supplied by some government or other organization abroad, but not for the dosimetric equipment needed to measure the radiation. This situation tends to arise because scientists are not a party to the planning of a hospital or a radiotherapy center. As a result, the physicist often has to make do with insufficient and inadequate measuring apparatus. There is also the problem of calibrating dosimeters at a standardizing laboratory in another country. Another problem is the difficulty of servicing. This applies to both the radiation machines and to the ancillary equipment. Usually equipment has to be imported, and the local servicing organization is inadequate. It is rare for a hospital in a developing country to have its own workshop, and certainly not of a standard needed for the precise work often required in a radiotherapy department and for radiation physics equipment.

Shortage of supplies and components links up with what I've already said about a poorly developed infrastructure and the lack of servicing. It is difficult for people from developed countries to imagine themselves in a situation in which a new battery for an instrument is simply unobtainable, or components of a particular kind are unavailable. Furthermore, since many of these items have to be imported, there is often a long delay due to customs difficulties before they can be obtained from the manufacturer.

What about the impact of the computer on that little group? It is difficult to see what impact the computer can have on the points in this group unless it be to persuade the scientist that he does not need to make measurements, since he can calculate everything. This mistaken point of view has already been dealt with under the previous section. The computer itself will, of course, come under the general heading of equipment and may be subject to the same general difficulties. However, perhaps because computing carries a certain prestige that other equipment and activities lack, ways and means will be found to overcome these difficulties and have computers supplied and serviced, and this in turn will pave the way for an overall improvement.

Now my final obstacle was under the heading of computing in the absence of a large computing center. Let us assume that computing in developing radiotherapy centers will be carried out via a link with a big computer rather than through a dedicated machine in the radiotherapy center itself. This is not the place for me to argue the alternatives, but it will be assumed that a large computing center able to serve many peripheral stations and to provide a service in many different spheres will be more advantageous and economically preferable to setting up isolated machines that are dedicated to a particular function. The shortage of these large computing centers is, however, an obstacle. One must presume that they will be needed for purposes other than radiotherapy and will therefore be made available on more general grounds.

HANSEN:

I'd like to open by giving a few general comments about the structure of the World Health Organization (WHO) and the regional office in the Americas which is called the Pan-American Health Organization (PAHO). The World Health Organization is a decentralized structure, and it's moving more in this direction every year. There are six regions of the WHO, one of them being in the Americas and the other regions serving other parts of the world. There's a representative in every country, with some exceptions, who has responsibility for all the work of the WHO or PAHO in that country. There may be from one to a dozen experts working in various health areas—nutrition, water supply, communicable disease control, etc. Radiation is one of the programs of the WHO, and we have a relatively modest activity in this area. Our efforts are directed at all areas in which radiation affects health, which includes diagnostic radiology, radiation therapy, nuclear medicine, and radiation protection. Approximately three tenths of one percent of the WHO budget is dedicated to radiation. This is the priority that has been established by the countries that use our services.

Basic ingredients to programs are equipment, some help to provide basic equipment, consultants, experts from the WHO staff or from outstanding institutions, and training fellowships. In almost any program that the WHO supports, those are the basic ingredients. The policy is to collaborate with the IAEA in some of the programs that have been mentioned—for example, the TLD intercomparison study.

Another activity in which we are cooperating is the secondary standard dosimetry laboratory. There are a number of these throughout the world—Singapore, Bucharest, Teheran, Mexico City, Buenos Aires. These laboratories have the potential, and in fact are being used as nuclei, for improving radiotherapy in a broad scale. Monographic courses are being given in some of the centers, and organizational plans are being made by which it is hoped that services can be given to a number of outlying centers. So this potential exists, and it is possible that computerized treatment planning could, at some time, be incorporated through these existing facilities.

I believe that most of us consider developing areas as being a spectrum, and at least as far as my own understanding is concerned, I realize there are very good centers in some cities in some parts of the world, and these may parallel some of the best centers in other parts of the world. The problem that exists is, as a person moves away from one of these centers, the quality falls rapidly. This is true also in the United States, I might add. The infrastructure probably is the biggest problem, and the gap that I see is not so much in the people who know something about computers. In some cities there are large computational facilities, at least in this part of the world. The gap is between the people in radiotherapy departments who will communicate with computer specialists; there is almost a complete lack in most countries of this type of person. If I were to step to the board and write the names of various countries and the number of medical radiation physicists in the country, except for several large countries where the numbers might be between fifteen and thirty, the numbers would be zero or one for almost every other country of which I have knowledge. This is a very serious problem.

With regard to financial support, I think, realistically, that international organizations will not have a lot of support to lend to computerization in radiotherapy. I hope this wouldn't chill the enthusiasm too much, because I believe that the technical and moral support that could be obtained may be useful in finding independent funding.

HENDERSON:

I haven't heard any reference to what have been called turnkey systems. Is this included in your thoughts, or is there any place for such systems as opposed to built-up computer systems in the developing centers?

M. COHEN:

I think I know what you mean. The trouble is, I'm not convinced there is such a thing as a turnkey system. There's a pseudo turnkey system—that is, turnkey if the user happens to have the same radiation equipment and therefore the same isodose curves as the input data that is available in the software of that particular turnkey system. If he doesn't, then he is in difficulty. Either he uses a software that is really inappropriate—data that are inappropriate for his equipment—or he tries to modify a turnkey system without the knowledge of how to do so. However, if there is a radiotherapy center that happens to have the right radiation equipment to fit in with a system that's available from elsewhere, and provided that the system is supported from elsewhere, then this would seem to be a good solution. It's expensive, but no doubt a good solution.

CUNNINGHAM:

I just wanted to refer to a little finding which, if my memory serves me correctly, came out of that last Vienna panel that Dr. Cohen referred to and was rather interesting and bears directly on the discussion. If I remember correctly, Jan Van de Geijn drew a map of the world on which he spotted the location of known large radiotherapy centers—that is to say, centers that had at least high voltage equipment—and then he approached one computer manufacturer, and said, "Where on this map does your company have large computer installations?" and the resultant map showed a very high correlation, indeed, between the location of advanced radiotherapy centers and the location of computer centers, and therefore potential use of computers in those nations. It may be that the next step would be communication between these two groups of people.

HOUDEK:

Most likely the majority of us without great computer experience started in a similar way. We had available radiotherapy equipment and access to a computer center. This is essentially what Dr. Cunningham is saying, that there are centers where they have a computer and a radiotherapy facility available. I think we should concentrate on these centers, where this coincidence already exists.

ROSENOW:

As Monty Cohen pointed out, there are two very controversial points of view that he and Ted Sterling hold, and, as is often the case, the truth may lie between these points of view. I wonder if some of the obstacles mentioned by Monty may be overcome by establishing partnerships between developed centers and developing centers. I believe that this would be the only way of really helping developing centers. Certainly the training, and appropriate training, would be facilitated. After a phase of training there could be a postal exchange of information—that means the developing centers could send prepared patient data to their partner center, and the computation could be done in this center and sent back by post. I don't think the turnaround time has very high priority in such developing centers. This postal interchange of data may be very well suited to bring the developing center up to the standards necessary when it takes over any systems. And I also think, in respect to failures of the computer hardware, that such a procedure should minimize the problem of the developing center, since it can go back again on the procedure of postal exchange of data if needed.

M. COHEN:

I think Dr. Rosenow's suggestion is excellent, and I would certainly go along with that. In my own defense, since everyone will assume that I am against computerization at all in developing countries, that wasn't really the purpose of my remarks. I'm merely taking the view that these countries do have certain difficulties, underlying difficulties, that the developed countries, the big industrialized countries, simply don't have. It doesn't get you anywhere to pretend that these obstacles don't exist. It's better to face squarely the fact that these problems exist and to say, "Well, how do we tackle these problems?" rather than just pretending that they don't exist. With all due respect to our chairman today, he said that we ourselves some years ago started off this game in a small way. That's perfectly true. But most of us started from a highly developed technological base which doesn't exist in most countries that we're talking about.

HOUDEK:

If there already exists computer technology, and it is utilized, it does not seem to me possible that they would have difficulties in using it also for radiotherapy purposes. However, I admit, and we all did in all our contributions, that where the problem ends up always is in training. Training is the major thing. If people are trained, then they can cope with obstacles. If they are not trained, they will never manage them.

CLIFTON:

I have listened to what Ulf Rosenow has said. As somebody who comes from a nation with a reputation of being colonializers of one sort or another, and also from an institution which had sister institutions in what might now generally be called developing countries, I may say that the one thing we must realize is that all these developing countries, quite rightly, have a very strong nationalistic tendency. Therefore, anything one does must not appear paternalistic. And it is very much a question of going there and teaching and helping the people there to do the job. They are not interested in big brother from across the Atlantic coming to lend a helping hand. They want to be taught there, on their own premises, with such materials as they have available.

GHILEZAN:

I think it is not only the question of hardware. There is also a psychological problem. In general, in the developing centers, the older people are the chiefs of departments and they are quite resistant to new methods and associated changes. For this reason I think that the study tours through the advanced centers, organized in part by the IAEA, should be expanded. Afterward, recommendations can be made to the respective governments on how to implement the new methods.

WRIGHT:

I would suggest that there is another method that many of us are using to get this partnership that Ulf Rosenow mentioned, and that's in training our residents. Many of these residents are going to "developing centers." Perhaps they're in our own country, or perhaps in another country. I suggest that resident training programs should have more emphasis on the computer aspects in treatment planning.

JAMESON:

If you consider simply the data base of a machine, machine-data for a dose-computation plan, how do you handle this? Does the developing country have the facilities to make something of it or not? Do we have the same quality of data and the same quality of planning in the developing country? Do we have to take out a team of people and train them in a big facility to calibrate, for example, a machine, or do we simply take programs over? How do you go about this sort of thing?

HOUDEK:

It's my opinion that the organization of training programs is best suited to international agencies like IAEA and WHO. Since these agencies are international organizations and the different countries are members of these organizations, there should be no real obstacles of nationalism involved.

ABEDIN-ZADEH:

Although this program in the IAEA has low priority, there's a chance of technical assistance being awarded to developing centers in the developing countries. At the same time other kinds of assistance—for example, a study tour within some advanced centers—has been organized by the Agency. The Agency carries on such technical assistance, fellowship awards, and study tours.

HANSEN:

I believe that "natural" arrangements are extremely beneficial and perhaps in the long run may prove to be more beneficial than aid from the international agencies. International agencies can try, can plant seeds, can create a nucleus here or there, but probably the long-term natural relationships will make a big effect.

STOVALL:

We have an association with two hospitals in Mexico City. I think this is an example of how a lot of us could help, if that's the right word, some of the centers in developing countries on a one-to-one basis. This has been very rewarding for us also. I was recently down there and I think I helped them some on their computer work, but on the other hand, I looked at their TLD system and the phantom that they're using for TLD mail service. It is much better than the one we're using. And so we'll very likely copy them in this respect. There can be a mutual exchange and let's not always think it's a one-way street.

HOLT:

It has been my impression that in many instances it is not a shortage of equipment but rather a shortage of trained personnel. It seems to me one of the means of supporting these countries would be to set up a mechanism for education, either by an exchange of scientists from knowledgeable centers or to bring some personnel from these countries to a center where they can spend a residency and go back to utilize what they have learned in their own center.

VII. Summary and Conclusions

Session XII: Panel Discussion. "What have we learned and where are we to go in the next five years?"

Chairperson	*Panelists*
J. R. Cunningham	J. S. Clifton
	L. Davis
	H. Frey
	W. Siler

CUNNINGHAM:

The order of this session is somewhat open to the panel members. The intent is that each of the members of the panel, now taking their places at the table, will have a chance to make some summarizing coments on sessions that have taken place during the week. Each member has covered at least one or two of the sessions, and I'd like to give them each a chance to make some comments about those sessions.

FREY:

In the radiobiology section, I was especially impressed by the paper of Dr. Kirk in which he showed that treatment schedules with equal CRE or equal NSD do not necessarily have equal tumor effect. And he pointed out that this applies, especially to short—under-fractionated, as it were—treatment schedules. I think this implies that a considerable amount of caution has to be exercised in deriving different schedules on the basis of these. I think we will not get an improved insight into them if authors continue to suppress the basic time-dose information in their papers and report only rets or something of this sort. I believe the authors of these concepts are the first to say that these need to be continually checked, and we can't check them without the basic data.

The other big source of improvement in radiation therapy in the next five years will be an increased tolerance on the part of radiotherapists to complications. If a surgeon finds a tumor in a patient which he can cut out and gets a reaction which requires that the patient get a colostomy, he feels he has been a failure. It is unreasonable to expect to have a very low level of complications. The worse complication of all, of course, is recurrent tumor.

As for the use of machines, I think everyone here is aware of the recent unfortunate accident which occurred with a non-computerized Cobalt machine in this part of the country. If this happens with a machine under computer control, the impact on further research is going to be pretty drastic. This points out the need for very strict fail-safe procedures, both hardware and software.

With the change of administrations in the United States, we'll be able to depend less on government support for our efforts than we could in the past. Computer systems are going to have to pay for themselves. What we must do is find ways to add radiotherapy capabilities to existing computers, and the most obvious targets are the nuclear medicine computers, which are being used increasingly in all hospitals for the support of gamma cameras. In the next five years we'll probably find a fairly small cheap package which we will be able to add to a nuclear medicine computer so that it can be used for radiotherapy as well.

One of the most exciting diagnostic techniques that has occurred in the past year or two is computerized axial tomography. It gives us the information we want in the form we want it. It gives us a density matrix for the patient. But I think that right now we're going to have a very hard time getting any part of this away from the neurosurgeons; these things are still in very short supply. However, we should all make a concentrated effort to get some kind of data-accession capability from these machines, so that we can do far better planning. This is more satisfactory than ultrasound, because it gives us the densities rather than simply the shapes of the contours.

There has been considerable controversy here concerning record and verify versus control. To me, doing record and verify and stopping there is like doing a culture in sensitivity on an infection and then failing to give the proper antibiotic. One computer manufacturer has told me that the additional cost to add the control option—once one has gone as far as record and verify—varies from something like 5 percent of the overall cost for a Clinac 4 and 2½ percent for a Clinac 18. This does not include the cost of the room. For anyone to stop short of control is rather foolish.

One thing that has really impressed me was the very large number of errors that have been shown by people like Chung-Bin in setting up a patient—14 percent of all patients—an incredible number for us to think about. I mention only half in jest that there is some kind of Heisenberg's uncertainty principle here, and that merely observing this phenomenon suffices to change it.

SILER:

I'd like to talk, more or less in a general way, about three points, because this conference has taken place not in only this conference room but in innumerable hallways and rooms and over dinner tables and beers. There have been three threads, I think, running through the whole thing, although not exactly with the same people.

First of all, I think it was made especially clear by the therapists and physicists here that the name of the game is better radiotherapy, not improved technology. The question is, how can the computer help? Well, certainly it can calculate doses, there's no debating that. But I think it can also help in training. In addition to this kind of link—the personal link—there's also the possibility of training films—the kind that show the spurious authority of the computer as a way of teaching how to do radiotherapy and use the computer as sort of (a) a gimmick and (b) a high-powered dose calculator. It's not technology for its own sake, but the need for better delivery of radiotherapy and health care.

The second thing that became very clear on the first day of the conference was that there was one hell of a generation gap here. There was a split right down the middle between the old guard, the people that went to the first Vienna conference, let's say, and the bright young cats that have come up and are doing their thing here. I talked to a number of the old guard and to the new guard, trying to get a feeling as to why this split was there. The initial dissatisfaction was voiced by the old guard, and I guess, I'm a member of that. It seems that the split is real and that it is coming, in part at least, because of the shift in emphasis from developing new ideas, toward the implementation of ideas. The ideas are getting increasingly complex and the implementation increasingly hard. The younger cats who are actually the ones doing a lot of the implementation work have a little impatience with the old guard, who are long on theory and short on licking the real problems that you have to deal with. The old guard, for their part, are impatient because the new guys are not interested in ideas and implications and what other people did back in 1959 or so, but are trying to get on with their immediate job. For the old guard I see very real danger here, and that is in disregarding the problems of implementation of some of these complex ideas.

For the new guard I also see two dangers, and I'm reflecting the viewpoints of others. One is that by disregarding what has taken place in the past and not paying attention to the literature, you may well be going just a degree and inventing the wheel. Even worse, you may be inventing a wheel that is somewhat out of round, or reinventing the flat tire, which is kind of sad. This field now has a substantial literature and substantial experience. This was not true in 1959.

Another thing that is becoming obvious, and the need here was voiced by everybody, I think, that I talked to, and that's the need for increased lateral communication on these complex and vexing problems, so that people around the country are more aware of what others are doing. This is particularly acute because in some places you have different aspects of the problem, and the whole thing has to be pulled together and integrated.

CLIFTON:

Perhaps I have the best opportunity to be brief, simply because, in his wisdom, Jack allocated me a panel that did not in fact meet. Therefore, I felt my only justification for being here would be if I devoted some thoughts to the title of this panel, part of which is "Where do we go in the future?" and I don't know quite what I can suggest here other than that my reaction from what I've heard this week has two parts.

First, let's stop and think. Second, let's go back to the drawing board. I would next like just to mention three topics which occur to me and which come from the various discussions we've had in the different sessions.

First, we've had a tremendous amount of discussion about validation, both in terms of dosimetry programs and tumor registries. While we have used computers as a tool to disseminate programs and information on radiation dosimetry, we have to accept that it is time we stopped saying that the computer is just a tool to do a job, and that we need to know nothing about how it does its job. If we are ever going to validate, we have got to put sound computer science into what we do, particularly when it comes to the development of programs. I think we may have to go back and restructure many of these long, straggly programs that we've developed over the years.

Secondly, we have had a great deal of discussion about two interacting problems—of training and of the errors in setting up a treatment. I think there is a possibility that, in terms of the use of computers in radiotherapy, until now we have missed the boat altogether. I'm reminded of the situation with the airlines where we can usually survive if the pilot misjudges the runway and lands from ten feet up—all that happens is that the aircraft goes for a heavy landing check. But if he forgets to put the undercarriage down before he lands, we're all in trouble. To get over this, of course, the airlines have simulators—computer simulators—and they train their experienced personnel over and over and over again. This is something we don't do. What's more, we train our technicians on the basis of putting one in tandem with another, and the net result is that the first person trains the second and so on, and all the errors propagate. One of the uses of computers in radiotherapy that we have not examined at all is the question whether we can use them to develop practical, simulated training techniques. One is struck with the limited amount of data that has come out on the measurement of errors that occur: 14 percent or so is the figure mentioned by the people in Chicago.

There were also very significant figures from the Marsden, and one notes the difference in error-rate between the two teams. What struck me was that a number of these errors were quite small in magnitude, and only a few errors were major. I think we might well reduce them to a very low level indeed if we concentrate on training, rather than the concept of automated set-up and so on. We have to accept that right now the trained technician can probably set up as well as we can with a computer, and this situation will prevail for a good many years to come.

COLLINS:

One aspect that has not been touched upon here falls within my other interest, as some of you may know: legal aspects. Of course, there has been concern for your responsibility, for all our responsibilities, for the material that we provide which is based on computer operation. But more important than this, I suggest that within the next five years an aspect may develop which is, do you dare treat without computer verification? To disagree with Monty Cohen, I think not 37 percent but 100 percent need treatment-planning unless you bring in an excuse from your mother. By this I mean suppose the patient has had a recurrence: that's too bad, the plan's a geographic miss. Where's your plan? I'm not thinking solely of the dose-distribution diagram except insofar as this has the anatomy, the tumor, and the dose you delivered. Is that correct? Or can you refute the patient's contention? Or another example: the patient has had a recurrence and needs retreatment. You receive a letter from another institution: "Please provide the data, this patient needs further treatment." I see a good number of these cases that come to me in consultation, and I divide them into two groups—those in which I would rather be the plaintiff's attorney, and those in which I would rather be the defendant's attorney. I could say that in the two cases just mentioned, I'd rather be the plaintiff's attorney.

Now with this, then, it's not merely a matter of whether you can calculate accurately or not, or whether if by eye you might hit the tonsil, but rather what is your record, and does it give the patient his expectation? You know there is informed consent, and that means that the patient didn't know that there is another way of doing it, that there is more to be offered. Or there is the injury involved on the basis of failing to meet the standards of the community, and the standards of the community today extend from San Francisco to New York and from Wisconsin to Houston. I think this is an important factor in looking forward to the next five years. We must rely more on this, and it will not be a gimmick. I think it is for the betterment of treatment.

DAVIS:

I would like to open a new topic for discussion, since, at least at this point, we're considering where we go during the next five years. For many of the people attending this conference, where we go over the next five years is dependent on available funds and other support they might have. In line with this it might be helpful in addressing to some funding agencies the sense of this meeting. I'd like to introduce a resolution for consideration. This resolution was drawn up aimed provisionally at funding agencies in the United States, but it can be modified so that it is more general.

"Whereas developments in computer assistance in radiation oncology now promise major gains in cancer research, training, patient management, and community services, as well as opportunities to multiply the effectiveness of the health research and service manpower now in short supply, and thus produce fiscal economies and improved patient care, and whereas the Fifth International Conference on the Use of Computers in Radiation Therapy represents the international leadership in the field, a strategic plan for the development of computer assistance in radiation oncology consistent in format with that utilized in the National Cancer Plan should be prepared by Conference representatives to afford the most authoritative recommendations in the cancer area to the Director of the National Cancer Plan, to appropriate program areas, to the appropriate program director within the National Cancer Institute, and to other concerned individuals."

CUNNINGHAM:

Dr. Davis' intent in presenting this item, as a resolution, is to see if the meeting will agree to have that statement included in the proceedings of the meeting. It is intended to be a statement that might be usable by delegates to this meeting in their own country after they return.

VIII. Contributed Papers

1. The Thomas Jefferson University Hospital Radiation Therapy Departmental Computer System

J. D. Steben
R. Wu
N. Suntharalingam
C. Mansfield

Introduction

This is a progress report of the implementation of a PDP-11/45 Departmental Computer System for Radiation Therapy and Nuclear Medicine by the computer group in Medical Physics (Radiation Therapy). The present system consists of 16 K core, 1.2 M words disk storage, 2 Dectapes, magtape, line printer, 611 scope, Calcomp plotter, and grafatron (rho-theta) tracer.

The computerization effort consists of several people at present, within Medical Physics, involved part time in developing and testing programs and other software. It is planned to add another full-time person. Hardware maintenance is under contract with Digital Equipment Corporation.

As will be discussed below, the computer has so far provided a major resource for dosimetry and treatment planning, and has been used considerably for data reduction in radiation biology research. It also has been used on a pilot study basis for clinical research examinations of patient records, as discussed below. It is hoped to implement the use of the computer for treatment verification on a BBC 45 MeV Betatron (6) and a Clinac-4. These usages will be further described in succeeding paragraphs.

Treatment Planning Computer Utilization

Basically, TJUH has used the external beam treatment-planning programs developed by Cunningham et al. (2, 3). These use scatter-air-ratio summations to calculate doses. The programs include:

CBEAM (rectangular fixed fields with wedges and patient contours) usable in both fixed-SSD and isocentric setup modes.
PBEAM (rotations; one- and two-isocenter)
IBEAM (irregular beam program for isodose calculations)
IRREG (irregular beam program for point calculations)
A special version of CBEAM which just reads and adds beams (doses) stored in a file is used for electron beams.
A program TIMER (written at TJUH) is used to calculate treatment times and/or monitor units, using scatter-air-ratios.

For brachy-therapy, treatment-planning is presently done for intracavitary and interstitial radium sources using a program derived from Cunningham's ISODOS, and for interstitial iridum sources using a program developed at TJUH.

Various radiation-treatment protocols have been developed, and beam properties of treatment machines have been studied. These activities are expected to continue.

Patient Records Computer Utilization

We purchased from Meditech the MUMPS and MIIS operating systems with about 100 application programs developed by Tufts – New England Medical Center (4) and translated into MIIS language by Meditech. The systems are now being used in research-oriented patient-retrieval studies. General clinically relevant information on extent of disease, diagnosis record, summaries of radiotherapy treatment, surgery chemotherapy, hormone therapy, and subsequent follow-up records of breast cancer patients are being fed into the disk via the two time-shared terminals with the purpose of long-term evaluations of treatment effectiveness in mind. Our plan is that complete records of individual patient or statistics of the entire patient population may be retrieved by personnel such as secretaries, medical students, or physicians with minimal instructions.

Further developments may include:

1. extending to other anatomic sites,
2. daily routine scheduling and billing,
3. letters to referring physicians.

System Development

In the past, the TJUH PDP-11/45 has been operated largely as a single-user, single-purpose system. With a core-size limitation of 16 K, dosimetry and most other general applications have been run under

DEC-supplied DOS-V8, while patient records have been mainly run under two user MUMPS. A MIIS system, also obtained from Meditech, will replace MUMPS for patient records analysis. The goal of the system development is a departmental computer for the Radiation Therapy and Nuclear Medicine Department which will also serve radiation biology and medical physics requirements related to the Department. Medical physics measurements indicated include ultrasound studies related to patient contour and internal structures, isodose measurements, and their digitization. An approach to live data acquisition and subsequent analysis will also be worked out for Nuclear Medicine imaging. Additional core has been ordered (an increase to 32 K) and should arrive at any time. This will permit a beginning of multitasking operations. These will initially be undertaken using a time-sharing operating system, SDOS developed by Wachtor (1) at Rush-Presbyterian Hospital (Chicago). A fairly ideal projected size which we plan for the TJUH system to attain is 48 K (or 64 K) core and two RK05 disk drives. Floating point hardware will be added to expedite treatment planning, and about 6 terminals will be connected. This should allow effective resource-sharing using an operating system of the sophistication of the RSX-11/M, incorporating also memory segmentation for the greater reliability afforded by user-file core-area protection. The major question at this time is the means of achieving dynamic resource-sharing between MUMPS and the other applications, a nontrivial but interesting software project.

It seems unfortunate that to date, so far as we know, the dialects of MUMPS existing for the PDP-11 each require a special operating system limited to MUMPS. This greatly restricts other uses of the system. Although other users have made at least some efforts to cope with this problem (5) the present project seeks a more comprehensive solution which would not exclude program development in higher level languages, including FORTRAN. At the same time, and all day, the computer should be available for patient records and activities, machine scheduling activities, etc., hopefully under MUMPS (MIIS).

One nontrivial approach to achieve this would be a system-alternation technique with common keyboard-interrupt servicing, in which MUMPS (MIIS) and SDOS alternate with roughly one-second time slices. Information would be swapped between the systems via special ascii I/O with dectape (or magtape). The bookkeeping would necessitate unique device-assignments (i.e. SDOS and MUMPS on separate disks) and controller-status checking. Other more sophisticated techniques are possible.

REFERENCES

1. Chung-Bin, A., Wachtor, T., and Hendrickson, F., "Verification of Patient Setup, Treatment Planning, and Information Retrieval with

PDP-11/45 Computer," *RSNA 59th Annual Meeting Abstracts*, p. 107 (1973)

2. Cunningham, J. R., Shrivastava, P. N. and Wilkinson, J. M., Computer Calculation of Dose within an Irregularly Shaped Beam," *Dosimetry Workshop—Hodgkins Disease*, AAPM, RPC, Cooperative Hodgkins Disease Clinical Trial, NCI, Chicago, Ill. (1970).
3. Johns, H. E., and Cunningham, J. R., *The Physics of Radiology* (3rd ed. C. C. Thomas, Springfield, Ill. (1969)
4. Neurath, P. W., Bloedorn, F. G., Munzenrider, J. E. and Pedrazzi, M. G., *Cancer, 33*, 1653 (1974).
5. Seymour, R., personal communication (1974)
6. Steben, J., and Suntharalingam, N., "Computer Assisted Entry, Verification and Recording of Treatment Parameters for 45 MeV Betatron" (this conference).

2. Rush Radiation Oncology Computer System

T. Wachtor
A. Chung-Bin
F. Korzeniewski

Introduction

It is felt by the authors that the Department of Radiation Oncology at Rush-Presbyterian-St. Luke's Medical Center has a computer system developed in a clinical environment uniquely tailored to meet the needs of a modern radiation therapy center. The computer is able to satisfy the day-to-day requirements as well as the research needs of a dynamic department.

Hardware and Operating System:

The basic hardware of the Rush Radiation Oncology system is a PDP 11/45 computer with 28 K core memory and 2.5 megabytes of disk storage. The PDP 11/45 is a 16 bit/word computer with significant add-on features. Two of the more important add-ons are a floating-point processor for fast arithmetic, which works in parallel with the C.P.U., and a memory-management unit that allows extension of memory to 124 K words along with hardware-protection fields within memory.

The PDP 11 family of computers is bus-oriented. That is, all internal communication is accomplished via a master-slave relationship between devices over a 56-line connector. An important result is that it makes for relatively easy design, construction, and debugging of specialized hardware devices.

The operating system currently supports eight user terminals. All terminals have complete access to all resources of the computer. Resources of the computer are managed by a modified version 4-disk operating system (D.O.S.), as provided by Digital Equipment Corp. D.O.S. version 4 was modified to allow an effective time-sharing among the users. Currently the resident operating system code occupies about 3 K of core memory. The rest of core memory is divided between I/O Buffers/System work space, and one user's area, in conjunction with a core image disk file which allows the user program to be swapped between the user area in core and the disk files. Individual user programs are allowed to reside for a short period of time in the user area. When the period of time is up, the user area is written to disk, and a different program is brought from disk to core user area. This swapping between user programs depends on a dynamic priority system that involves initial priority set, actual run-time used, time spent residing on the disk, and type of input/output performed. Currently, the swaps are forced by keyboard, line-printer, and plotter input/output.

The necessity of monitoring real time events in a time-sharing computer is achieved by user programs installing subroutines into a chain of routines located in system-work-space keyed to the clock interrupts. That is, every fiftieth of a second this chain of routines is executed by the operating system. These routines can then monitor a (slow-moving) real-time process without the main program being in core.

To those unfamiliar with DEC's D.O.S., the main software features are (1) an assembler, (2) a text editor, (3) a Fortran compiler, (4) a linkage editor, (5) an interpretive basic compiler, (6) a peripheral interchange program, and (7) a command input (somewhat similar to batch processing). Although the basic operating system is similar to DEC's D.O.S. version 4, modifications have been made to allow both D.O.S. 4 and D.O.S. 8 versions of the above program to operate.

The operating system has several different versions. Basically they run the gamut of operating on a 16 K PDP 11/20 through various upgrades to a 28 K PDP 11/45 with floating-point hardware. Used in 16 K of core memory, each terminal appears to have an 8 K D.O.S. system available to it. When used with 28 K of core memory, each terminal appears to have a complete 16 K D.O.S. system available to it.

Unfortunately, the memory-management unit is not implemented in any of the above systems, hence these are unprotected operating systems. Obviously, running programs of dubious reliability is extremely trying on all concerned. Work is progressing on a D.O.S.-4, D.O.S.-8, compatible operating system that will take advantage of the memory-management unit. However, the present system allows rapid changeover to the PDP 11/20 C.P.U.

Application

The growth and design of the Rush-Presbyterian-St. Luke's Medical Center system has been strongly influenced by the actual requirements of the department—that is, the medical staff, physics staff, and administrative personnel. Application programs can be broken roughly into three areas of interest. These are dosimetry, treatment assistance, and patient-data management.

Dosimetry

A fairly extensive package of programs to assist in dosimetry is available to the physics section. These include a program to handle external beam dosimetry, the M. D. Anderson RADCOMP program to handle implant dosimetry, and an iridium wire inplant dosimetry program from Jefferson Medical School of Philadelphia.

Smaller utility programs calculate scatter-air ratios, effective tissue-air ratios for rotation type treatments, nominal standard dose for ordinary and split course treatments, and monthly tables of dose versus time for various Cobalt units in the area.

Primary input into these programs is digitized data fed onto a terminal. Primary output is the Houston incremental plotter or the terminal in the case of simple calculations.

Treatment Assistance

Treatment assistance at the Rush Radiation Oncology Department means the interaction of computer and treatment personnel to ensure more consistent patient treatment. Toward this goal a large package of programs and hardware have been developed. The general uses of these programs are monitoring and verification. Monitoring requires the hardware and software to convert analog and digital signals from the therapy units to meaningful physical parameters, such as 180 degrees for gantry rotation, and the recording of such values in a file where they are available later. Verification involves retrieval of these prerecorded treatment parameters and their comparison to the parameters set during a patient's treatment. Any discrepancies then have to be resolved by conversation with the treatment machine operator. We are currently monitoring and verifying two therapy units. One is a specially modified Theratron 80, the other is a computer-prepared Varian 4 MeV Linear Accelerator.

Patient Data Management

Patient data management falls into two general categories. The first is a general long-range project. The second is a group of short-range special studies. The general long-range project involves gathering demographic, treatment, and pathologic information on all patients entering the department. The type of information, and its acquisition is the subject of another paper. However, a few points should be covered here. Without the file structure inherent in a system like MUMPS, a method of multiple access to shared data had to be developed. All data on active patients is stored in one large contiguous file. The file has its own directory structure, space-allocation scheme, and I/O routines. The I/O routines allow a read of data at any time. However, if a file update is required and the file is already opened for update by another user, the I/O routine automatically requests a swap to the disk for the period of one second. Upon return to core, the I/O routine again examines the file and either requests another swap if the file is still open for update or goes ahead and does the requested update. The update is performed by opening the file for update, which automatically locks out interference by other users. Upon completion of the update the file is closed, releasing it to others. When additional file space is requested or if a directory is to be updated, it is the calling program's responsibility to raise its priority high enough so that other users are locked out of the computer until this critical operation is completed.

Short-range special studies usually contain small amounts of selected data for a relatively small group of patients. The input and analyzed data varies so much from study to study that usually a different set of Fortran programs are developed for each study. However, use is made of a package of subroutines that perform general tasks, such as computation and printing of a survival table.

Teaching-Research

At any institution teaching has a valuable role. Here at Rush the computer system is being used in the teaching of a short three-week course on computer basics to medical technology students, residents of radiobiology, and other interested personnel. The course involves a series of lectures on basic computer structure, followed by lectures and labs on the use of the BASIC language. The multiple terminal usage of the BASIC language is valuable here.

While this course is too short to learn any practical programming skills, it is felt that a fundamental understanding of how a computer operates will better enable medical personnel to formulate problems and data bases suitable for computer solution and manipulation.

Easy access to a computer with the capability of Fortran allows for computer-assisted research. Currently, a research project based on the Cohen Radiobiological Call Model is being programmed on the computer. Another project is the determining of N.S.D. isodose curves. Easy access to the computer also allows the Department of Nuclear Medicine at Rush to get some experience in the uses of a computer in its department before any decision on in-department computer capability is made. This has involved a modest patient file and reporting scheme, coupled with several programs to analyze various diagnostic data.

Future Goals

Goals of the Rush-Presbyterian-St. Luke's Medical Center System cover a wide area. Fundamental to the goals is the development of a protected operating system. In dosimetry, implementation of a more interactive computing program based on the methods of Cunningham will be developed. In particular, the program should be capable of performing calculations for complex dynamic treatments. This will mean not only more accurate dosimetry but one more easily used. Toward this end, a graph-pen input with plotter output that will work over phone lines is desired. Treatment assistance will be enhanced by increased system reliability. Moreover, dynamic forms of treatment will be investigated. Toward this end, a dual-processor configuration featuring a PDP 11/45 communicating with a PDP 11/20 via direct-memory interfaces will be developed.

There are no major plans for data management. However, there will be increased effort at gathering additional information during the patient's treatment in the department. Chiefly, more programs will be written to utilize existing data in a useful fashion.

Conclusion

In conclusion, our computer developments in a clinical environment have shown that a single computer can meet the needs of a Radiation Oncology Center. In summary, these needs are a comprehensive dosimetry package (on line/interactive), a treatment monitoring and verification system (a real-time process), and the maintenance of an information system.

3. A Support and Dissemination Center for Users of Dedicated Computers in Departments of Radiation Oncology

C. S. Chui
J. Hahn
S-N Yu
L. J. Lidofsky

Until a few years ago, a radiotherapy department desiring computer support had in practice three options, namely to make use of

(a) a major computing center,
(b) a timesharing service, or
(c) a small special purpose, minicomputer.

The latter has appreciable limitations resulting from its small memory size, short word length, and the lack of generalized software support, with the consequence that programs had to be written in assembly language, not in a higher-level compiler language.

In general, most departments did not have major computing centers available. Even if they did,

(a) Radiotherapy applications, particularly treatment planning, are preferably done in an interactive mode. Typically, major computing centers are batch-oriented and do not support interactive computing.
(b) If a time sharing service was selected, the typical input/output hardcopy device supported was a teletypewriter, which placed an undesirable limit on the man-machine communication process.

In either case—that is, whether a major batch-processing computer center or a large time-sharing system was used—the computer was not owned by the radiotherapy department, and there was a charge for service which was normally linear with use. This tended to discourage use, with the result that a therapist might be reluctant to request additional plans for a patient.

Developments in computer technology which have taken place during the past few years have provided radiotherapy departments with new options. The advent of medium and large-scale integrated circuits has resulted in the cost of computer hardware dropping at the same time that computing power has been increasing. One can now purchase, for a cost of approximately fifty to one hundred thousand dollars, a medium-sized computer system.

Computers in this price range can be purchased with Central Processing Unit power, memory size, and speed closer to the capabilities of the large computers of the mid-1960's (e.g., the IBM 7090 series) than to the mini-computers of the same period (e.g., the Digital Equipment Corporation's PDP 8). Moreover, high-level languages are now available on low-cost dedicated computers, which are superior to those available at that time. The cost of such a system can be justified in a large department of radiotherapy, particularly if the computer system will be used for other purposes in addition to treatment planning, i.e. patient data base, patient scheduling, and, potentially, therapy machine verification and control.

A computer system is, in general, a highly dynamic entity. In some sense the most successful systems are those whose specific use may not have been anticipated at the time they were purchased. Because of this it is advisable to select a computer that is general purpose—i.e., designed for general scientific calculations and research—rather than a turnkey device whose future growth capability is suspect.

There are a number of computers with the hardware capability of handling a radiotherapy department's needs. The purchaser need not be excessively concerned with the specific hardware minutiae of a given manufacturer's product. He should rather be in a position to take a large number of additional factors into account.

In general a machine should be chosen for which as many efficient, high-level language translators as possible exist, and at least one flexible, powerful operating system. (Here too, the availability of more than one operating system can be used at different times for different functions.)

One should take into account not only the computer support provided in the past (not promised) by the particular manufacturer but also the existing and potential user's group. In this regard few things succeed as much as success! A computer produced in large quantities implies not only a manufacturer capable of providing the financial support for additional system software, and improved translators, but in addition promises large user groups with the concommitant development of user-developed software. Also, a machine sold in large quantities frequently results in additional software being available from independent systems houses. Finally, a general-purpose machine with high production gives incentive to independent peripheral suppliers to provide the purchaser with additional—and typically lower cost—sources of memory, disk and tape drives, and other input-output devices, some of which may not even be available from the computer manufacturer.

Having presented the case for purchasing general-purpose computers with a maximum of growth capability, diversified software, and a flexible operating system or systems, which will potentially be manufactured in a large quantity, we must now acknowledge a possible significant drawback of proceeding in this manner. The problem relates to the specific user-required radiotherapy application programs. Selecting a computer on the basis of our indicated criteria provides no assurance at all of having available flexible, adaptable, user software, without the need to write it oneself. Furthermore, even if programs exist (and they do) for the user's application, he may not have easy access to them. The Laboratory of Computer Science at the Mount Sinai School of Medicine,working with its Department of Radiotherapy, has therefore attempted to develop and act as a dissemination center for radiotherapy programs for use with dedicated medium-sized computers.

To further these ends and to establish communication between users of dedicated computers in departments of radiotherapy, we have sponsored or cosponsored a series of invited meetings attended by radiotherapists, physicists, and computer scientists who were either already using medium-sized computers in radiotherapy or who were interested in such use. The first two meetings, cosponsored by the Ontario Cancer Institute, were held at Mount Sinai in December of 1972 and May of 1973 respectively. Each was attended by approximately forty people, representing approximately twenty institutions. At the first meeting Mount Sinai was requested by the participants to assume a coordinating role for users of dedicated computers in radiotherapy and to serve as a communications center for information relating to both hardware and software available for such use.

A third meeting, cosponsored by Rush-Presbyterian-St.-Luke's Medical Center, took place in Chicago in December of 1973, and a fourth, again at Mount Sinai, in June of 1974.

Over the interval spanned by these four meetings there has been apparent a growing commitment to the use of dedicated medium-sized computers in radiotherapy. At last count at least fifteen institutions had made such commitments.

The laboratory of Computer Science at Mount Sinai has attempted to develop and modify existing radiotherapy computer programs, for their own use and for the growing number of users of medium-sized computers in radiotherapy. To assure flexibility and adaptability, the laboratory set as goals that programs

(a) be modular, so that a user can readily generate a system tailored his needs,
(b) be usable by radiotherapists, or physicists with exposure to computer science,
(c) make use of input/output techniniques that are accurate and easy to use and that provide a maximum amount of information to the user.

To achieve these goals one of our major decisions was to insist that as much of each software application package as possible be written in FORTRAN. This was done so that the resulting programs could easily be transported to the large number of computers provided by a variety of manufacturers. Input/output device drivers, some parts of which must necessarily be written in assembly language, were documented in a manner that clearly specified all parameters to be passed so that users with unique machines and/or unique input/output devices might readily "patch" their own assembly language routines into the system.

General features of the applications programs we are developing are that each must be segmentable so that each segment can fit into 16 K, or smaller, core memory.

The interconnection of these programs to provide a complete functioning system must unfortunately be operating-system dependent. Our experience to date has been, however, that the change from one operating system to another is not difficult once the system is understood.

The American Cancer Society, for the calendar year 1974, is providing funds to the Laboratory of Computer Science at Mount Sinai to serve as a "Support and Dissemination Center for Users of Dedicated Computers in Radiation Oncology."

More specifically, the Laboratory of Computer Science has been charged with serving as

(1) A repository for computer programs and systems relating to the use of dedicated medium-sized computer systems in radiation oncology;
(2) A center for the development of computer programs and the program modules not available from other sources; and
(3) A dissemination center for the programs and information available through 1 and 2 above.

We recognize this as a unique opportunity to be of aid and assistance to the growing group of computer users in radiotherapy.

In particular, the American Cancer Society has accepted an innovative concept relating to the dissemination of computer programs for radiotherapy. They have recognized that the *installation* of computer programs by users not familiar with the programs can be time-consuming and costly. To reduce this time and cost the American Cancer Society has provided limited funds so that staff from Mount Sinai can travel to a user's site and oversee the installation there on his specific hardware configuration. This is a major innovation in helping a user's group become operational.

We are now in the process of implementing our role as a program repository and dissemination center. At the present time we basically have two sets of radiotherapy planning programs. The first of these is concerned with external beam therapy and was provided by Jack Cunningham of the Ontario Cancer Institute. The second is concerned with dose calculations from implanted needles and was developed at Mount Sinai. We have in addition received communications from several groups telling us that they have programs that they would make available. We as yet have not obtained them.

After receiving but before distributing programs, it is necessary to determine needs for modifications or adaptations. These occur at several levels. First, one must make the program work, which means that drivers may have to be written either to incorporate I/O devices which we have and others do not, or to replace I/O devices that the program supplier has and we do not. For both of these categories, of course, we have had no problems with the needle program we wrote, although we did have to make some adaptation to the programs from Cunningham. There is a possibility that drivers will have to be written for other places if they either lack an I/O device or have a substitute device. If the device is relatively simple, it is probably easier for us to write the driver, given a description of their device, than for *them* to write the driver, given a description of *our* program. If we don't believe that to be the case, we distribute the description of what the driver is to accomplish, what the host program expects to receive or pass in the way or parameters, make that available to the user, and then request that when he has written a driver that works, he make it available to us so that we can distribute it to others.

Before distributing programs, we test as many options as we can think of, both for our own and for others' programs, in order to assure that the program will work in the way we think it should. At this point we have a program we believe works as the originator intended it to. Of course it may be that for our own purposes we will want to change something about the program so that it suits our concept of how an easy-to-use program should operate. In doing this, however, *we do not change the physics.* Our intent at this point is not to create new radiation physics techniques—to calculate doses, for instance—but rather to make the techniques that already exist easier to use, as well as generally available. To date we have made only one installation—at Rhode Island Hospital, where we made an initial installation of some of Dr. Cunningham's programs. By the end of September we will have made a complete installation there as well as in several other hospitals in the Northeast area.

In summary, if our program is successful we hope to provide a portion of the radiotherapy community with the best of all possible worlds. The therapist can choose a computer system which he feels is optimal from a hardware, software, and local service point of view (among other criteria), and be provided with a set of programs which will enable him to begin using his system quickly. If in the future he desires to change these programs, and we believe that he may, it is our hope that the approaches used to develop the programming systems will make this a relatively straightforward task.

4. Application of a PDP-11/45 Computer in Treatment Monitoring and Verification of Daily Patient Setup in Radiation Oncology

T. Wachtor
A. Chung-Bin

We are currently using a PDP 11/45 computer to monitor and verify all patient treatments on a Theratron 80 teletherapy unit. Monitoring of patient treatment is simply recording the machine position and some dynamic factors during treatment. Verification is the use of previously monitored and stored data to assist the teletherapy unit operator in delivering accurate treatment. Verification, therefore, has to be an interactive process, in partnership with the operator. In addition to providing more accurate treatment, this stored data is currently being analyzed in the hope of improving operator action.

First some detail on the actual work involved. Before the program could be used, certain interfacing had to be done. It was essentially of two types: one to the operator of the Theratron 80 and one to the Theratron 80 itself. Interfacing to the operator is a Hazeltine 2000 remote terminal, driven by a DEC DC11A transmitter-receiver. It is driven at 1200 Baud, which is fast enough so that the operator doesn't have to wait for messages to come out. The software is driven by a modified DEC keyboard driver. We have modified it quite a bit, because we are running in a time-sharing environment.

Constructing an interface with the operator is simple; it turns out, however, that communication with the operator is one of the main problems of treatment-monitoring and verification. The other interfacing is with the Theratron-80 itself. We have AECL-installed Computer Instruments Corporation high resolution film potentiometers (series 7800 and 205) attached to the ten motions of the Theratron-80. Across the pots we put a -10 to +10 voltage from two supplies. The wiper voltage which is from -10 to +10 volts is brought to a semiconductor-specialist LM 201 operational amplifier. The output voltage of each drives an API micro-amp meter. This enables us to eyeball the condition of the pot and op-amp. The output voltage also goes to the DEC AD01D A/D converter. We have sixteen channels on this. Ten bits and sign per channel gives an effective resolution of + or - 1024. On these channels we have the ten parameters associated with the T 80. Actually this takes eleven channels, because gantry rotation requires two channels. We also monitor beam on and beam off and the gantry rotation direction. We also have the ability to monitor the transit dosimeter, though we have not used it yet. The integer value from the A/D converter is converted into an actual physical variable — for example, gantry rotation equal to 350.1 degrees. This information is the type stored. The A/D integer is converted to the physical variable via the below equation:

Y=A*SQRT(X+1024)+B*(X+1024)+C

This equation is of a modified translated, rotated parabola. We choose it because unfortunately not all of the potentiometers are as linear as desired. Our collimator X pot was quite nonlinear. Most of the others, however, were quite linear, meaning that the coefficient A is very small. We have a small file containing these constants. A logical unit number assigned to a particular motion points to the correct conversion constants in a table of constants and to the A/D channel number in a table of those numbers. So much for interfacing. One of the more important parts of a monitoring program is the storing of the information. A description of the file structure follows.

On an RK03 1.2 million-word disk we have allocated a 578 block contiguous file, which we call the main patient file. Reading from the file is done through an open-I (that is, open for input) routine, so that many programs can be read from the file simultaneously. Writing to the file is through an open-U (that is, open for update), so that only one program at a time can write to the file, which is normally just the monitor program itself. After every write to the file, however, the file is closed, thus allowing multiple users to write to the file. During any critical file-update process where there is any possibility of conflict, the requesting program first sets its priority so high that it cannot be swapped out until it has completed its file update. This allows apparent, simultaneous entry of data from different sources.

Inside the file, the first block, which is called block zero, is the bit pool block. In this block we describe the total number of blocks in the file, the number of blocks in use, and the number of free blocks. Then each block in the file corresponds to a bit in this block. Therefore, we can allocate blocks to a certain patient, then free them when the patient is finished and the data are moved to magnetic tape for permanent storage. Blocks 1 through 5 are the first five directory blocks. They are chained serially, and another block can be added when necessary. These directory blocks contain an entry for each patient in the file. This entry contains an indicator with the patient's status and what machine he is being treated on. Also, it has a Radix-50 packed name, hospital number, and physics number. The physics number, an invention of the Physics Department, is assigned by our secretary when the patient first walks in the door. This gets around the problem of many out-patients not having a hospital number at the time of their first treatment. In the file, for each patient, are as many treatment blocks as needed. They are chained together and contain, in an interlaced pattern, field records and treatment records. The field record pertains to a particular setup in a patient treatment and contains information on what type the field is (i.e. fixed, rotation, etc.) what the effective tissue-air ratio is, wedge angle if present, and blocking information. The treatment record itself is larger, and there is one treatment record for each patient treatment. These records also contain pointers to the next treatment. The treatment information is the date of treatment, time of day, time of beam-on, ten Theratron-80 parameters of that treatment, and other dynamic information that varies with the type of treatment, such as beam stops on an arcing type of treatment or direction of rotation in a rotation type. Also, the ten Theratron-80 parameters are recorded again at the time that the beam actually goes on. By recording the information twice, we are also trying to monitor what the operator is doing. We also have demographic blocks in the file which contain the full name, mailing address, phone number, social security number, and various other data, such as age, race, and sex. This information is entered by a label program. When the patient walks in the door, the admitting secretary of the department obtains the information from the patient and enters it into a remote terminal, in this case a teletype. For her troubles the computer later prints out eight gummed labels that can be attached to the various charts and forms associated with the patient. Also, from this we are able to generate the daily and weekly admission lists. Currently, some pathological type of information is being stored in the demographic block. It will be used to form the basis of an information storage and retrieval system.

Now let us go into the monitor program itself. It is written in PDP assembly language. There is a kernal of resident subroutines and data, then four overlays. Each overlay is brought in by a DOS tran, which is considerable faster than doing Fortran-type call links. The maximum size of the kernel and the largest overlay is only 2952 words. Not counted in this is the system and all the I/O overhead. I am confident, however, that when going through the effort of dedicating a unit to monitoring a machine that all of this can be done internally by a program in a much smaller space, and that the whole program could fit in a minimal configuration 4 K machine. The small size of the program is due in some part to the fact that all messages to the operator are kept on the disk until needed, as are the conversion factors. This saves approximately 1300 words of core storage. Since we are running a time-sharing system of our own design, the complete monitor program is swapped out of core and written to the disk on all keyboard I/O and when the program requests to be swapped. This occurs when the program is monitoring slow events, as when the beam goes on or off. While the main program is on the disk, a small subroutine running off the computer clock interrupts every 50th of a second and periodically checks the beam status. If it determines that something significant has happened, the system is notified and the main program swapped back into core. With this time-sharing system, according to my rough estimate, the program utilizes perhaps one percent of the total central processor time in an eight-hour day. Most of that is disk I/O wait time.

Now we will go through the program. The first thing is to open the files and initialize certain variables. Next, a message is printed to the operator, and the computer waits for an answer. The computer spends most of the day waiting for something to happen. The first thing that must be done is to get the operator's initials. We only allow certain operators to run the program. The next thing is to get the patient's physics number. With the physics number a directory search is done for the patient. If nothing is found, the operator is asked if this is really a new patient, one not already in the computer. Many times the physics number is typed incorrectly. If nothing is found, the operator is asked to inform the admitting secretary of that fact, since all patients walking into the department for consideration of treatment should have been entered into the computer at that time.

If during the directory search the patient is found, his name and hospital number are printed and the operator is asked if this is correct. Again, this is done to ensure against typing errors. If the data are not correct, the program goes back and re-asks for the physics number. In either case, when the patient's identity is established, the program asks for the number of the field that will be treated. Then the string of field records for the patient is searched. If that field record is not found, a new field record is allocated, and filled in with information from the operator. Then a treatment record is allocated and the date, time of day, operator's initials, and the ten static parameters are recorded. The program then waits for the beam to go on, records the dynamic type factors, and asks the operator if there will be another field for this patient, or if he has finished treatment for the day.

If the field record for this field is found, we assume that this is at least the second treatment. We locate the first treatment record and move the static information associated with it to a temporary space. If at any time during the search a treatment record is found which says that it is the new standard for treatment, its static information is placed into the temporary area and then used as the basis for comparison. We describe the type of treatment to the operator, and ask her if this is really the field that is going to be treated at this time. If it is not, the program asks again for the field number. If it is the correct field, a treatment record is allocated and the static-type information recorded from the Theratron-80 along with date, time of day, etc. Then we match these static parameters to those associated with the first treatment, assuming that the first treatment was correct. The comparison is by arbitrary standards we have chosen, such as arm rotation on a fixed field within five degrees. Outside this range we call it an error; inside that range, it is correct. If at this point any serious errors are detected, we tell the operator of those errors and ask her what is to be done about them. The operator is given four options. (1) She can say, "No, I am right and the computer is wrong," in which case the computer proceeds to wait for the beam to go on. (2) She can say that the field has been changed and that henceforth this should be considered the new standard of treatment, in which case the computer proceeds as in the case of the first treatment for that field. (3) She can say that she has made an error in the setup, in which case the computer waits for her to correct the setup. Or (4) she can say that actually the wrong field number was typed in, in which case the program clears what has been done so far and goes back to ask the field number. In any event, a point is reached where the operator and computer are satisfied. The computer waits for the beam to go on, and then records the dynamic information (time). When the beam goes on, we re-record the static information. This allows us to record corrections and therefore errors made by the operator. At the end of the treatment, the dynamic-type parameters are matched against what is considered correct, and the operator is informed of any inconsistencies. We do not actually stop the treatment when errors of this type are detected. It was decided that this would accomplish little, and the patient might be frightened. At the end of the treatment the operator is asked if this patient's session will continue or is finished, or if the patient's course of treatment is finished—in which case a "finished therapy" flag is set.

Besides the Theratron 80 monitor program itself, several other support-type programs are necessary The MESLD program loads part of the file with messages, which can be printed without storage of the message in the code proper. The SETPAR program determines the constants necessary to convert the analog/digital values to actual numbers having physical meaning. The label program inputs the demographic information. The update program provides some information on patients not treated on the Theratron 80. The DKTOTP program deletes patients from the main file and stores them on magnetic tape. Even if the information is not permanently stored, it is necessary to delete patients from the relatively small file. The PFUTIL program is a generally useful utility program. It is able to initial, save, restore, and modify the patient file. Naturally, besides these large programs there are a host of subroutines.

I would like to bring up some of the problems and points of interest that we have run into. Most of the problems encountered are ones relating to the operator. There is a very serious problem on a fully motorized unit such as ours—extremely slow setup. All motions have to be set up sequentially, and are limited by the speed of the motors that drive the motion. The slow setup combined with a heavy patient load leads to a number of problems. Number one is that the operator, all too often, initiates the program too soon or too late. When the program is initiated too soon, the parameters recorded are not those of the actual treatment setup and, obviously, are the wrong parameters. When the program is initiated too late, dynamic-type information, such as the initial arm position on a rotation-type treatment, will be recorded incorrectly. Secondly, when the operator is rushed, there may be error in the operation of the remote terminal keyboard itself, which means that the format must be checked for each response typed in. Also, at each point of information entry to the keyboard, the operator must be given an easy way to exit from that point and go back to a previous point in the program. If the task is not made easy, the operator may say "The hell with it" and not bother to correct trivial mistakes. Another type of problem is of a computer crash, especially in one having a home-grown operating system. When there is a crash in the middle of a treatment, the data recorded will be incomplete, Therefore, the next time around the computer has to recognize incomplete data and be able to recover from this without confusing the operator with erroneous information.

5. A Proposed Scheme to Implement a Transverse Section Transmission Scanner for Radiation Therapy Treatment Planning

V. Smith
R. J. Baker

Introduction

The first commercially available unit for computerized axial tomography, the EMI Scanner (8) has gained wide acceptance for the visualization of small differences of density within the cranium. Another instrument has been described (10) which eliminates the need for a constant-path-length water bath around the patient and has extended the concept to include every part of the body.

So far, computerized tomography has been used almost exclusively as a diagnostic technique in neuroradiology, but the technique has an obvious application in radiation therapy. Computer programs that calculate dose distributions, taking into account tissue inhomogeneities, have been available for many years. Until the development of the Computerized Axial Tomograph (CAT), however, no good technique existed to determine the distribution of densities within transverse body cross-sections, necessary as basic input to the dose calculation programs.

Cost Factor

Even though commercially available CAT's capable of transverse-section body tomography are now beginning to appear on the market, their high cost (approximately $300,000) probably places them out of consideration for a department of radiation therapy. The purpose of our investigation was therefore to determine whether a system could be developed for radiation therapy treatment-planning at a reasonable cost. We determined that considerable cost savings could be accomplished partly by simplifying the technique as much as possible, and partly by making use of equipment which probably already exists in many large departments. Considerable simplicity of mechanical design can be achieved by using a multi-element detector in a fan-beam geometry. This eliminates the need for translational motion, and suggests the possibility of using a therapy simulator to provide rotational motion of the X-ray source and detector about a patient lying on the simulator couch.

Detector System

The detector assembly must be sensitive along a length of about 50 cm, have a linear resolution of about 0.5 cm, and be capable of handling count rates up to 10^6 counts/second or greater. This latter requirement also places constraints on the readout instrumentation.

Many schemes are possible to implement the above, but we shall single out one example. A group at the University of California has described a multiwire proportional chamber for biomedical applications (9). A single-wire version of this chamber has been constructed and is being applied to computerized tomography for pion therapy treatment-planning by workers at Stanford University and the Univeristy of California (1). This position-sensitive line detector consists of a pressurized xenon gas proportional chamber enclosed by an aluminum cylinder 50 cm long, 0.5 mm thick, and 15 cm in diameter. Position readout is derived from the delay of pulses induced in a helical wound delay line that serves as a cathode plane. Another parallel cathode plane opposite the delay line is defined by an open electromesh grid. The cathodes are raised to a positive high voltage with respect to the cylinder wall, which generates a drift field and collects ionization produced outside the high field region. The total gas thickness is 3 cm, which yields approximately 30 percent detection efficiency at 75 psig working pressure.

Timing pulses from the detector are processed by NIM modules, including preamplifiers, zero cross discriminators, and a time-to-amplitude converter (TAC); and the event is stored in the computer memory.

Boyd used a ^{241} Americium radiation source in his preliminary experiment (1), which gave relatively low count rates compared to those possible from a diagnostic X-ray tube. He indicates that by using the arrangement above with a 100 MHz ADC and pil-up rejection, count rates of 2×10^5 counts/second could be handled. At this count rate the density distribution in a body cross-section could be determined to ± 5 percent precision in a total scan time of less than one minute. Boyd suggests that the basic proportional counter design could be modified to give parallel readout with multiple anode wires, each connected to an inexpensive 10-MHz 16-bit scaler. Such a system could handle 10^8 counts/second and provide good density precision with very brief scan times.

Position-sensing proportional chambers in a variety of configurations are now available commercially.

Reconstruction of the Density Distribution

The problem of reconstructing two-dimensional distributions from multiple one-dimensional projections has received attention by workers in many fields. Gordon has assembled an extensive bibliography (6). A bewildering array of different algorithms have been used which can be grouped in several different ways. One possible grouping is

(1) Direct matrix inversion techniques.
(2) Algebraic reconstruction techniques (ART).
(3) Convolution and fourier transform techniques.
(4) Iterative least squares techniques.

The first of these is probably not feasible for the purpose under consideration here, because the inversion of large matrices requires too much run-time on the processor. Dehnert and Boyd have published an intercomparison of some of the other available techniques (4). They implemented on a PDP 11/45 computer an iterative method (5), a convolution method (2, 11), and an ART method (7), modified to use the Goitein cell-fraction table. They concluded that the convolution method was best if only limited time was available, but that the modified ART gave even better results when five or more iterations were performed. The performance of each technique is to some extent determined, however, by the noise present in the data and the choice of damping factors used in the iterations. There is reason to suspect that a combination of techniques may be desirable.

Budinger has examined various iterative and convolution techniques with regard to the reconstruction of radionuclide distributions from gamma camera measurements (3). This report includes a listing of computer subroutines to implement four different algorithms. For the purpose under consideration here, however, the routines would have to be modified to allow for fan-beam geometry.

Summary

Many large departments of radiation therapy already possess a treatment simulator and a PDP 11/45 or other mini computer. The preceding discussion has indicated that with a relative modest additional outlay of approximately $10,000, a detector and associated instrumentation could be purchased to implement the basic data acquisition system for computerized tomography. In addition, position readout and control of the angular rotation of the treatment simulator would have to be provided.

Obviously the implementation of a system such as we have indicated would not be without problems, but we feel that both the detector technology and the reconstruction algorithms have been developed to the point where this could be brought to a practical reality.

REFERENCES

1. D. Boyd, J. Coonrod, J. Chiu, D. Lim, B. Macdonald, and V. Perez-Mendez, *Science, 21* (1), 184-187 (1974).
2. R. N. Bracewell and A. C. Riddle *Astrophys, J. 150* (2), 427-434 (1967).
3. T. F. Budinger and G. T. Gullberg, *Three Dimensional Reconstruction in Nuclear Medicine by Iterative Least-Squares and Fourier Transform Techniques*, Lawrence Berkeley Laboratory, University of California, Report LBL 2140 (January 1974). Available from the National Technical Information Service, U.S. Department of Commerce.
4. J. Dehnert and D. Boyd, *A Comparison Study of Some Computer Reconstruction Techniques*, High Energy Physics Laboratory, Stanford University, Report 276 (July 1973).
5. M. Goitein, *Nucl. Instr. Methods, 101*, 509-518 (1972).
6. R. Gordon, *A Bibliography on Reconstruction from Projections*, available from Mathematical Research Branch National Institutes of Health, Building 31, Bethesda, Maryland 20014.
7. R. Gordon, R. Bender, and G. T. Herman, *J. Theor. Biol. 29*, 471-481 (1970).
8. G. N. Hounsfield, *Brit. J. Radiol., 46*, 1016-1022 (1973).
9. S. N. Kaplan, L. Kaufman, V. Perez-Mendez, and K. Valentine, *Nucl. Instr. Methods, 106*, 397-406 (1973).
10. R. S. Ledley, G. Dichiro, A. J. Lussenhop, and H. L. Twigg, *Science, 186*, 207-212 (1974).
11. G. N. Ramachandran and A. V. Lakshminarayanan, *Proc. Natl. Acad. Sci., U.S., 68* (9), 2236-2240 (1971).

6. DIDOS: A Matrix-Based Dose-Planning System

T. Gustafsson
U-B Nordberg
K Liden

1. INTRODUCTION

The two-dimensional automatic dose-planning system for external beam-therapy DIDOS is based on a library of matrices of measured dose-distributions on disk or tape. The system thus enables the use of flat as well as wedged fields for all types of treatment units, beam energies, photons, or electrons. Correction for oblique incidence and all sorts of heterogeneities can be performed. Calculations are made for the whole cross-section of the patient in a grid with 3 mm spacing, and the resultant dose-distribution is plotted together with a sketch of the cross-section, with as many details as are desired, and in five colors.

1.1 Goals

It is our intention to achieve an automatically optimizing or, alternatively, an interactive, multisectional dose-planning system. Today the system already allows for multisectional dose-planning at levels where the distribution of absorbed dose can be considered approximately the same as in the principal plane of the beam. Our intention is, however, to extend the validity outside this region by applying a correction-function.

With our present computer equipment, a remote terminal at the clinic, we have to run the system as a remote batch job, and a self-optimizing program for selecting the field parameters has therefore seriously been considered (7). Should the equipment be replaced by local computer, a matter that is under consideration, the great advantages of an interactive dose-planning system make a self-optimizing program unnecessary.

The use of film as a recording medium has the advantage of recording the absorbed dose simultaneously at all points of the distribution during a period of time corresponding to that of a normal patient-irradiation. Many fields can be measured during a short period of time (4). Therefore there is no need for making a special wedge-correction program, which gives another source of error. The resulting wedged fields are directly recorded. The density-matrix of measured points also contains a lot of information which makes calculations in the dose-planning program itself much easier and faster.

1.2 Related Systems

The dose-planning system operates in close connection with the medical records system, enabling an adequate exchange of information between the system for documentation of external beam-therapy, BEKO (1), which handles all parameters concerning external beam treatment—anatomical, physical, as well as technical— and the system for patient-records and follow-up, RUFS (2). Among other advantages, this means that any dose-plan for a patient can be reproduced on demand.

1.3 User-Oriented Output

Great efforts have been made to create a form of presentation meeting the user's needs, since in our opinion the introduction of automatic dose-planning must not in any way reduce the service now being given to the physician. On the contrary, the service has been extended to assist the physician with additional data concerning the dose-distribution. The dose-plan is therefore plotted in full size on an incremental plotter in five colors, i.e. in the same manner as our manual plans. The physician should neither be forced to fiddle with knobs and look at small CRT-displays (3) nor have to deal with line-printer maps.

2. COLLECTION OF DATA

2.1 Dose Distribution

2.1.1 Film dosimetry. The distributions of absorbed dose in planes through the central axis of the beam, parallel to the field edges, are recorded by means of films. The naked film is exposed in a polystyrene phantom and without any tilting, to the central axis. We use a low-sensitive graphic film (such as Gaevert T51P). The film-density is kept linear to absorbed dose by appropriate film-processing, giving a density between 1.5 and 2.0 for 200 to 300 rad with a normal haze of 0.04. The energy-dependence is taken care of by calibration to absorbed dose along the central axis and at the absolute dose-maximum point. The validity of this calibration for 8MV X-rays and ^{60}Co has been confirmed. The transverse beam profiles at 2, 10, and 20 cm, measured with film and with an ionization chamber, showed very good agreement.

The energy variation across the beam at a fixed depth thus seems to have a rather small influence on the dose-density calibration. In fact, if a correction for this energy variation should be done for the ionization measurement, the two profiles would be brought even closer together. The ionization chamber had a fairly good energy response.

2.1.2 Energy calibration. The film is scanned and its density digitized in matrices with a cell-size of 3 mm and punched on paper tape. The punched paper tape containing all the digitized data of density from the scanned film is then read into the computer by the calibration program, ATLAS. The input data is checked thoroughly for any abnormal values, which are corrected automatically, if possible. This is done in a data-bounding procedure, where isolated erratic values, i.e. values that differ significantly (positively or negatively) from all their surrounding elements, are replaced by the mean density of the surroundings. The average background density is subtracted afterward. The central axis depth-dose (CADD) and the absolute dose-maximum for wedged fields are punched on cards and used for calibration of the density scan into a normalized distribution of absorbed dose. The maximum value on the central axis is set to 100 percent.

The calibration is done as follows: a least-square fit to the density values is made along the central axis, starting at the maximum value. Although the function differs for different beam qualities, it is parabolical over the first part, the shoulder of the density curve, and an overlapping 3rd degree polynomial fit down to maximum calibration depth. The calibration curve is arrived at by comparing the density function with the CADD values down to the smallest CADD value. The calibration function is then linearly extrapolated to zero density. The position of the central axis in the density matrix is computed automatically for wedged fields as well as for unwedged fields but can be given as input data. The corresponding column of density values, which is used for calibration purposes, can, however, be shifted at will.

The depth for certain dose values, for example 70 and 80 percent for linear accelerator X rays, is compared to the correct depths for these points, and should the mean error exceed 1.5 mm, the CADD

CADD is shifted this distance in relation to the density matrix, and a new calibration takes place. If the difference is less than 1.5 mm, this amount is stored for future shifting of the plotted isodose curves.

Each density value is then replaced by the normalized absorbed dose value, which is calculated according to the calibration function.

The dose-distribution matrix is plotted as a contour map with 10 percent level-spacing, together with the density-dose calibration curve. These plotted isodose charts were in use for manual dose-planning a long time before the automatic dose-planning system was used routinely.

2.1.3 File structure. Each field is labeled with a code-number describing the treatment unit, radiation quality, SSD, filter, field width, and equivalent square area. To keep the number of dose matrices required within practical limits, only a limited number of equivalent square fields for each field width are stored. This division into classes or areas is individual for the treatment units and is done so that the maximum error in the central axis due to this classification is less than 1.5 percent. The dose-distribution matrix is then packed into 1/3 word (12 bits)-format, sorted, and stored on mass storage. The 200 most common fields are stored on disk and the rest on magnetic tape. The file has the same code number as the sorting key. The total field atlas consists of about 600 fields and covers all the different high-voltage treatment units, photons as well as electrons.

2.2 Anatomical Cross-section

2.2.1 Sonic pen. The sonic pen digitizer (Graf/Pen) consists of two microphones, each 50 cm long, one for x- and y-direction and a spark-emitting pen. The time difference between the firing of the spark by pressing the tip of the pen against the surface of the table and the reception of the ultrasonic wave by the microphones is measured digitally, and these values represent the coordinates. They are automatically punched on paper tape as integers with four digits, corresponding to a resolution of about 0.13 mm. The practical limit, however, lies in the bluntness of the tip of the ball-point pen. No analog-to-digital converters are needed, and there are no moving parts.

The sonic pen is interfaced to a teletype so that alphanumerical information can be entered on the keyboard. This information is punched on the same paper tape as the information from the sonic pen.

2.2.2 Manual procedure. Areas have been outlined on the working tablet (50 cm × 50 cm). These boxes are assigned different meanings, and they are used for so-called menu-picking. They correspond to light buttons on a CRT-display. When the operator points in one of these boxes, a coordinate pair is punched as for any other point on the tablet, but the computer program recognizes this point as a box coordinate and the program flow is branched according to the significance of the box. The contours are traced in single-shot mode—i.e., one coordinate pair is transferred to the teletype each time the tip of the pen is pressed against the tablet. The planning suggestions can be entered as mentioned above, but can also be altered by adding corrections on punched cards, such as beam-angle, field-weight, and entry-point as well as the field-matrix itself.

The system allows for 50 fields, 7 heterogeneity areas (the effective density is entered on the keyboard), and an unlimited number of other areas of interest in the dose plan. Free text can be transferred from the keyboard to the plot. Most boxes can be activated in arbitrary order. Boxes labeled, for example, "points of interest" or "entry point favorability" have been reserved for a possible self-optimizing program.

3. DOSE COMPUTATION

3.1 General Principle

The patient matrix has a maximum size of 150 × 100 elements (45 × 30 cm) and one field 100 × 120 elements (30 × 36 cm), all in core memory. Because of the small cell size, which can be achieved with film as the recording medium, no interpolation is necessary which reduces the computation time considerably.

One field at a time is read from the disk and added cumulatively to the patient dose-matrix, so in principle any number of fields could be used. The corrections for oblique incidence and for inhomogeneity are made by the isodose-shift method (5), and these corrections are performed along the columns of the field matrix. If the depth in the patient exceeds 30 cm, the field matrix is extrapolated. The computation time does not increase significantly with correction for heterogeneity, and it is the same for photons as well as electrons. No extra measures have to be taken for wedged fields, since these are recorded as separate fields.

3.2 Coordinate Systems

There are two main coordinate systems, the patient's and the field coordinate system. The dose is computed only for discrete grid points in the patient matrix.

3.3 Correction for Oblique Incidence

This correction is done with the isodose shift method, using an effective depth, the distance for shifting the isodoses, which is the true distance multiplied by an appropriate factor that is 0.5 for an 8 MV linear accelerator, 0.75 for a 33 MV betatron, and 0.67 for cobalt units—all equipment at normal SSD's, 0.5 for Caesium used at extremely short SSD's and 1.0 for electrons.

3.3.1 The build-up region. The correction performed from the surface down to dose maximum, however, is that of "effective SSD method" (6).

3.4 Correction for Heterogeneities

This correction is, as mentioned above, also done with the isodose shift—i.e., the effective depth is computed cumulatively along the columns in the field matrix and the dose at the corresponding depth is added to the patient dose at that particular point.

4. PRESENTATION OF THE DOSE PLAN

4.1 Line Printer Output

Important dose parameters, such as maximum, minimum, and mean absorbed dose in the target volume and the critical organs, are calculated. Furthermore, the area encircled by the different isodose levels is estimated as well as the integral dose. This information, together with parameters of beam geometry and data necessary for patient setup, is printed on a separate sheet and could also be written on magnetic tape for transfer to the BEKO-system.

4.2 Color Plot

The plotter tells the operator which color to select according to the color code. The shifting of pens is done manually but is very easy and can be done quickly on our plotter. The patient outline, other anatomical details (except for lung tissue) and text are drawn in black. Lung tissue is drawn in blue and the target area (-s) in red. The isodose-lines are drawn in green, representing each 20 percent level outside the target area and every 5 percent level involving the target area. The geometrical field limits are drawn in yellow and diverge through the whole cross-section. If a field weight is less than 100 percent, the percentage figure is marked in red at the entrance of the field. The density values for lung and bone tissue are given in the same color as the corresponding contour, so that they will not be mistaken for dose values, which are green. The field axis is drawn with a broken line.

4.3 Isometric Presentation

An isometric display of the dose distribution can be ordered if desired. This presentation, which is in fact analog, is of value for visualization of the relative dose distribution between target and nontarget areas, and for warning of hot spots outside the target volume.

5. HARDWARE AND SOFTWARE SPECIFICATIONS

The system is run in remote-batch mode on a UNIVAC 1108 at the University Computer Center from a UNIVAC 9200-II terminal. This terminal is equipped with a card reader, a paper-tape reader, line printer, and incremental plotter. Transmission capacity is 4800 baud.

The program is written in Fortran V and occupies, after segmentation, 42 K words of core storage. The average turn-around time for a dose plan is about 30 minutes, and the CPU-time around 30 seconds. In that time, the dose is calculated in about 10,000 grid points.

6. CONCLUSION

The average cost for a dose plan, single section, is 40 Swedish crowns, based on the prices at our university's computer center (roughly $9.00 U.S.A.).

REFERENCES

1. Gustafsson, Th., Moller, T. R. and Nordberg, U.B., *Computer Programs in Biomedicine, 3* 135-144, (1973).
2. Moller, T. R., Johnsson, J. E., Sundstrom, A., and Gustafsson, Th., "Computer-Based Patient Record and Follow-Up System for Radiotherapy," these proceedings.
3. Cunningham, J., (contributions to) "Discussions of Response to Precirculated Questions," *Proc. Fourth International Conf. on the Use of Computers in Rad. Ther.*, (Uppsala, 1973), p. 47.
4. Gustafsson, Th., and Nordberg, U. B. "Accurate Computer-Aided Evaluation of Beam Flatness for Accelerators," *Third Int. Conf. on Medical Physics* (Goteborg 1972).
5. Nordberg, U.S., *Acta Radiologica, 11* 113-128 (1972).
6. ICRU Report 10d: "Clinical Dosimetry," *NES Handbook 87*, National Bureau of Standards, Washington, 1963.
7. Hope, C. S. and Cain, O., *Computer Programs in Biomedicine*, 2 221-231 (1972).

7. A Computer-Assisted Method for Computing Machine Time for Square and Rectangular Fields on Teletherapy Machines

W. D. Renner

Introduction

A computer can best ease any computational task which is repetitive. The routine calculation of machine time can be laborious if some attention is not paid to simplifying the task. The following method was developed for situations where a dedicated computer is not available, but computer support from another site can be supplied. The method is intended to simplify the calculations of machine time for square and rectangular fields on any therapy machine. Furthermore, since the computer can be at a remote location, it would only be necessary to mail the printout periodically to the therapy center.

M. J. Day has discussed the equivalent field method (1). The method is applicable to most therapy gamma-ray energies, and the field-size correction factors in air for ^{60}Co have been found to obey closely the same rule well within acceptable error limits. These two observations have been taken advantage of in producing the computational system presented herein.

To use the system, one merely picks off the equivalent square value for a rectangular or square field from a wall chart. The printout is then referred to and the column that is headed by the same (or close) equivalent square value is found. By going down the column to the appropriate depth, the dose rate in rads per minute or rads per monitor units may be directly read. This number contains the machine output, field-size air-correction factor, backscatter factor, and percentage depth dose. The dose rate obtained is then divided into the dose that the therapist desires to give at that depth. Another division is required if an attenuating tray or wedge is used that would change the dose rate. All of this may be done on a standard form that is added to the patient's chart.

It will be necessary to replace the printout periodically to account for the decay of a ^{60}Co source or a change in calibration of an accelerator. To avoid this, a permanent printout could be obtained with the output not multiplied in. However, this would require an additional multiplication for every patient calculation, defeating some of the advantage of a simple and less error-prone computational method.

To summarize, the advantages of this computer assisted method of calculation are:

1. The elimination of the need to interpolate between columns and rows of a table, a usually time-consuming and error-prone procedure. The increment of equivalent square in the printout was purposely chosen to be small, so that interpolation between columns would be unnecessary—that is, there is really no significant difference between two adjacent columns.
2. The number of arithmetical operations necessary to reach an answer are reduced to the minimum.
3. The accuracy of the computation has been maximized so that the calculation of machine time is not the limiting factor in the overall accuracy of the treatment.
4. A technician can easily perform this task for the physician.

Mathematical Method

The computer program can use as a data base percent-depth dose tables, tissue-air-ratio tables, or tissue-maximum ratio tables.

For depth dose calculation the following equations are used depending on the data base:

$$D(P) = \text{OUTPUT}\ (t, Wo, \text{DIST})\left(\frac{\text{DIST} + C}{\text{SSD}+d+C}\right)^2 \text{FSC}(Wt')\ \text{BSF}(Wd)\ \text{TMR}(d, Wd) \quad (1)$$

$$Wt' = Wt\ \text{FSSD}/\text{SSD} \quad (2)$$

$$\text{TMR}(d, Wd) = \left(\frac{\text{RSSD}+d+C}{\text{RSSD}+t+C}\right)^2 \frac{\text{BSF}(Wt)}{\text{BSF}(Wd)}\ \text{FFD}\ (d, Wt, \text{RSSD}+t) \quad (3)$$

$$D(P) = \text{OUTPUT}(t, Wo, \text{DIST.})\left(\frac{\text{DIST}+C}{\text{RSSD}+t+C}\right)^2 \text{FSC}(Wt')\ \text{BSF}(Wt)\ \text{FFD}(d, Wt, \text{RSSD}+t) \quad (4)$$

Equation 1 is calculation of the dose at depth d for field-size Wt measured at the surface. Output is the calibrated output at equilibrium depth t, field-size Wo and distance DIST. C is a correction term that may be applied to all inverse-square-law calculations. FSC is the field-size correction factor normalized to field size Wo. BSF is the back-scatter factor or analogous equivalent when using a TMR table and is normalized accordingly.

TMR is the data base stored or is calculated from equation 3 if the data base is not a TAR or TMR type table but rather a percent-depth-dose table. Wd is the field size at depth. FSSD is the distance at which the field sizes of the FSC table were measured at. SSD is the source surface distance for which the printout is being made and RSSD is the distance the percent-depth-dose table is normalized to.

Equation 4 is used only when RSSD = SSD and is a direct use of the percent-depth-dose table. Isocentric calculations are done using equations 2, 3, and 5 as is appropriate:

$$D(P) = \mathrm{OUTPUT}(t,\mathrm{Wo},\mathrm{DIST})\left(\frac{\mathrm{DIST}+C}{\mathrm{SAD}\pm S+C}\right)^2 \mathrm{FSC}(\mathrm{Wt}')\,\mathrm{BSF}(\mathrm{Wd})\;\mathrm{TMR}(d,\mathrm{Wd}) \qquad (5)$$

S is the distance from SAD at which the calculation is to be done. S only takes on values of 0 and S = (–d+t) in order to calculate the depth dose at SAD and the percent-depth-dose respectively.

TAR, TMR, and percent-depth-dose tables are stored in the same array. The FSC and BSF arrays should be filled with unity values if this is appropriate. An interpolating polynomial is used to interpolate all data points in between values of the stored table. As extrapolations often result in large errors, it is important that enough data be stored in the program to make extrapolation unnecessary.

The accuracy of converting one SSD to another is subject to the same limitations of the TAR, the same basic assumptions being involved.

REFERENCE

1. Supplement 11, *British Journal of Radiology*, 1972

ACKNOWLEDGMENTS

The author appreciates the discussions and help he received from Dr. S. R. Amtey, Ph.D., LL.B., Chief of the Medical Physics Division, West Virginia University Medical Center. This work was supported in part by a West Virginia University School of Medicine Institutional Research Grant.

8. Source Vignetting and Scatter-Air Ratio Dose Calculation in Teletherapy

J. F. Drew
J. C. F. MacDonald
D. J. Dawson

Introduction

The calculation of dose at depth within a large irregular beam using scatter-air ratios is well established. Measurements in the outer region of a large beam from a Theratron 80 in this Clinic consistently gave lower values than those calculated by an established computer program (1, 2). The PC 12 (Artronix) planning computer system has a program (PC BEAM) for calculating isodose distributions using scatter-air-ratios. This also gave larger values in the outer regions of large beams than were measured.

The assumption that the primary intensity remains at 100 percent (3) was made in both these papers. In an attempt to determine the difference between the measured data and calculated results, an analysis of the primary-beam profile was undertaken. This report is a summary of that work and establishes a technique to compute dose values correctly.

Measurements in this report were made with a Baldwin Farmer 0.6 cc ionization chamber with a build-up cap mounted on a remote controlled drive. The output was read on a Keithly 610 C electrometer. The Cobalt unit is an AECL Theratron 80 and all measurements were taken at 100 cms source-axis distance (SAD). The chamber was positioned on the axis and scanned across the field perpendicular to the central axis. Measurements were stopped 2 cm. from the beam edge.

Primary Beam Measurements

A simple model of the primary beam profile from a Cobalt 60 teletherapy unit assumes that only the inverse square law and penumbra affect the profile of an otherwise uniform beam. In most units, penumbra can be assumed to have no effect more than two centimeters inside the geometric edge of the beam; this report is concerned with that part of the beam which is not affected by penumbra.

Several authors (4, 5, 6) have noted that the primary dose decreases with distance from the central axis at a rate greater than would be expected by inverse square considerations alone. It has also been noted (5) that the off-axis variation was not identical for two apparently identical AECL Theratron 80 cobalt units.

Table 1 gives the results obtained from measurements of a Theratron 80 primary beam. The data shown are for three beam sizes along a principal plane (a plane that contains the beam axis and is parallel to one side) with the inverse square dependence removed. It is apparent that there is a considerable decrease in the primary-dose profile in the outer region of large beams.

Figure 1 is a schematic drawing of an AECL Theratron 80 collimator and source. The collimators are hinged at a distance of 1.43 cm. from the face of the source. The spacing between the collimator faces is adjustable and may be set to suit the source diameter. The source used for these measurements has a diameter of 1.5 cm, is 1.67 cm high, and is enclosed in a source drawer of depleted uranium.

Consider the point A in the outer region of a large beam (Fig. 1a). It cannot "see" the entire source, since the collimator hinge blocks a portion of the top of the source. Therefore, gamma rays from this part of the source BCD will be vignetted by the collimator hinge. As the point A is moved farther from the central axis, more of the source is blocked in this way, and a reduced primary dose is expected.

It is seen from Figure 1b that the hinge spacing may be increased to a point where no vignetting occurs. Although the section BCD of the source is not obstructed by the hinge, the gamma rays would be attenuated in passing through the source drawer.

Table 2, column 2, gives the results obtained from a scan with no collimator present and indicates the effect of attenuation by the source drawer. Column 3 gives the results for a collimator present with the hinge spacing (2.46 cm) sufficient to ensure no source vignetting. The difference between these two scans is probably accounted for by scatter from the collimator. Column 4 gives the results for a hinge spacing of 1.93 cm (which was the original spacing for a 1.5 cm diameter source). A significant drop is observed which is accounted for by source vignetting.

Primary Beam Calculations

The primary beam intensity at a point (x,y) off a principal plane and away from the beam edge may be calculated using a primary beam profile from a principal plane. Let M(x) be a modifying function describing the measured primary beam profile in a principal plane, with the inverse square law dependence extracted and excluding geometric penumbra. As the effect of adjacent hinges on the primary beam is independent of each other, the value of the modifying function M(x,y) at the point (x,y) is the product of the two components M(x) and M(y), then:

$$P(x,y) = M(x) \bullet M(y) \bullet (ISL) \bullet P_o \tag{1}$$

where P(x,y) is the primary beam intensity at the point (x,y), (ISL) is the inverse-square-law dependence, and P_o is the primary-beam intensity on the axis. Extra terms need to be added for points in the penumbra.

Table 3 gives a comparison between calculated and measured values of the modifying function taken at 40° to a principal plane for the case of a 40 × 40 cm beam. Agreement is better than 1.5 percent.

Scans for varying source-detector distances established that the modifying function may be scaled with source distance. In addition, Table 1 establishes that it is not strongly affected by the field-size setting; therefore, only one modifying function need be determined, and this may be used, with no more than a small error, to calculate the primary-beam intensity for any given field size or source distance.

Dose Calculations Using Scatter-Air Ratios

The calculation of the absorbed dose at a point (x,y,d) using scatter-air ratios is well established (7). For a uniform beam

$$D(x,y,d) = D_A(d) \cdot [T(d',0) + S(d)] \tag{2}$$

and

$$S(d) = \sum_{i=1}^{n} S(d,r(\theta_i)) \frac{\Delta\theta_i}{2\pi} \tag{3}$$

where:

D(x,y,d) is the dose at a point (x,y) within a phantom depth d,
$D_A(d)$ is the "reference dose" in air on the central axis,
T(d′,0) is the zero area tissue-air ratio at depth d′
d′ is the slant distance from the surface along the ray joining the source to the point of calculation
S(d) is the total scatter-air ratio at the point (x,y,d),
$r(\theta_i)$ is the distance from (x,y) to the geometric edge of the beam at an angle θ_i,
$\Delta\theta_i$ is the angular width in radians of the sectors used in the summation of S(d), $r(\theta_i)$,

$S(d,r(\theta_i))$ is the scatter-air ratio for depth d and radius $r(\theta_i)$, and n is the number of sector used to describe the beam.

In the case of a nonuniform beam, equations 2 and 3 must be modified to correct both the primary dose at (x,y,d) and the amount of scatter produced by the nonuniform beam. In the case of a large Cobalt teletherapy beam, the nonuniformity is described by the inverse square law dependence (ISL) and the primary modifying function M(x,y), and so:

$$D(x,y,d) = D_A\,(d)\;[(ISL)\cdot M(x,y)\cdot T(d'0) + S(d)] \tag{4}$$

and

$$S(d) = \sum_{i=1}^{n} \frac{\Delta\theta_i}{2\pi} \sum_{j=0}^{\infty} (ISL)\cdot M(u,v)\cdot \Delta S(d,r_j) \tag{5}$$

where

$\Delta S(d,r_j)$ is the differential scatter-air ratio for a volume element a distance r_j from (x,y) with coordinates (u,v).

Table 4 compares measured data with results calculated with and without a modifying function to an angle of 40° to a principal plane. Calculations of the dose distribution over the range of 5 to 15 cm depth with any size beam show that the use of the modifying function produces agreement better than 2 percent to actual data.

Conclusions

This study has led to a number of conclusions that are important in the computer calculation of large beam dose distributions. These are:

1. The source-collimator geometry of the Theratron-type cobalt unit may influence the primary-beam contribution to the dose near the periphery of a large field. Changes of source size or collimator should be followed by a reexamination of the primary-dose profile. This is necessary regardless of the method of calculation.
2. The calculation of dose distributions using scatter-air ratios must include provision for a modifying function to take into account the effects of source-collimator geometry.
3. This modifying function must be evaluated from measurements of the primary-dose profiles of the therapy unit in question. There is evidence that similar units with the same source-collimator geometry may have the same modifying function.
4. The parameters used in other methods of calculation such as a

field equation (8) or decrement lines (9) must also be evaluated for the unit in question. Care should be also exercised in the use of published or borrowed isodose distributions for large beams.

5. The established values of scatter-air ratios neglect this effect and so underestimate the values for large radii. However, the error will be small as the scatter from the periphery of a large beam is small.

REFERENCES

1. Cunningham, J. R., Shrivastava, P. N., and Wilkinson, J. M. presented at the Dosimetry Workshop, Hodgkin's Disease, Chicago, Illinois, Sept. 17, 1970.
2. Cunningham, J. R., Shrivastava, P. N., and Wilkinson, J. M., *Computer Programs in Biomedicine, 2* (1971).
3. Johns, H. E. and Cunningham, J. R., *The Physics of Radiology*, 3rd ed. Springfield, Illinois, 1969.
4. Cundiff, J. H., Cunningham, J. R., Golden, R., et al., presented at the Dosimetry Workshop, Hodgkin's Disease, Chicago Illinois, Sept. 17, 1970
5. Cox, R., Almond, P. R., and Lampiere, V., *Radiol., 106.* 213 (1973).
6. Drew, J. F., *Br. J. Radiol.* In Press.
7. Cunningham, J. R. *Phys. Med. Biol., 17,* 42 (1972).
8. Sterling, T. D., Perry, K., and Katz, L., *Brit. J. Radiol., 37,* 544 (1964).
9. Orchard, P. G., *Brit. J. Radiol., 36,* 756 (1964).

Table 1.
Theratron 80 In-Air Dose Profiles for Three Field Sizes (with Inverse Square Dependence Extracted)

Distance from Central Axis (cm)	Field Size 20 × 20	30 × 30	40 × 40
0	1.000	1.000	1.000
5	0.998	0.998	0.998
8	0.984	0.989	0.993
10		0.980	0.989
12		0.967	0.980
14			0.968
16			0.956
18			0.926

SAD = 100 cm.

Table 2.
Theratron 80 In-Air Dose Profile Measured with No Collimator and with Two Collimator Hinge Settings (with Inverse Square Dependence Extracted)

Distance from Central Axis (cm)	Collimator Removed	With Collimator Hinge Setting 2.46 cm	1.93 cm
0	1.000	1.000	1.000
5	0.997	0.998	0.997
8	0.995	0.993	0.990
10	0.993	0.989	0.980
12	0.989	0.980	0.964
14	0.986	0.968	0.938
16	0.980	0.956	0.902
18	0.976	0.926	0.848

SAD = 100 cm Field Size = 40 × 40 cm

Table 3.
Theratron 80 In-Air Dose Profile in a Plane at 40° to a Principal Plane (with the Inverse Square Dependence Extracted)

Distance from Central Axis (cm)	Measured	Calculated
5	0.998	0.998
10	0.989	0.984
15	0.973	0.961
19	0.944	0.934
22	0.917	0.905

SAD = 100 cm   Field Size = 40 X 40 cm

Table 4.
Comparison of Measured Data and Calculated Values with and without a Modifying Function Using Scatter-Air Ratios

		Dose Relative to Central Ray	
Distance from Central Ray (cm)	Measured	Calculated without Modifying Function	Calculated with Modifying Function
10	0.961	0.973	0.961
12	0.947	0.961	0.947
14	0.929	0.947	0.928
16	0.905	0.930	0.899
18	0.874	0.909	0.869
20	0.835	0.884	0.831
22	0.786	0.850	0.783

40 X 40 cm   Depth = 10 cm   SAD = 100 cm
40° to Principal Plane

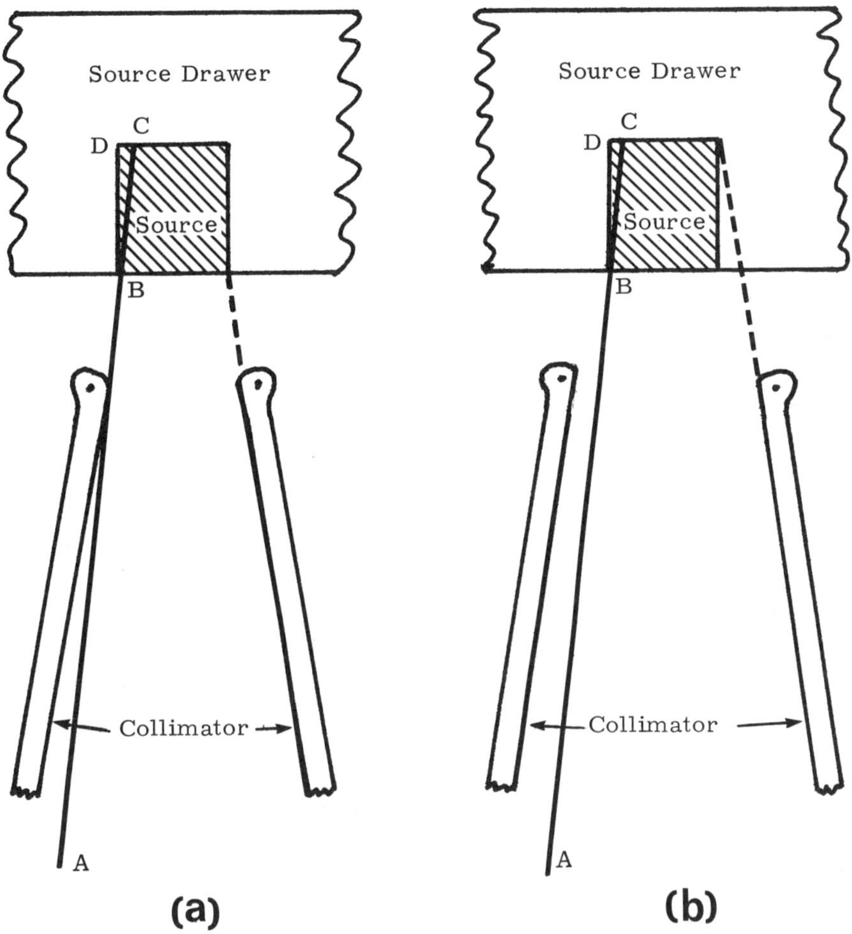

Figure 1. Theratron 80 Source-Collimator Geometry

9. Application of a Low-Cost Computer Graphics Terminal to Radiotherapy Treatment Planning

D. G. Jameson
P. Crossland
J. L. Haybittle

Introduction

The project was started in April 1972 at the Middlesex Hospital, London, and Addenbrooke Hospital, Cambridge, and was financed by the Dept. of Health and Social Security (London). The objective was to develop a low-cast graphics terminal and explore the feasibility of using this equipment for radiotherapy treatment-planning. The project was divided into three main stages.

1. Commissioning of hardware.
2. Development of system software and applications packages.
3. Testing in a clinical environment.

The first two stages are at an advanced state of development, and the third stage will be started very shortly. The aim now is to provide an initial evaluation of the project by April 1975.

Hardware

The hardware design of the terminal is based on a Varian 620L mini-computer, and the list of interfaces and peripherals used are as follows:

Varian 620L mini-computer—8K core.
Communications interface to GPO modem operating in asynchronous mode at 1200/75 baud.
Stabletron vector-generator driven by direct memory access.
Hewlett-Packard 1310A Display oscilloscope.
Fast-paper-tape system.

Calcomp 565 Incremental Plotter.
Function box for drawing on oscilloscope screen - (designed and interfaced by P. Crossland).

This assembly of hardware provides a graphics terminal capable of drawing absolute and relative vectors on the screen of a refresh oscilloscope, with a resolution of 1/100th inch. Data are transmitted to the host computer at 75 baud over an ordinary two-wire dial-up telephone network, and graphic and alphanumeric information is received from the host computer at 1200 baud. The display information is buffered in the Varian 620L and drawn on the oscilloscope screen at a refresh rate of 50Hz. The host computer is a Univac 1108 operated by Scicon Ltd and using the Exec 8 operating system.

Software

The development of the software has taken place in two main sections: the code concerned with activity in the terminal, which is in assembly code, and the code resident in the host computer, which is standard Fortran IV. Since this cannot be simply divided into the operating system and the applications packages, it is better to consider the two applications of the terminal separately.

1. external beam treatment planning.
2. interstitial and intracavitary dose calculations

External beam treatment-planning. The terminal runs under the control of a program, GRAFIX, which requires 3K core. The activities GRAFIX controls are listed as follows:

1. Housekeeping procedures to provide a dynamic system of buffers for alphanumeric and graphic display.
2. Polling of all devices in the terminal, since there is no priority interrupt system.
3. Alphanumeric symbol generator.
4. Control of graphics and alphanumerics in local mode—i.e. writing and drawing on display screen either with the keyboard or function box.
5. Control of graphics and alphanumerics in remote mode—i.e. by a set of control characters transmitted from the host computer. These control characters controlled the following functions:
    (a) initiation of loading of graphics information
    (b) erase loaded graphics
    (c) erase alphanumerics
    (d) erase local graphics

(e) force local graphic point transmission
(f) force teletype printing
(g) dynamic display editing.

6. Establishing connection between terminal and host computer, and decoding of graphic streams.
7. Drawing of various symbols and messages on the display screen indicating the state of the terminal.
8. Control of hardcopy device.
9. Vector drawing routines.
10. Screen image dumping and loading by paper tape.

The terminal can be used both as a graphics terminal and as a V.D.U. and has the ability to display graphics and alphanumerics simultaneously.

In the host computer there is a set of Fortran IV programs which comprise the following:

1. Patient-data input/edit program—EDIT.
2. Dose computation program—DOSE.
3. GRAFIX LIBRARY (precompiled graphics package).

The runtime-edit program will provide the interactive features of the system to input data and to edit the data for any subsequent reruns of a treatment plan.

The dose-computation program is a comprehensive system providing almost all the features considered important in external beam-planning. These are listed as follows:

1. Wedge and plain fields.
2. Fixed field and rotation plans.
3. Isocentric and fixed SSD plans.
4. Inhomogeneity corrections.
5. Build-up region corrections.
6. Parallel section calculations off the central axis.
7. Effect of compensators on dose distribution.

The program uses a semi-empirical formula for computing the doses, developed by R. L. Thomas at Addenbrooke Hospital, and has the twin advantages of being fast and requiring the storage of only a small set of numbers. The accuracy of the formula has been tested in the following way:

Doses were compared at 0.5 cm intervals along cross-plots for several fields, both plain and wedged. A score at each point was computed as either the difference in calculated and measured doses expressed as a percentage of the central axis dose at the depth of the plot, or the distance in mm, measured along the cross-plot, between the point and a position where the measured dose was the same as the calculated dose at the point under consideration. The lower of these two values was chosen, unless the distance exceeded 5mm, in which case the dose difference was used.

For plain fields 95 percent of the scores were $\leqslant 3$, and 83 percent were $\leqslant 2$. For wedge fields the corresponding percentages were 91 and 78 respectively. The highest score values occurred either outside the beam at a depth or at the beam edge near the surface on the hot side of wedged beams. In the latter case, the distance criterion often could not be applied, because the calculated value was greater than the measured value at the peak of the crossplot.

The GRAFIX LIBRARY has a set of routines in Fortran IV which provide the contour plotting package and also have provisions for labeling contours. The library also contains routines for scaling, and controlling the terminal display remotely, including erasure of a graphic component of a picture, if corruption occurs during transmission, and automatic retransmission of that component.

Interstitial and intracavitary dose calculations. The system is divided into three parts in the same manner as the external beam calculation system:

1. Data input and editing program—ZPLAND.
2. Dose calculation program—RTPG.
3. GRAFIX LIBRARY.

At the present stage of development ZPLAND is an independent assembly code program that runs in the terminal and requires approximately 4K words core. This program draws a picture, in perspective, of the radiation sources on the display screen; the three-dimensional information of the source positions being derived from radiographs. This picture can be rotated about the X, Y, and Z axes so that the shape can be examined in detail. A plane, representing where the dose calculation will be carried out, can be made to move through the picture of the implant and can be stopped wherever required. At this stage in the program, the three-dimensional coordinates of the source positions and the plane position are calculated and listed as the program output.

The task now remains to incorporate ZPLAND into GRAFIX to provide a data preparation and editing program for interstitial and intracavitary applications. The difference between this work and the external-beam planning program is that the data input and editing routines reside entirely within the terminal.

The dose computation program provides for filtered, linear, point, and Cathetron sources and for various radioisotopes. The GRAFIX

LIBRARY routines provide graphical output in a manner similar to that used by the external beam planning system.

Choice of Host Computer

The host computer used in this project is a Univac 1108 run by Scion Ltd, Milton Keynes, about fifty miles from London and Cambridge. Before we made this choice, a version of the external-beam program designed for operation on a teletype was benchmarked on several machines: D.E.C., PDP 10, and Atlas II. Control Data CDC 6600 and 6400 were considered but not benchmarked.

The PDP 10 system was too slow, and the running costs rose rapidly with the complexity of the plan. The CDC machines required that the terminal should either simulate a CDC 200 user terminal or a teletype operated at 110 baud. Our graphic terminal was designed to appear to the host machine as a medium speed alphanumeric visual display terminal. To modify the terminal to simulate the CDC 200 user terminal would have meant a major change in the project proposals. The Atlas II was used for a major part of the program development because this machine is used at Cambridge in the Computer Aided Design Centre and is orientated to graphic work, after which the programs are transferred to the Univac 1108. It was a deliberate policy of the project that the Fortran programs should be written in ANSI Fortran IV so that they could be transferred from one manufacturers equipment to another. One version of the external-beam program has been run on an IBM 370, ICL 1906, Atlas II and Univac 1108, and the transfer has required minimal program alterations.

The facilities used to access the Univac 1108 are:

1. A dedicated port operating at 1200/75 baud for the graphic terminal.
2. Back-up at 110 baud for teletype.

The time to complete a run once the data is prepared is less than one minute. The computation being completed in 10–20 secs and the remaining time taken up producing the graphic information and drawing on the screen. The cost of the computation is approximately $2.00–$3.00.

The provision of back-up facilities at 110 baud is a very useful feature with output in the form of character plots for external-beam plans and dose matrices for interstitial calculations. This feature has evolved during the development of the project because some of the early versions of the dose-computation program were written before the graphic facility was available.

Problems Experienced during Development

The vector-generator was the only piece of hardware built to order, and there were a number of technical problems, initially, such as noise on the display traces, which took some time to rectify. The communications interface had been designed to meet Bell Telephone specifications, and when it was operated on the GPO telephone network, the data error rate was too high. This was finally corrected by modification to the receiver circuits of the interface.

Because of shortcomings in the original specification of the terminal, there is flicker on the display screen when one attempts to draw a picture with a large number of vectors. The flicker is because the whole picture takes more than 20 msec to draw, and the refresh cycle gets out of phase. The drawing speed is related to the speed of the vector generator and the cycle time of the computer, and these problems can be overcome when the hardware is upgraded. The 8K core of the graphic terminal holds both the display buffers and the GRAFIX programs, so that the servicing of the refresh display and the operating system both have to be handled by the single central processor.

Operating the System in Other Centers

The project was developed at two major radiotherapy centers in England, so that the system was designed from the beginning to meet the requirements of more than one department.

The project timetable aims to complete the experimental phase by April 1975. If it is considered successful, a development phase will be started, and the system will be set up and evaluated in other centers. The ability to transfer the programs from one host computer to another has been mentioned above, and there is particular interest in running on ICL 1900 series machines, since the Regional Hospital computer centers in the United Kingdom are equipped with these machines.

The setting up of a computer system in any department necessarily involves establishing a data-base for the treatment machines, and this has been successfully done in four hospitals. The back-up facility on the teletype has also proved useful because it has allowed other hospitals to gain experience of the system, and their comments have proved valuable to us in program development.

10. Radiation Treatment Planning on a Multitasking Computer System

D. Ingram
A. Todd-Pokropek
J. S. Clifton
P. J. Mulvey
D. Mayhew

Introduction

A computer system has been designed and installed to investigate the advantages of using real-time multitasking software to support a number of clinical areas simultaneously. Three areas currently being investigated are radiation treatment-planning in radiotherapy; data collection, analysis and display in nuclear medicine; and clinical data analysis in neonatal intensive care. This paper describes briefly the computer configuration and the software organization, and explains in detail the implementation of treatment-planning procedures with the system. The benefits of using modular systems are discussed.

Computer Configuration

The principal components of the system are based on a PDP 11/45 central processor. In addition to the main disc storage of 2 × 1.2M word-moving head cartridge discs, a 128K word fixed head disc has been installed and a system of virtual memory (by software) implemented to handle matrices too large to fit in available core store. A CAMAC coupler has also been interfaced to the system. This is a simplified peripheral processor with autonomous access to core which can handle sixteen different input-output operations (CAMAC tasks) simultaneously.

A video disc system has been developed for on-line display, capable of supporting up to 60 terminals (1). This is based on a fixed-head disc unit with four head stations, each station containing sixteen read/write heads. Each track will refresh a 625-line noninterlaced video monitor, and may be loaded with character information (26 rows of 50 characters) or with a 400 × 260 bit matrix of graphical information. The output of tracks can be mixed, and this feature is utilized to produce both color and grey scale displays. The video signal may be driven over distances of up to 1 Km using a single coaxial cable. Data from the terminal keyboard (or joystick) are transmitted back to the computer on the same cable, via a multiplexor, during flyback time. Utilization of 19-inch domestic television sets results in a very cheap terminal that can display a full-size patient outline. Distortion can be reduced to a negligible level by minor adjustments to the sets.

Software Organization

The PDP 11/45 processor runs under the manufacturer-supplied RSX 11/D operating system, which provides an event-driven multitasking environment with a priority-interrupt structure. Opportunity thus exists to interleave computational loads with those interactive processes which consume little processor time. The practicability of refreshing interactive displays directly from core memory is limited, since the idle time from one application area must be exploited in order to process another area's demands. However RSX 11/D is not a time-sharing executive, and simultaneous direct interaction by a number of users cannot be handled efficiently. Therefore an indirect method of control of the system had to be devised to enable multiple users to communicate with their program areas, to facilitate interleaving, and to establish and maintain the correct order of priority for processing efficiently any combination of application tasks that might be active at a given time. This has been achieved by writing a special piece of control software called the task driver, which not only simplifies interaction with but also prevents abuse of the operating system. It functions as a single privileged task, running at the highest level of priority, monitoring all other tasks that are active, and allocating priorities.

Each task contains a set of tables that define both the logical structure of the procedures it performs and a complete specification of required interaction with the user—file processing, computation, and display. Individual operations are performed by program modules written mainly in FORTRAN. The tables are interpreted by the task driver. Active applications tasks build up a queue of requests for service. The task driver interprets the next step or sequence of steps defined in the tables until it has to pass control back to the application task for initiation of I/O or execution of a program module. At this point it will proceed to service the next request from the queue, if one exists, or suspend activity. Error-bound checking, macro-command processing, and free-format input routines are other facilities provided within the task driver.

The individual tasks that make up an application task are constructed in modular form and can be entered and reentered in any sequence convenient to the user. Internal flags within the table structure ensure that illogical sequences will not be permitted (e.g. a dose distribution cannot be computed before appropriate treatment fields have been set up). Procedures common to several application areas—e.g. the generation of graphical displays—have been developed as separate utility tasks, which may be activated by demands from the applications tasks or the task driver.

Radiotherapy Treatment-Planning

The treatment-planning application itself, based on the previous system developed at U.C.H. (2, 3), is divided into four independent tasks, dealing respectively with:

(1) Input of patient details and opening a planning file
(2) Specification of treatment fields
(3) Dose computation
(4) Display of computed plans and organization of the library of completed plans

(a) **Task 1—setting up the planning file.** The file structure provides for the reading and storage in standard form of the body outline, tumor outlines, and critical organ positions. A number of such patient profiles may be stored. All planning data are identified in the system at all times with the patient name, number, date, etc.

(b) **Task 2—specification of treatment.** Size, position, orientation, weighting, and wedge angle if required are entered for each field specified, together with parameters defining the treatment machine to be used.

(c) **Task 3—Dose-matrix computation and storage.** For external-beam planning, dose-computation modules utilize the decrement line system. Correction can be made for body curvature, lung inhomogeneity, and the use of wedge fields. The file contains a dose-matrix for each field specified. Computation of a single field dose-matrix of 15,000 points takes approximately 10 seconds. If a subsequent change is made in the specification of a field, the dose-matrix for that field is recalculated. Field matrices are summed using weightings defined by the user, and the resultant composite dose-matrix is stored along with component field descriptors.

An advantage of separating dose computation in this way is that different computational algorithms can be introduced within the same overall task structure. Also, the organization of operational tasks and files makes possible the computation of the dose matrix for one field in parallel with interactive specification of the next field, thus improving response time of the system. For long-term storage only the finally selected plans are saved. Sufficient information is held with each plan to permit later amendments and to allow doses from new planned treatments to be added to those delivered previously.

(d) Task 4—Display of Results and Archives of Plans. Patient and tumor outlines, fields, and dose distribution contours are stored on three separate tracks of the video disc. Three outputs from the video disc are utilized to write respectively patient outline, field information, and contour dose distributions. These three sets of information can thus be displayed in separate colours. Changes in field position or size can be made without recourse to rewriting the entire display. Information on the video disc may be read back into the core store. This facility allows selected displays to be taken from the disc, saved, and subsequently reproduced as hard copy. Full-size plans can also be generated directly using the STATOS V electrostatic plotter. A library of past plans is being built up, to be held in on-line storage as a teaching aid and guide to evaluation of treatment technique.

The Treatment Planning Terminal

The proposed display terminal consists of three 19-inch domestic T.V. receivers. The availability of the video disc system permits a number of useful innovations. The center monitor of the three units is to be used for planning, and may be either color or black and white. The second and third displays will be used for comparative optimization and three-dimensional presentation. A completed plan can be transferred to another track on the disc and displayed on the second monitor while a new plan is determined using the central monitor. Thus a maximum of three plans can be directly compared at any one time. For three-dimensional presentation, dose computation in two planes at right angles can be presented on two adjacent screens.

Future Developments

The major effort in the initial phase of the project has been the development and organization of the basic system software. In each of the clinical application areas a number of future developments are envisaged. For radiation treatment planning these include the application of video mixing to generate a composite display of the calculated dose distribution superimposed on a radiograph, and the use of multiple-color displays (developed for the nuclear medicine application) to present dose distributions. In addition, the development of macro command processing and specialized input systems to expedite operator interaction are to be further extended, and the utilization of the CAMAC coupler to implement the monitoring of treatment is being studied.

Conclusions

It is possible to support a number of clinical areas on a real time multitasking system. The modularity of the software necessary for successful operation provides a number of advantages for radiation treatment planning. Alternative procedures can coexist within the same overall structure (e.g. different algorithms can be used to calculate a dose distribution matrix). It is flexible in operation in that the user may move freely from one section to another with only internal flags constraining his possible range of options at each point. A batch-processing facility for planning can be introduced in parallel with the interactive procedures making use of the same set of tasks.

The display system allows terminals to be widely distributed within the hospital, each connected by a single coaxial cable to the central computer. As a benefit of the low cost of the individual terminals it has been possible to design a radiotherapy terminal using multiple screens with immediate benefit over conventional systems with a single display.

Acknowledgments

This work is supported by a research and development grant, A/C 334/B94/13 provided by the Department of Health and Social Security.

REFERENCES

1. J. S. Clifton, A. Todd-Pokropek, D. Ingram. *Display Systems for Medical Applications*, Brit. Computer Soc., University College Hospital, London (March 1974).

2. J. S. Clifton. Computer Assisted External Beam Dosimetry with Special Reference to Correction Calculations and Presentation of Data, *I.A.E.A. Technical Report*, 57, 63 (Vienna 1966).

3. J. S. Clifton. *Developing a Computer Service for Radiotherapy in Medical Computing: Progress and Problems*, ed. M. Abrams, British Computer Soc. (1970), 121–132.

11. A Coordinate System for Computer Beam Angles and Determination of Indicator Angles for a Patient Setup in Radiation Therapy

S. M. Brahmavar

Introduction

In recent years the use of computers in treatment planning has become an integral part of modern radiotherapy. The increasing use of computers in radiation treatment-planning has resulted in the use of different coordinate systems to define the radiation beam angles that describe the beam positions used in radiation treatments. The existence of different coordinate systems in computer treatment-planning is due to a particular choice made by the computer specialist writing the programs for the large time-shared computer, or chosen by the manufacturers of the dedicated mini-computer planning systems. In many instances such coordinate systems are chosen without regard to the gantry coordinate system used on the rotational therapy unit. The computer beam angles as given by the digital printout need to be translated into (a) actual gantry beam positions and (b) the indicator angle readings of the therapy unit before the patient is set up for treatment.

A Coordinate System for Computer Beam Angles

At this time there is a need to standardize all the parameters used in patient treatment and treatment-planning. A standard system of coordinates for computer beam angles is proposed. Such a standard system of rotation coordinates will specify that

(a) all rotations shall be scaled from 0 to 359° irrespective of the range of rotation desired,
(b) the rotation scale shall read zero when the radiation beam is directed vertically downward, and

(c) viewed from the point on the axis of rotation on the patient contour, the rotation scales shall increase from 0 to 359° in anticlockwise direction.

The need for such a standardization is spelled out by Joy (1), in the HPA radiotherapy physics topic group in the proposed code for a standard system of coordinates for radiotherapy apparatus.

Determination of Indicator Angles

When such a standard system of coordinates for computer beam angles is utilized, simple formulae could be developed to translate the computer beam angles (CBA) into the indicator angles (IA) that will be used in the patient setup and treatment.

The formulae to obtain the indicator angle from the computer beam angle are given here for two widely used rotational therapy units with vertical gantry rotation indicators. These formulae are:

Theratron 780 (AECL): *Cobalt 60 Unit* (1)
: $IA = 360° - CBA$

Clinac 4 (Varian) : *Linear Accelerator* (2)
: If $CBA < 180°$, then $IA = CBA + 180°$
: If $CBA > 180°$, then $IA = CBA - 180°$

These formulae will be valid for all therapy units that use identical gantry rotation scales. The routine use of these formulae at our institution has helped to minimize the confusion between the medical physicist, dosimetrist, radiation therapist, and technologists.

ACKNOWLEDGMENTS

The article by Joy (1), HPA radiotherapy physics topic group, was published just after the abstract of the present paper was submitted to the program committee of the Fifth International Conference on the Use of Computers in Radiation Therapy. The author wishes to thank Won C. Park, M.D., Robert A. Grugan, M.D., John P. Sullivan, M.D., and Said M. Zubi, M.D. for encouragement and help during this work.

REFERENCE

1. Joy, A. R., *Phys. Med. Biol.*, *19* (2), 213-219 (1974)

12. A Technique for Superimposing Cross-Sections of the Pelvic Bone Structure on Calculated Radiation Isodose Curves for Gynecological Curietherapy

J-C. Barral
R. Mampey
H. Regis
L. Bousquet

Introduction

Several programs for calculating radiation isodose lines for gynecological radiotherapy are now in existence. None of these programs, however, associates the isodose contours to the anatomical structure of the patient under treatment. The work presented in this paper is a preliminary approach to this problem: it concerns a representation which associates each isodose contour in a given plane with the corresponding cross section of the pelvic bone structure.

Method

The method consists of storing the coordinates of a typical pelvic structure in a file in the computer memory and then adapting this model to the individual morphology of each patient. Once the model has been adapted, both the outline of the bone structure and the isodose lines are drawn for each of the cross sections selected by the user.

The spatial coordinates of the basic pelvis type were calculated using two orthogonal Xrays of the pelvis of a skeleton on which lead references points had been placed. Four references points are used to define a system of real (S2) and virtual (S1) axes on the pelvis type. The model is corrected by adjusting the S2 coordinates of the pelvis being examined with respect to the S1 coordinates of the reference pelvis in memory.

Utilization of the Program

To obtain the pelvis cross section of each patient, it is necessary to locate certain bone structures on two orthogonal Xray pictures taken in certain defined positions. The points used as references are used as follows:

I Upper frontal angle of the first sacral vertebra
II S1-S2 axis
III Upper limit of the left cotyloidian cavity
IV Upper limit of the right cotyloidian cavity

With these four points, the stored pelvis type can be adapted to resemble the pelvis of the patient;

V Upper apex of the pubis
VI Midpoint of the front edge of the fourth lumbar vertebra.

Points II, V, and VI enable the construction of the Fletcher ganglion plan passing through VI and the middle of II and V.

It is also necessary to locate the various radiation sources on each X ray.

Results and Conclusions

All cross sections in the horizontal, saggital, and frontal planes can be calculated for a given reference point on each X ray. It is also possible to plot the section of the oblique Fletcher lymphatic plane. The program can also generate the cross sections and isodose lines in a plane passing through a reference point in a bladder or a rectal probe.

The program reported in this paper is now in routine use in the Centre Claudius Regaud. The remaining problem is to locate the contours of the affected organs, i.e. the bladder and the rectum.

13. Interactive Treatment Planning in Radiotherapy

G. Gell

Environment

The division of readiotherapy in Graz is part of a central department of radiology in a large general and university hospital with 3000 beds. The division has three staff radiologists, one radiation physicist, and two residents, and is equipped with (besides conventional X-ray therapy) one Siemens Gammatron serving a population of 1.8 million people. This machine runs 12 hours a day, with very little time left for planning and measuring.

The department has a PDP 15 computer with DECtapes, fixed-head disk, Calcomp plotter, two teletypewriters, one Tektronix display with joystick and hardcopy unit, and a graph pen for analog input. The computer is used for nuclear medicine, radiation-therapy planning, and documentation.

Programs and Algorithm

Doses are calculated according to the formula of Richter and Schirrmeister (4, 5), based on previous work by Pfalzner (3).

$$D(x,y)=D_L \bullet (f/(f+x))^2 \bullet k(x) \bullet F(u) \bullet ((f+x)/f)^2 \bullet A_o)m(x)$$

where

A_0 = field area on body surface
D_L = dose on the surface
$D(x,y)$ = dose at the point x,y
$u = y \bullet f/(b \bullet (x+f)$
k(x), m(x), F(u) are empirical functions (polynomials).

The functions k(x), m(x), f(u) were fitted to the measured dose-distributions for our machine as published by the IAEA (7) and checked with some later measurements in our division,

In the actual computation these functions are not evaluated for each point of the cross section separately; at the beginning the program calculates tables for different values for x and u with the given beam parameters (f,b,A_0) and then interpolates for each point of the plan.

Normally doses are calculated on a one cm grid. The program handles coplanar fixed and rotational beams (with corrections for oblique incidence) as well as radioactive implants.

The programs are written in FORTRAN IV and structured in several overlays to fit into the 16K memory of our computer.

The system runs in two modes, normal and special. Normal operation is designed to be used by an operator for routine calculations and assumes most parameters (f, grid size, plot mode, etc.) to be constant. The "special" mode allows for variation of most parameters and is used by a physicist or radiotherapist for interactive iteration of field data to get the optimal beam configuration.

Planning Procedure

(a) Medical data. A radiographer takes the contour of the patient with a special device and inserts some anatomical structures from a cross section atlas (6) with the aid of X-ray films and fixed points, taken from the patient (e.g. caput femoris, os pubis, spina iliaca ant. sup., etc.), and if possible the target area. For routine calculations, the radiotherapist enters the beam data in a therapy form that is sent to the computer together with the contour.

(b) Computer planning. (1) *Input of patient contour.* The patient contour-data are entered in the computer by means of a sonic digitizer (graph pen). As the operator presses the pen on distinct points of the contour these points appear on the screen of the display together with an audible signal. After the display the contour can be corrected immediately.

(2) *Input of beam data.* Beam data and data for radioactive implants are entered on the keyboard of the display (or of the teletype if a hardcopy is desired).

(3) *Calculation of dose distribution within the cross section.*

(4) *Display of dose distribution on the screen* (this step is omitted in routine use without interactive planning). At this point the radiotherapist (physicist) can produce a screen-size hardcopy in about ten seconds simply by pressing a button, changing the field data, and

starting with step 3. When the final configuration is found, the user proceeds with step 5.

(5) *Isodose-plot and numerical data.* The isodose plan of the dose-distribution is plotted in life size (or with any desired enlargement factor) on the plotter. Some additional numerical data (e.g. the dose-values of the isodose lines, the maximum dose, etc.) are printed on the TTY.

For routine calculation the operator performs steps 1, 2, 3, 5 and they take from 8 to 15 minutes, at least half of which time is needed for plotting.

Interactive planning is necessary in 5-10 percent of the cases. The interactive planning cycle (steps 2-4) takes 2-5 minutes. This task was greatly improved by the introduction of the display with hardcopy unit, because it is difficult to remember and to compare several dose distributions (if seen only on the display) and the plotter takes too much time for interactive planning.

The dose-calculations are performed routinely for every radiotherapy (CO^{60}) patient—on the average three patients per day (2).

Third Dimensional Representation

In addition to the isodose map it is possible to produce a three-dimensional representation of the dose-distribution where the dose is plotted along the z-axis over the contour in the x-y plane (1). This is useful to clarify the isodose map in instances with very high local dose-gradients (e.g. addition of doses from external beams with doses from radioactive implants) or very small gradients, where the exact localization of an isodose line may have no physical significance. Besides that, it is easy to explain the meaning of isodose lines (and their dependence from a reference scale) with the aid of a three-dimensional representation.

Future Developments

In the near future we plan the introduction of wedge-filters (not used thus far) and inhomogeneities. Another project is the storage of the cross-section atlas into the computer and the automatic fitting of these data to the patient contours, taking into account some fixed points (of the skeleton).

ACKNOWLEDGEMENTS

We wish to thank the Osterreichischer Forschungsfonds and the Jubilaumsfonds der Osterreichischen National Bank for supporting this work.

REFERENCES

1. Gell G., *Meth. Inf. Med.*, *12* (4), 204 (1973).
2. Gell, G., Kahr, E., *Strahlentherapie*, *146* (5), 511 (1973).
3. Pfalzner, P. M., *Radiology 79*, 439 (1962).
4. Richter, J. D., Schirrmeister, D., *Strahlentherapie*, *126*, 177 (1965).
5. Richter, J. D., Schirrmeister, D., *Brit. J. Radiol.*, *40*, 479 (1967).
6. Takahashi, S., *An Atlas of Axial Transverse Tomography and Its Clinical Application* (Springer, Berlin-Heidelberg-New York, 1969).
7. Webster, E. W., Tsien, K. C., *Atlas of Radiation Dose Distributions*, *1*, IAEA (Wien, 1965)

14. Automated Computer Input of Dosimetry Data Using the "Grafatran" Device

P. N. Shrivastava

The purpose of this paper is to present data on the accuracy, reproducibility, and convenience in savings of time and money in using the Grafatran device for automated input of dosimetry data and the dedicated computers like the Rad 8 and PC-12.

The common belief has been that the Grafatran was not accurate enough to input beam data for multiple-field planning or for automated digitization of spatial coordinates needed in dose calculation for shaped field and intracavitary brachytherapy. Our efforts show that with proper calibration, not only is the Grafatran device very accurate and reproducible, but also that it adds to convenience in computerized dosimetry. It reduces human errors resulting from tedious measurement and from teletype input errors caused by improper input format.

The data are presented with reference to three applications:

(1) Applications in intracavitary radium treatment for cancer of the cervix.
(2) Input of isodose beam data for multiple-field treatment planning.
(3) Dosimetry for irregularly shaped fields.

Our computer system is a Rad 8 PDP 8-I computer with a memory of 8K, 12 bit words. All of the programs described are written in FORTRAN II, which also demonstrates that these computers can, indeed, be programmed in FORTRAN for complex and long dosimetry calculations.

I. Applications in Intracavitary Dosimetry (Programs CSM and CSMDIS)

For accuracy the Grafatran device is fixed on a table and used over a light box. The positions of the sources are input into the computer by placing the Grafatran at the ends of radium sources and pressing the key "R" for "react" on the teletype. The procedure is quick and easy compared to manual digitization.

The accuracy of the method in using the Grafatran has been compared with that of hand calculations. Differences in coordinate values are small and the percentage of difference in the length of the source calculated by the two methods is generally less than 1 and at most 2. Ten consecutive measurements of coordinates of the same point with the Grafatran allowed a standard deviation of 0.5 mm.

The advantages of this system are:

(a) The coordinates of tube ends are automatically read by using the rho-theta transducer resulting in a great saving of time and effort.
(b) The program is in Fortran so that it can be understood universally and altered according to individual needs.
(c) It can be used with the small 8k, PDP8/I computer which is being increasingly utilized for therapy planning at many centers.

II. Applications in Beam Isodose Data Generation (Program BMIN 23)

The BMIN 23 Program is used for digitizing isodose data for storage on DECtapes. The isodose curves are placed on a set of fan lines originating at the source and diverging like the radiation beam. The original program (Digital Equipment Company) required 47 fan lines and five depths for complete storage of data. The isodose values at the intersections of the fan lines and the depth were manually obtained and input through the Teletype Scope System. In the BMIN 23 Program, the Grafatran is placed at the intersection of the isodose line with the fan line and the key "R" on the teletype is pressed to "read." An "o" is typed if a particular fan line does not intersect a given isodose curve.

After the intersects of the isodose curves between 100 and 10 percent are read by the Grafatran and the distances of such intersects from the surface are printed out by the computer for verification, if necessary. When all 23 lines have been read, the computer generates from these data all of the percentage dose values required for storage on the Rad 8 Computer for multiple-field treatment-planning. The accuracy of this method is very good.

The great savings in time and cost in generating 300 curves for storage on the DECtapes by using the BMIN 23 Program at the cost rate of $10.00 per man hour are shown on the following table.

Method	*Time for Data Reading*	*Time for TTY Input*	*Man Hrs. per Curve*	*Cost for 300 Curves*
RADS	2 X 2 hr.	0.5 hr.	4.5	$13,500
Beam 47	2 X 0.6	0.3	1.5	4,500
Beam 23	2 X 0.3	0.2	0.8	2,400
Present	0.2	0	0.2	600

III. Dosimetry in Irregularly Shaped Fields (Program ANYFLD)

Coordinates of up to 40 corners may be required for calculations of dose in "Mantle" fields. The use of the Grafatran to directly input this information into the computer results in savings of time and yields greater accuracy, reproducibility, and savings of cost as shown below.

	Time Sharing Computer		*Rad 8 Using Grafatran*
Manual coordinate digitization	15 Min.		-0- Min.
Making paper tape	20 Min.		8 Min.
Paper tape input	1.7 Min.		.5 Min.
Entering coordinates w/Grafatran	-----		2 Min.
Program execution and output time	8 Min.		30 Min.
Average number of errors Teletype input	3		1
Correction time for error	3 Min. (On-Line in Edit Mode)		1 Min.
Computer cost	66 CPU	$1.98	
	Connect Time	1.66	
	Personnel Cost @ $6.25/hour	5.00	$4.40
	Total Cost per Sample	$8.65*	$4.40

*Plus $1.20/day storage charge.

15. A Mathematical Model for Time Optimization of Treatment Regimes in Clinical Radiotherapy

J. Kirk
T. E. Wheldon

Introduction

The aim of radical radiotherapy of cancer is the total elimination of malignant cells. In practical radiotherapy, however, the choice of treatment regime used to irradiate the tumor is limited, since the biological damage to normal connective tissue included within the treatment volume must never exceed tolerance. Since radiation damage to normal tissue is of prime importance, considerable effort has been devoted to attempts to assess and evaluate the effects of that damage. To that end, Cohen (1) has developed a semi-empirical biological model, while Ellis (2) in his NSD concept and Kirk, Gray, and Watson (3-8) with their Cumulative Radiation Effect (CRE) have presented empirical descriptions of the biological effect of radiation. On the CRE system, the biological effect in normal connective tissue is measured on a scale of accumulated subtolerance radiation damage, the CRE. The CRE system will be used in the following analysis.

By using this system the effects on normal tissue of various treatment regimes can be easily assessed and compared. Any specific level of effect can be achieved for fractionated radiation by a variety of of combinations of the dose per fraction, number of fractions, and time interval between fractions. However, treatment regimes which have equivalent effects on normal tissue will in general have different effects on neoplastic tissue, because of its different cell kinetic properties. It may therefore be possible to find a regime that will inflict maximum damage on the tumor.

The primary objective of this contribution, by means of the mathematical model to be described, is to establish whether such an optimum regime exists and whether it offers a significant improvement on, or differs greatly from, those in current use.

The Mathematical Model

Radiation damage and repair in tissue is very complex and, for this preliminary investigation into the optimization of treatment regimes, the simplest possible assumptions on the mechanisms of damage and repair are adopted, so that only the essential elements of the biological system are considered.

It is assumed the the CRE system provides an adequate description of the effects of fractionated radiation on normal tissue. From Kirk et. al. (3) the CRE, R_F, achieved by a fractionated schedule can be written as

$$R_F = D \bullet N^{-0.24} \bullet T^{-0.11},$$

where

D is the total dose.
N is the number of fractions, and
T is the total treatment time.

It is more convenient for the present purpose to put the dose and time, which are both dependent on the number of fractions, as dose per fraction, d, and the time interval between fractions, t, so that the CRE equation becomes

$$R_F = d \bullet N^a \bullet t^{-b}, \quad (1)$$

where

$d = {}^D/N$, $t = {}^T/N$, $a = 0.65$ and $b = 0.11$.

Since no description like the CRE system has been proposed for neoplastic tissue, it is necessary to define a criterion for assessing the effect of radiation on that tissue. As previously stated, however, the aim of radiation treatments for cancer is to reduce the population of malignant cells to as low a level as possible. Thus it is natural to choose the fraction of tumor cells surviving as a measure of the curative effect of the radiation treatment.

The fraction of the surviving cells, σ, following a single dose of radiation d, can be described by the well-known multi-target formula

$$\sigma = 1 - (1 - e^{-d/D_o})^n, \tag{2}$$

where

D_o and n are constants characteristic of the type of cell irradiated and the radiation quality employed.

In general, tumors demonstrate a rather complex growth pattern, but for simplicity it is assumed for this model that the tumor population is growing exponentially. Therefore, the growth in the population of malignant cells can be written as

$$Q = Q_o \cdot e^{\lambda t} = Q_o \cdot e^{\frac{0.693\, t}{\tau}}, \tag{3}$$

where

Q_o is the initial tumor cell population,
Q is the number of cells after a time t (days),
λ is the fractional growth rate, and
τ is the doubling time (days).

After a treatment schedule of N fractions, each of d rads, separated in time by t days has been given, the resulting surviving fraction of tumor cells just prior to the $(N+1)^{th}$ fraction can be written as

$$Q/Q_o = \sigma^N \cdot e^{N\lambda t}, \tag{4}$$

where σ can be replaced by the expression in equation 2. The possible choice in the values of d, N and t which can be used in equation 4 is restricted according to equation 1 for a specific level of the CRE, since the level of damage which can be inflicted is limited by the biological effect generated in normal tissue. Equation 1 can be rearranged to make N the subject, and when that expression is substituted in equation 4 for N and σ is replaced from equation 2, equation 4, which describes the surviving fraction of malignant cells after radiation, becomes

$$Q/Q_o = \left[1 - [1 - \exp(-d/D_o)]^n\right]^{R^{1/a} \cdot d^{-1/a} \cdot t^{b/a}} \cdot \exp[\lambda \cdot R^{1/a} \cdot d^{-1/a} \cdot t^{1+b/a}]. \tag{5}$$

Only two variables then remain to be determined: d and t. An optimum treatment schedule can be found when Q, the surviving number f malignant cells, is minimized. This condition is satisfied when the derivative of Q with respect to d and t is zero.

The procedure required to determine the values of d and t, which correspond to a minimum in Q, although straightforward in principle is rather cumbersome. The mathematical methods required can be found in any textbook of advanced calculus dealing with maxima and minima of functions of more than one variable. Attention is confined to physically admissible solutions (i.e., positive and non-zero roots). It is found that for the optimum value of d, which at this stage need not be made explicit, and the extrapolation number, n, t is proportional to the tumor doubling time, τ. This relationship is shown graphically in Figure 1, where a family of lines is given for the various values of n likely to be of practical interest. It is also found that the optimum dose, d, bears a linear relationship to the parameter D_O for any value of n. A corresponding family of lines is shown in Figure 2 for this relationship.

Thus, in summary, from a knowledge of three items of information concerning the tumor tissue—the doubling time, τ, the extrapolation number, n, and D_O—and from a knowledge of the desired biological effect (usually tolerance) to be generated in the normal tissue necessarily included in the treatment volume, described by the CRE, an optimization procedure can be developed to obtain values of the variables d, N, and t of the optimal treatment schedule. This procedure is summarized in Figure 3. It therefore appears that an optimal schedule exists which will minimize the surviving tumor population.

It is instructive to take a typical example that will give some idea of an optimal treatment schedule predicted by the model. Suppose a tumor has a doubling time of 70 days. This tumor doubling time is the average found by Tubiana (9) for epitheliomas and is typical of many tumor doubling times. The parameters of the cell survival curve (or multi-target formula) selected as typical values are $n = 2$ and $D_O = 150$ rads. From Figure 2, the optimum dose per fraction, d, is 345 rads. From Figure 1 the optimum time interval between fractions, t, is about 24 days. If the CRE for tolerance of normal tissue were 1760 reu, the number of fractions required would be 21. The optimal treatment schedule would thus be a total dose of 7245 rads in 21 fractions over a period of 480 days. This optimal treatment is extended over a considerably longer time than that normally employed.

The mathematical model used in this preliminary investigation into optimal schedules is greatly simplified and doubt could be cast on various aspects of it; nevertheless, there are grounds, as shown in the above particular case, for thinking that radiation treatments could be improved by employing schedules lasting considerably longer than those presently used. It would seem that investigations of such schedules are warranted. Retrospective surveys of protected schedules, where these exist, could be carried out to see if any evidence for an improved curative effect exists, and animal experiments could be contemplated and designed to test the validity of the above suggestions.

In order to see (1) whether optimal schedules proposed on the basis of this mathematical model demonstrate any significant improvement in curative effect, assessed as the surviving fraction, Q/Q_O, of malignant cells, over those currently used in clinical practice, and in order to investigate (2) the way in which the surviving fraction, Q/Q_O, varies with dose per fraction, d, and the time interval between fractions, t, in the region of the minimum of Q/Q_O for schedules that achieve the same CRE for normal tissue, the surviving fractions, Q/Q_O, for a variety of schedules have been computed. For this analysis, the same tumor-doubling time, τ, of 70 days and the same parameters for the multi-target formula, n=2 and D_O = 150 rads, as those used in the above example, were chosen as typical average values.

The variation in the surviving fraction of tumor cells, Q/Q_O, with the dose per fraction, d, for values around the optimum dose of 345 rads, when the time of separation between fractions is kept constant at its optimal value of 24 days, is shown in Figure 4. It can be seen from this figure that a deep nadir is found with a minimum value of Q/Q_O, of about 1.1×10^{-13}.

In an analogous way, the variation in the surviving fraction of tumor cells, Q/Q_O, with the time of separation between fractions, t, for values around the optimum time of 24 days, when the dose per fraction is held constant at its optimum value of 345 rads is shown in Figure 5. It can be seen from this figure that a marked nadir is again observed, with, of course, the same minimum value of Q/Q_O, but in this case the depression is shallower and wider. This suggests that greater latitude is possible in the time used between fractions than in the value of the dose per fraction without seriously affecting the resulting survival fraction of malignant cells.

It is instructive to compare the surviving fraction of tumor cells for a conventional schedule with that for an optimum schedule which achieves the same CRE. As a particular case, the same doubling time and multi-target parameters as those used above were employed. A frequently used schedule in radical radiotherapy is one of 6000 rads given in 6 weeks, with 5 fractions per week given at daily intervals. The surviving fraction of tumor cells from this schedule, which achieves a CRE of about 1760 reu, is approximately 3.3×10^{-10}. When this surviving fraction is compared with that of the optimum schedule of 1.1×10^{-13}, it can be seen that the surviving fraction is significantly smaller, by a factor of 3000. The level of surviving fraction from the conventional schedule is indicated by lines on Figures 4 and 5, in order to give a measure of the extent of the nadirs in these figures.

As a further measure of the effectiveness of the optimal schedule for this particular situation, the total dose that would have to be given on a conventional schedule in 6 weeks, with 5 fractions per week given at daily intervals, to achieve the same surviving fraction of tumor cells as that found for the optimal schedule has been computed and found to be 7450 rads. On a conventional daily fractionation scheme, this dose would exceed normal tissue tolerance. Thus the optimal schedule would seem to offer a significant improvement in curative effect over schedules currently in use.

Conclusion

This mathematical model for the time optimization of treatment schedules is of necessity greatly simplified, with the gross features of damage and repair of normal and tumor tissues described by the minimum number of variables. However, in its role as a model for preliminary investigation, it incorporates the essential elements of the cell kinetics of tumor growth and an empirical description of the biological effects of radiation on normal connective tissue, using the CRE system. It serves to demonstrate that optimum treatment schedules exist and that longer intervals between fractions than those customarily used are proposed. This feature of the model, in particular, merits further investigation.

Other aspects of a clinical situation, such as obstruction of possible malignant spread, may contraindicate intervals as long as those suggested, but for a well defined tumor longer treatment times should be entertained. The optimum schedules suggested seem to offer a significant improvement on those employed in current clinical practice, and for this reason also deserve further consideration. The model at this preliminary stage is too simple, and the available data inadequate for the conclusions reached to be used as a numerical guide to clinical practice.

This work is continuing in an endeavor to develop a more realistic model, and further advances will be duly reported. A more complex and realistic model may well suggest that more complexly structured regimes should be used than the simple regular schedules reported here, but this simple model has served to indicate several points of interest for future study.

Beyond doubt, the role of time effects in radiation therapy is of considerable importance and has to date received less attention than it deserves. It is strongly urged that greater effort should be devoted to the temporal aspects of radiation treatments.

REFERENCES

1. Cohen, L. *Radiology*, *101*, 419-427 (1971).
2. Ellis, F., "The Relationship of Biological Effect to Dose-Time-Fractionation Factors in Radiotherapy," in Ebert, M., and Howard, A., eds., *Current Topics in Radiation Research*, *4* (North Holland Publishing Company, Amsterdam, 1968), pp. 357-397.
3. Kirk, J., Gray, W. M., and Watson, E. R., *Clinical Radiology*, *22*, 145-155 (1971).
4. Kirk, J., Gray, W. M. and Watson, E. R., *Clinical Radiology*, *23*, 93-105 (1972).
5. Kirk, J., Gray, W. M. and Watson, E. R., *Clinical Radiology*, *24*, 1-11 (1973).
6. Kirk, J., Gray, W. M. and Watson, E. R., *Clinical Radiology*, *26*, 77-88 (1975).
7. Kirk, J., Gray, W. M. and Watson, E. R., *Clinical Radiology*, *26*, 159-176 (1975).
8. Kirk, J., Cain, Olive, Gray, W. M., and Watson, E. R., *Clinical Radiology* (in press).
9. Tubiana, M. *British Journal of Radiology*, *44*, 325-347, (1971).

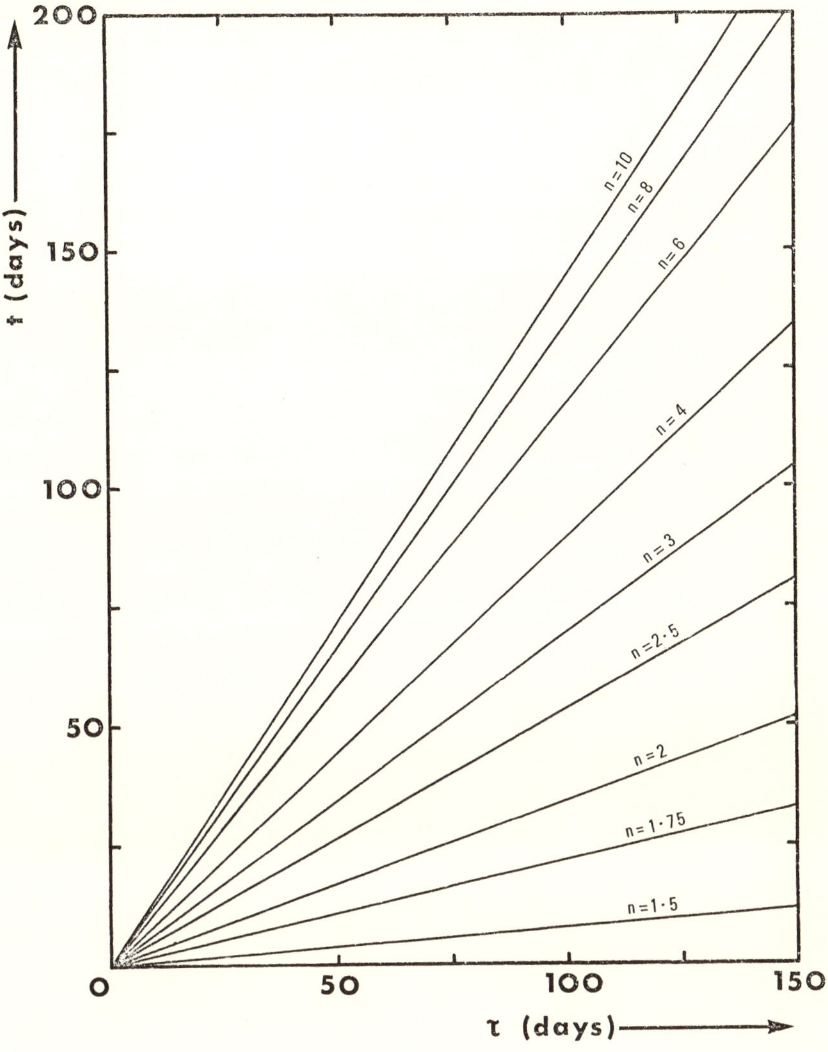

Figure 1. Relationship Between the Optimal Time Interval Between Fractions, t (days), and the Tumour Doubling Time, τ (days), for Various Values of the Extrapolation Number, n, Presented as a Family of Lines

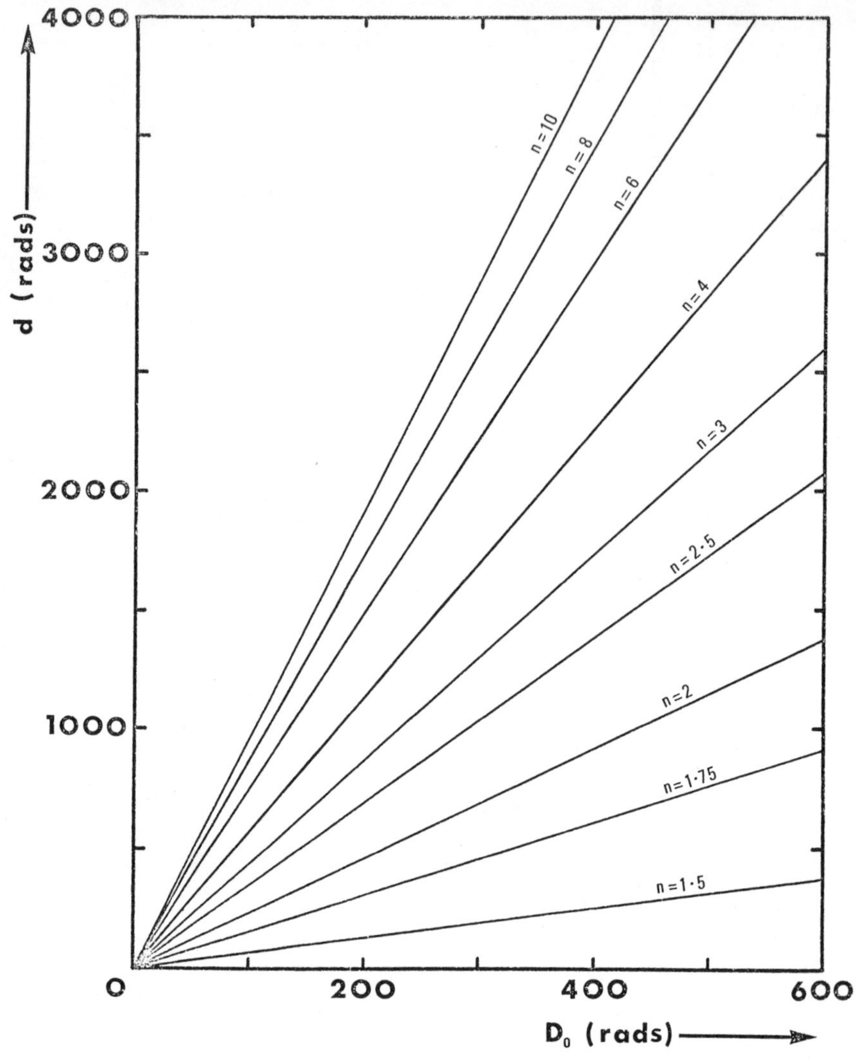

Figure 2

Figure 2. Relationship Between the Optimal Dose per Fraction, d (rads), and the Multi-target Parameter, D_0 (rads), for Various Values of the Extrapolation Number, n, Presented as a Family of Lines

SUMMARY OF OPTIMISATION PROCEDURE

Required Data	Method Employed	Resulting Information
Parameters from multi-target formula relating to tumour cells irradiated and radiation employed: $n\ ,\ D_o$	By graph based on equation of the form: $d = D_o \cdot f(n)$	Optimum dose per fraction: d
Tumour doubling time and optimum dose per fraction (from above): $\tau\ ,\ d$	By graph based on equation of the form: $t = \tau \cdot f(n)$	Optimum time interval between fractions: t
Value of CRE for tolerance, or other level of biological effect, to be generated in normal connective tissue occuring in the treatment volume, and optimum dose per fraction and optimum time interval between fractions (from above): $R_F\ ,\ d\ ,\ t$	From equations of CRE - system: $\left[\frac{R_F}{\rho} \cdot d\right]^{1/0.65}$ for example	Number of fractions: N

Figure 3. Summary of the Procedure for Obtaining an Optimal Treatment Schedule as Defined by the Minimum Value of the Surviving Fraction of Tumour Cells.
Data Required: — Concerning Tumour:
Doubling Time, τ, and Multi-target Parameters n and D_o;
Concerning Normal Tissue: Desired Biological Effect, CRE.
Resulting Information on Optimum Schedule: — Dose per Fraction, d, Time Interval Between Fractions, t, and Number of Fractions, N.

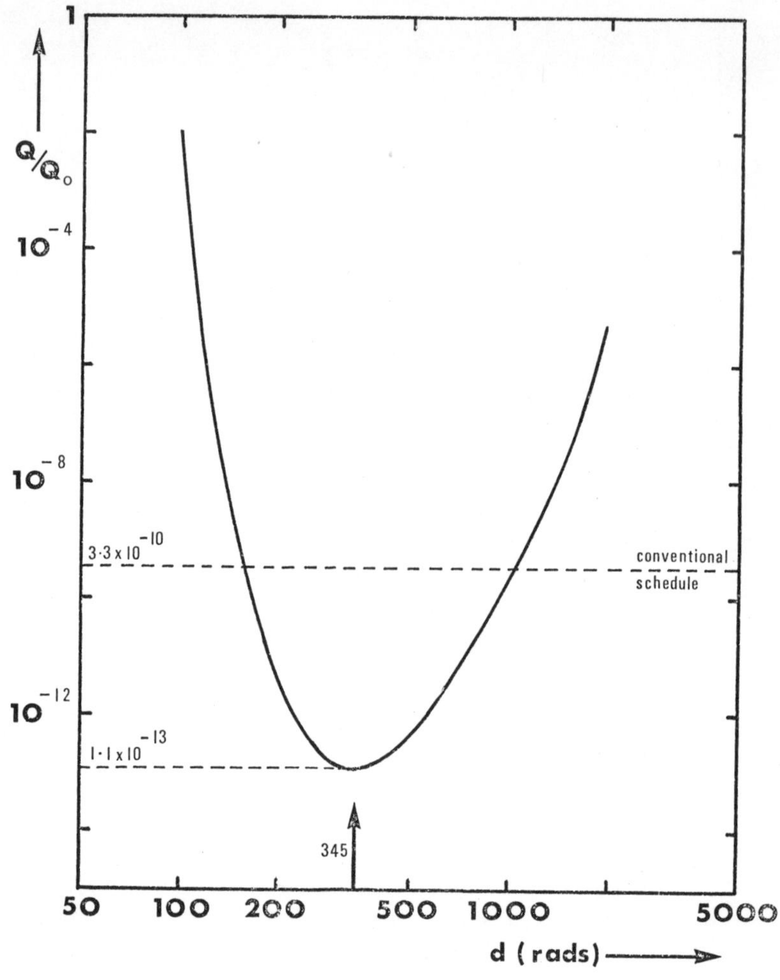

Figure 4. Graph of the Variation of Surviving Fraction of Tumour Cells, Q/Q_o, with Dose per Fraction, d (rads), when the Time Interval Between Fractions, t, is Held Constant at the Optimum Value. For this Particular Example, t = 24 Days, Tumour Doubling Time, τ, = 70 Days, Multi-target Parameters are n = 2 and D_o = 150 rads, and CRE = 1760 reu. The Surviving Fraction ($Q/Q_o = 3.3 \times 10^{-10}$) from a Conventional Schedule of 6000 rads Given in 30 Daily Fractions in 6 Weeks Achieving the Same CRE is also Shown.

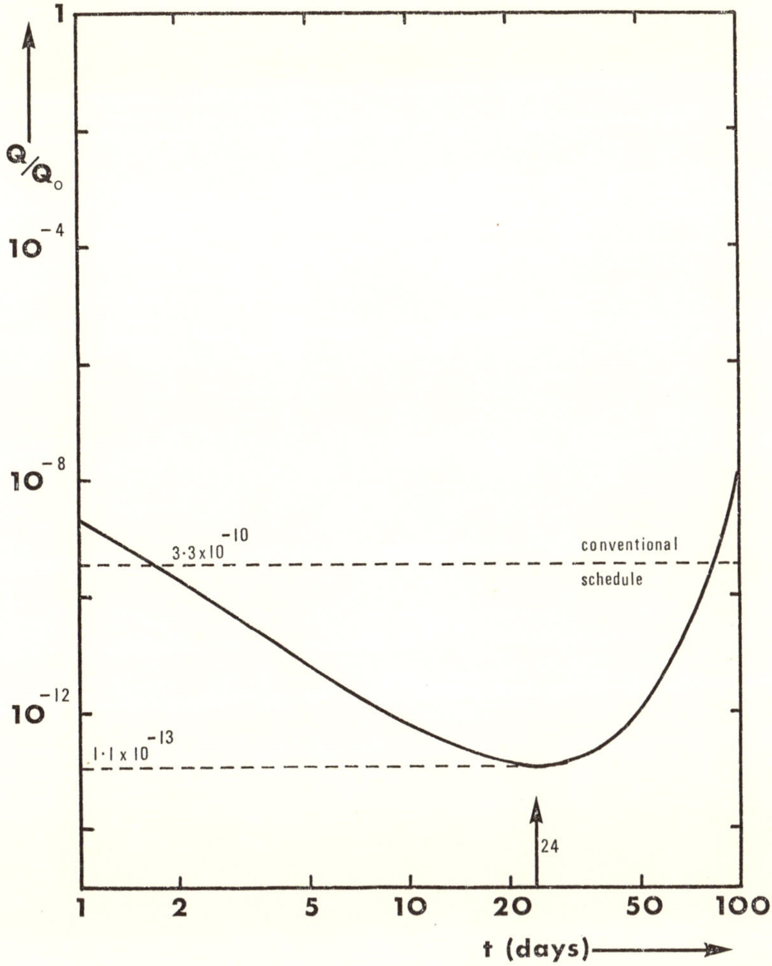

Figure 5. Graph of the Variation of Surviving Fraction of Tumour Cells, Q/Q_o, with the Time Interval Between Fractions, t (days), when the Dose per Fraction, d, is Held Constant at the Optimum Value. For this Particular Example, d = 345 rads, Tumour Doubling Time, τ, = 70 Days, Multi-target Parameters are n = 2 and D_o = 150 rads, and CRE = 1760 reu. The Surviving Fraction ($Q/Q_o = 3.3 \times 10^{-10}$) from a Conventional Schedule of 6000 rads Given in 30 Daily Fractions in 6 Weeks Achieving the Same CRE is also Shown.

16. Implications of Departmental Scheduling on the Operation of a Tumor Registry

D. P. Ragan

Since their inception, tumor registries have advanced from simple lists of patients with cancer all the way to computerized files of patients with tens of pages of information per patient. Several years ago the radiation therapy department of Mallinckrodt Institute of Radiology became disillusioned with the hospital-run, card-based tumor registry system. Its information was inaccurate, out of date, and insufficient to meet the needs of the medical staff. In 1968 a computer-based tumor registry with about twenty entries per patient plus complete follow-up, was instituted (1).

Motivation

When this system was reviewed two years ago it became apparent that the tumor registry would have to contain significantly more data at about the same cost in terms of dollars and manpower than the existing information system, while having far superior performance in terms of data retrieval. To accomplish this goal a computer system was developed capable of supporting the diverse functions carried out in the operation of the radiotherapy department. This is described in the companion paper "Diversified Radiation Therapy Department Computer Support." It was hoped that the system could cost-justify itself on the basis of billing and scheduling and at the same time provide cost-free tumor-registry capability.

Usage of a dedicated mini-computer in-house system provided the flexibility desired for the tumor registry. Successful performance of departmental operations boosted the credibility of computer systems. Finally, information was gathered and computer expertise was developed by performance of many miscellaneous department tasks.

System Description

The tumor registry, as developed over the past year and a half, is currently operating on an extended MUMPS PC system. It is a multi-user interpretive system with 120 million characters of on-line disk storage.

The computer system is capable of bisynchronous communications with the IBM 360 on the Washington University campus. It has a floating point processor and two printers. There are LINC tapes available for data and program back-up.

Data are contributed to the tumor registry from both Mallinckrodt Institute of Radiology and St. John's Mercy Hospital. Treatment data are obtained in the process of performing scheduling and other service functions for the department. These data are augmented by coding forms filled out by the treating physicians at the end of treatment. Follow-up information is obtained primarily from in-house follow-up visits or from referring physicians. There are currently over nine thousand patients, going back as far as 1950, with extensive follow-up.

Our particular design philosophy and hardware implementation has provided noteworthy things. In performing scheduling and related functions for the department it is possible to boost computer credibility and to accession a reasonable amount of data in the process. However, traditional MUMPS, although well suited for data accession and possessing a flexible file structure, is not particularly appropriate for large file-searching where presorting may not be appropriate. A brute force search of the tumor registry files takes hours. This was unacceptable for what had been hoped would be an interactive data retrieval system. In order to reduce these long search times, an inverted file structure known as bit mapping has been implemented (2, 3). An additional problem arose with accounting programs that needed to place fixed-decimal arithmetic capable of nine places of accuracy. A third problem came in the areas of providing a full set of ninety-six characters. This is needed for computer assistance in typing consult notes and scientific articles. Finally, it was desired to extend the I/O capability to accommodate such things as an optical-mark sense reader and therapy machine verification unit. In order to fill these needs, which went outside the traditional MUMPS capability, the manufacturer provided hardware bit-searching capability, extended arithmetic capability by utilizing a floating point processor, an improved I/O priority scheme for handling more rapidly seven-bit ASCII characters, and a generalized I/O format.

Bit String Searches

The most important addition to MUMPS has been the implementation of bit-map inverted lists in order to facilitate the rapid retrieval of patient records satisfying several search criteria. The first application of bit maps was reported by Terry Reagan (4). This was an application motivated primarily to facilitate sorting and to eliminate problems of being disk bound. We have extended this concept to eliminate the need for time-consuming traversing of the complicated tree structures in our data-retrieval file.

Bit maps are ideally suited for MUMPS implementation and can complement the tree-like MUMPS structures. A bit map is a file structure consisting of bit strings that correspond to individual responses where a given bit position in all strings corresponds to a different original patient record. Table 1 shows a sample set-up for four patients with various sites and pathologies. This list of patients and their data (A) is entered into the original patient file (B). This file is then used to construct the bit map file (C) for sites and pathologies. Each record is referenced by the search filed (1 = site, 2 = pathology) and the response (i.e. site = 3), and a given bit position refers to the same patient number in all bit strings. I.e., for patient 7303 the second bit is 1 where the response is true, and 0 where false.

To search the file, for example, for site = 2 and path. = 11, one takes BIT (1, 2) & BIT (2, 11) 1010 & 0011 = 0010, which says that the third patient is the only one with both conditions true. To locate the flagged records, an inverted file (D) is used that gives the patient codes when referenced by bit position. In the example, INV(3) = 7303, showing that patient 7303 was the only one to meet both requirements.

The bit map is specifically implemented in MUMPS by using strings of six bit ASCII characters, where each character represents five patients (one bit is always left on to ensure a valid character). One can sort 475 patients per 95-character string, or about 10,000 patients in 21 strings. Therefore, by using bit maps, a search can be made on 10,000 patients for a number (N) of conditions with 21 × N file searches as opposed to the 10,000+ searches needed in a straight file search. (The *and*'ing and *or*'ing of two bit-strings takes about the same time as the manipulation needed to find and compare the search field in two patient records.)

The organization of a bit map can be varied to meet the requirements of various types of information. For example, selection of all patients between the ages of 40 and 50 can be conveniently handled by the proper implementation of the bit-mapping technique. The software that was developed utilizes these inverted lists, allowing optimal searching of mapped criteria; subsequent searching of unmapped criteria or free language text provides maximum searching flexibility.

Status

The present tumor registry implementation is operational on a data base of nine thousand patients. Conversational input routines allow lay users of the system to input single or multiple search criteria. These users can also specify a variety of information to be tabularized on output. Work still needs to be done to make this process more straightforward and to expand the variety of available outputs.

The most important result of this work has been the demonstration that MUMPS is indeed capable of handling large file searches. In fact, turn-around time is faster in MUMPS than it was using multiple keyed PL/1 files on an IBM 360/65. Also, all of the MUMPS files needed for the system take less than one third of the space needed for the single IBM 360 file. Much work is left to be done in terms of data reduction; expanded arithmetic capabilities of extended MUMPS PC will become useful in this area.

It is believed that modern hardware/software combinations have progressed to the point where all medium to large radiotherapy departments should avail themselves of information-processing systems. The multi-user capability of modern systems makes data accession much easier than previously. The flexible high-level languages like MUMPS allow for versatile program development at minimal cost. Finally, rapid on-line retrievals can be accomplished in a timely fashion to provide rewards and motivation for system utilization.

REFERENCES

1. Rigdon, M, "Users' Manual: Radiation Therapy Information Retrieval System," Department of Radiation Oncology, Washington University, St. Louis, Missouri (1972).
2. Knuth, Donald E., *The Art of Computer Programming*, Vol. 3, *Sorting and Searching*, Addison-Wesley Publishing Company, Reading, Massachusetts (1973).
3. Selbmann, H. K. *Methods of Information in Medicine, 13*, 2 (1974).
4. Reagan, T., Private communication (1973).

Table 1.
How Bit Mapping Aids in Identifying Subsets of Patients Satisfying a Particular Set of Criteria. The Subscripts on Bit Are Bit (< search field >, < search field value >).

A.

Patient no.	*Site*	*Path*
7301	2	10
7302	3	10
7303	2	11
7401	3	11

B.

SPA
SPA(73) — SPA(73,1) = "2, 10"
SPA(73) — SPA(73,2) = "3, 10"
SPA(73) — SPA(73,3) = "2, 11"
SPA(74) — SPA(74,1) = "3, 11"

C.

BIT — BIT(1) — BIT(1,2) = "1010"
BIT — BIT(1) — BIT(1,3) = "0101"
BIT — BIT(2) — BIT(2,10) = "1100"
BIT — BIT(2) — BIT(2,11) = "0011"

D.

INV — INV(1) = "7301"
INV — INV(2) = "7302"
INV — INV(3) = "7303"
INV — INV(4) = "7401"

17. The Tufts-New England Medical Center Computer-Based Tumor Registry

R. E. Folland
P. W. Neurath
W. T. Powell

Introduction

Most tumor registries were founded just after World War II as part of new cancer control program of the American College of Surgeons. They wanted to determine the incidence of disease by diagnostic category, age, sex, and geographical distribution, as well as the effectiveness of different treatment modalities. Such data, averaged nationally, have been reported for a number of years by the American College, the American Cancer Society, and the National Institutes of Health (1, 2). Their figures are probably accurate for demographic purposes.

For the individual patient a tumor registry's most important function is to assure a regularity and continuity of follow-up visits. For the physician the role of the registry has been ill defined and its usefulness questioned.

The new tumor registry system at Tufts has been designed to meet several well-defined objectives resulting from the desire to improve upon an existing card-file system. As finally implemented, it represents a complete reorganization which utilizes computer facilities to achieve its aims.

Old System

A description of the original system is a logical point of departure and will serve as a basis for comparison. The old manual system consisted of the following: two card files—an alphabetical patient-index file, and an alphabetical tickler file for follow-up purposes—and abstract forms for each patient registered. The Medical Records Department routed to the registrar the charts of those patients discharged with a diagnosis of malignancy. The registrar then abstracted the chart on to the state registry form. Required information not explicitly or implicitly available from the chart had to be traced through written and telephone inquiries to the physicians concerned. Such legwork was both time-consuming and frustrating. Occasionally incomplete forms resulted. Since neither referring nor attending physicians received a copy of the abstract for verification, the system provided no way to audit the accuracy of the required data. The completed abstracts were filed alphabetically by year and by primary diagnostic category. Follow-up requests were initiated on each patient yearly, utilizing the follow-up tickler file. Follow-up and death information were entered on cards and abstracts upon receipt of such data.

This system provided the registry with the capability of answering specific queries for data. Statistical reports, listing the total number of cases within each diagnostic category by year, were generated sporadically upon request. With the exception of occasional special inquiries, registry data were neither analyzed nor disseminated; they merely accumulated.

Since the records of outpatients do not require completion of discharge summaries, and since they are neither audited nor processed in the same way as those of inpatients, outpatients have not routinely been registered by the tumor registry.

The manual system, because of the above procedures, had a number of shortcomings: low percentage (less than 50) of both registration and follow-up; a long delay (as much as three years) between admission and registration; questionably accurate data; inability to retrieve patient data by parameters other than diagnostic category and date of entry. Such criteria as department, treatment modality, and stage of disease were not readily available for study purposes.

The results of these multiple shortcomings have been twofold: probationary disapproval of the registry by an accrediting agency, and, more importantly, lack of use. The tumor registry facilities have been largely ignored by the medical staff. In contrast, the system has had two advantages. It has been both inexpensive to operate and has required absolutely no effort from the medical staff. It has also been fairly typical of the average hospital tumor registry. The accreditation problems of our registry were shared by those of most Boston teaching hospitals.

Objectives of the New System

The Cancer Committee of the New England Medical Center Hospital felt that a change was in order and set several goals to be achieved with the aid of a computerized information system:

a. Complete registration of all cancer cases treated at NEMCH whether in or out patients
b. Timely registration, within two months of admission at the latest
c. Yearly follow-ups of all patients registered, with periodic accounting of the results
d. Rapid, random data-retrieval capability
e. Issuing periodic comprehensive and informative reports.
f. Assurance of complete and accurate data
g. Capability to serve as a research resource to store specialized data, e.g. on protocol patients, for a researcher who wishes to do this at a reasonable pro-rated cost
h. Conformation to accreditation standards

Implementation

In order to meet these objectives, two major changes were effected. First a modest increase was in the effective Tumor Registry budget to include remuneration of medical and scientific staff. The second was an agreement by the NEMCH medical staff, especially groups treating over 90 percent of all cancer patients, to participate in the data collection task. It was agreed that the radiotherapy, tumor surgery, gynecologic-oncology, medical oncology, otolaryngology, and hematology departments would complete a simple one-sheet entry form on all newly diagnosed cancer patients.

Based upon such commitments, the objectives of the Tumor Registry have been translated into the system described below.

1. **Organization.** The first step has been to establish an Office of Cancer Management, under the aegis of the chairman of the Cancer Committee, administered by an experienced professional, to operate the Tumor Registry as well as to organize symposia and lectures and to coordinate grants.

2. **Registration.** A patient is entered into the system via input from two sources—his physician and his pathology report. Physicians of the oncologic departments previously mentioned, as well as individual practitioners who admit cancer patients, have agreed in principle to furnish a data sheet on each new patient. A primary task has been the definition of the content of that sheet. By necessity it is a compromise between the amount of information which would be optimally desirable but of excessive length and the amount which can be easily and quickly supplied and stored. The resultant entry form, which contains a minimal amount of adequate information, comprises a single sheet. The data included are:

a. positive identification and address of the patient
b. identification of physicians who referred the patient and provided the major therapy
c. date of admission
d. date of diagnosis of primary tumor
e. prior tumors, if any (i.e. other primaries)
f. diagnosis of current primary by site of pathology (histology)
g. extent of disease as one of six possible choices, stage of disease as an optional choice
h. dates and types of all major therapies given for the current admission(s)
i. cause of death and its relationship to the tumor
j. identification of the source of this information

No knowledge of code numbers is necessary to complete the form. However, answers must put a patient into one of several possible mutually exclusive and exhaustive categories. This classification must be understood by those who complete these forms, i.e. both the physicians and their staffs.

3. Usefulness of limited data. Clearly, this brief amount of information is not sufficient to describe a patient for such purposes as assessing optimal treatment. Rather, the data were selected to attain the eight objectives listed. An explanation of the philosophical concepts behind rapid random data retrieval may be in order here. The Tumor Registry does *not* aim to record, on each patient, all data that might be needed for future research programs. Instead, it allows for the selection of certain patients to meet specified parameters. The data stored are adequate only to define a specific group of patients from the total number registered. Should the researcher require further detail on these patients, he would have to examine their medical records. A list of patients meeting any combination of parameters for the data shown on the entry form or the follow-up form can be obtained in twenty-four hours or less when needed. These lists can be made manageably small by both the descriptors on file and the fact that they can be used in any combination. For example, consider that there are about 50 disease categories into which patients fall; further select a group by sex (two choices), age (three groups), and extent of disease (four groups); this selects one in $50 \times 2 \times 3 \times 4$, i.e. one in 1200 on the average. Even when distributions are not average in size, the system easily allows the selection of a well-defined group of less than 100 patients from a data bank of more than 10,000 patients.

4. Data sources. To ensure the accuracy of a patient's clinical data, his physician's participation in completing the form is essential. Only the physician knows the primary site, extent of disease, and past and present therapy well enough to *categorize* them precisely. Such categorization is essential for later retrieval. Medical record descriptors, being largely in medical jargon, a subset of natural English with all its nuances, do not usually permit a nonphysician such as a tumor registrar to classify the patient information for correct retrieval. To simplify the physician's task, the entry form was designed so that much of the identifying information can be completed by ancillary personnel. The major organizational problem in data gathering is the establishment of a routine in all oncologic departments. As long as one person in each department is responsible for completion of the entry forms, the input problem for perhaps 85 percent or more of all patients needing registration is solved.

5. Computer entry and verification. With the entry form, data are entered into the computer by registry personnel or, optionally, in a large department with its own terminal, by one of that department's personnel. Entry is performed in a conversational mode. The format of entries having a specific format are checked by the computer. All entries, even those entered in code, are printed on the terminal in English text for immediate verification. The final audit of patient data occurs when a copy of the computer-generated, typed summary of the patient's entry form is returned to the physician for his file.

6. Optional entry of research protocol data. The limited data base, adopted to make the hospital-wide system effective, need not be an obstacle to a particular physician or group wishing to record, analyze, and retrieve more detailed data. Special entry and follow-up forms can be designed for such users. If these special forms contain all the Tumor Registry information in *identical* format and categorization, other desired data can easily be added.

The radiotherapy department has had a computerized information system in operation since 1971. By utilizing its accumulated data base, the computer-programmed entry of nearly 3,000 radiotherapy patients into the Tumor Registry in early 1974 gave the registry system a large file to begin operations. There was one drawback. Some of the now-agreed-upon data for the registry was not in the radiotherapy files, making some data more incomplete than they would normally be.

7. Pathology reports. Registration by submission of the physician's entry form is by no means foolproof. Failure to furnish a form would simply leave the patient unregistered. Therefore, out of necessity, the system includes a second method of entry. The Tumor Registry receives copies of all pathology reports describing a malignancy. The reports include the patient's name and hospital number, date, attending physician, and pathology findings. These data are entered into a temporary file unless the patient is already registered. If, within six weeks of input of a pathology report, an entry form has not been received and entered by the tumor registry, the temporary patient entry is flagged as delinquent by a special program. A reminder letter and entry form for the delinquent patient is sent to his physician. Personal follow-up is made if necessary. By using this dual system of registration, the registry has a reasonable chance of achieving almost 100 percent coverage, even when a patient has been diagnosed elsewhere, because hospital policy requires a second, in-house pathology report before any major therapy is performed.

8. **Follow-up data collection.** Follow-up data have been kept extremely simple. For a patient still living, on the follow-up data and three single digit codes representing three multiple choice answers need be recorded on the line marked with X's. The first question concerns the progression or regression of the tumor. The only other requested data are therapy since the last visit and any planned therapy. Such follow-up data can be entered for any patient whenever it is received. To ensure that no patient is overlooked, however, each day a computer listing identifies all patients who have had no entry for over a year since their last follow-up (or six months since initial diagnosis). For each patient so identified, the computer produces a follow-up form that contains a brief summary, up to the last available status report, and room for the current entry. A copy is sent to the referring physician for him to update by entering the date, status, and therapy responses where indicated.

9. **Computer facts.** To store and manipulate data and to generate various forms of output, terminals connected to a mini-computer system are used. The computer is a Digital Equipment Company PDP 11/20, operating under MUMPS 11, a disk-oriented time-sharing system originally designed at Massachusetts General Hospital. The name MUMPS stands for Massachusetts Utility Multi-Programming System. The 1974 Status Report of the Laboratory of Computer Sciences, Massachusetts General Hospital, Harvard Medical School, on "Computers in Patient Care and Medical Education" has a brief up-to-date description of MUMPS and the MUMPS system on pages 54-57. A copy of that report can be obtained from G. Octo Barnett, M.D., Director of that Laboratory.

The PDP 11 computer has ~44,000 16-bit words of core with a map box to use all of it, two DECtape drives, and two moving head disks, each having a storage capacity of 60×10^6 alphanumeric characters or 30×10^6 16-bit words. The time-sharing system hardware and software allows twelve terminal users to be connected concurrently. The Tumor Registry presently stores data on about 3,000 patients and uses about 85 programs. Documentation and listings of these programs can be obtained from the authors upon request. The length of each program in characters is given in parentheses. Together, the data and programs occupy about 3×10^6 words or about 10 percent of the disk storage on a device, the total cost of which is approximately $30,000. Thus if disk usage is about 50 percent the storage costs amount to approximately one dollar per patient.

MUMPS is particularly efficient and cost effective, allowing many users to store and retrieve large amounts of data, as distinct from performing fast, high-speed mathematical calculations. This can be demonstrated from the following cost figures for the operation of a tumor registry utilizing MUMPS. Each terminal requires about $5,000 for installation. It costs another $5,000 per year for 40 hours per week of computer time and maintenance; $3,000 per year would amortize the capital cost of the central computer and the terminals. One terminal on such a system would be sufficient to register 500 or more new patients and to follow all patients in a typical 300-bed hospital. The registry system described has required a man-year of programming to establish. Further changes and improvements will require some continuing programming effort. The cost of the original program and the changes are, of course, largely independent on the number of patients registered.

Typically, in a large hospital these cost figures might work out as follows: To register 1500 patients per year, two terminals would be required at an annual amortized cost of $16,000 per year. Program changes would use a programmer half time, adding $7000. A registrar's and an assistant's salaries would be $20,000. With $5,000 to compensate a staff physician, the total would be $48,000, or $32 per patient registered, which includes lifetime follow-up.

If one considers that it costs about $10 to send out and collect a single typical hospital bill, and that the medical cost for each registered patient exceeds $1000, this cost appears reasonable. It is, in fact, a minimum expenditure for accessible information required if there is to be any real management of cancer treatment and should be included in the budget for normal operating costs.

10. Availability of data. With about 100 facts on each of many thousands of patients recorded, the registry has been designed to make information based on them available. One use has already been explained, viz. the automatic follow-up reminder. Several other types of reports have been planned for routine dissemination, and programmed accordingly. These include:

a. An annual report for each physician listing all of his cancer patients. The printout is arranged to first separate those patients still alive from those who have died and within these subdivisions to list them alphabetically by year of diagnosis. The age, sex, and diagnosis of each patient are also given. Survival tables summarize the data for all patients of a given physician.
b. A hospital-wide annual report of all cancer patients registered,

subdivided by major disease categories and showing the major therapy modalities for each category of patients.

c. A hospital-wide annual summary showing the total number of treatments by modality, i.e. the number of surgical procedures, the number of courses of radiation therapy, etc. given to new and previously followed patients.

d. For each department, the number of cancer patients treated by each physician in that department with survival tables for total number registered from that department.

In addition to these periodical routine reports, others, available on request, include:

a. the statistical search program, previously mentioned, produces a list of patients meeting any combination of specifications in terms of the data in the computer file. The list can contain not only the patients' names and/or numbers but also other pertinent data requested.

b. A geographical breakdown of all, or selected groups of, patients by zip code.

c. Survival statistics with life tables, survival rates, and their statistical significance for any specified group of patients, using an elaborate mathematical program known as the BMD program 76(3).

It should be emphasized that only trained medical records personnel with a knowledge of the frequently changed code words have access to these data. The terminal is located in the Office of Cancer Management. Therefore there is the same assurance of privacy and confidentiality as with the previous manual system. In turn, operating a computerized patient information system also requires the same kind of professional integrity and attention to security from the staff as a good manual medical records system does.

Conclusions and Prospects

The Tumor Registry described here is now operational. It has been designed to meet certain objectives that seem possible to attain. Whether the effort will be justified depends upon the amount of use the system will get. It is hoped that one result will be improved patient care by substantially more regular follow-up examinations. Administrative planning should be aided by both routine reports and the special listings that can be generated. It is the physician, wishing to review the results, who remains the key unknown factor. If he finds the tumor registry reports useful and requests them in substantial numbers, the system should quickly pay for itself in terms of medical education and improved methods of treatment. The same result will be achieved if substantial use is made of the possibility to implement research protocols.

Finally, this type of computer-based system lends itself particularly well to a joint registry effort by several hospitals, allowing users in each participating institution access to the combined data base without access to such identification data as the names of patients, doctors, and hospitals. Such a system would offer a tool for quality review to the participating hospital administrations if they agreed to exchange data. There is an urgent need to pool the large amounts of data needed if advances in cancer management are to be proven more rapidly than has been possible in the past. No one Boston area hospital treats enough cancer patients to have meaningful statistics on any except the most frequently occurring diagnoses. Several of the Tufts affiliated hospitals and/or departments are actively planning to form a pooled registry of this type. Its realization would be a significant milestone, both in cancer management and in cooperative endeavors.

REFERENCES

1. *1973 Cancer Facts and Figures,* American Cancer Society, New York (1973).
2. *End Results in Cancer,* Report No. 4. ed. Axtell, L. M., Cutler, S. J., and Myers, M. H., U.S. Dept. of HEW, Pub. No. (NIH) 73-272 (1972).
3. BMD Biomedical Computer Programs, ed. Dixon, W. J., Health Sciences Computing Facility, Dept. of Preventive Medicine and Public Health, School of Medicine, University of California, Los Angeles (May 1968 version).

ACKNOWLEDGMENTS

This work was supported in part by HEW grant 12178. The patient data collection system is based in part on those developed by W. Powers at the Mallinkrodt Institute, St. Louis, Missouri, and by T. Phillips at the University of California at San Francisco.

18. Integration of Treatment Planning with Tumor Registry by Means of a Cassette Tape for Each Patient

K. Inamura
S. Otani
A. Matsuoka
Y. Ueda
N. Furushima
Y. Kubo

Preface

A cassette magnetic tape for each patient was adopted as a memory medium in a radiotherapy department. The purpose was to combine treatment-planning with tumor registry, and, in the near future, to integrate several subsystems. Patients' data are gathered and stored in a cassette tape assigned to each patient throughout our system, named THERAC-II.

Hardware Configuration

Hardware configuration of the THERAC-II system is as follows:

(1) A mini-computer NEAC-M4 with 24 KB 8 bits as a central processor.
(2) A grafpen for input of anatomical data, and for input of position of radiation source in the case of brachytherapy. This device is used for computer input in both external beam therapy and brachytherapy.
(3) A function key board with numerical keys. This unit was spe-specifically designed for easy interaction between man and machine. It has several command keys.
(4) A graphic CRT unit for display of dose distribution, anatomical data, and position of radiation source.
(5) A digital plotter.
(6) A high speed input/output typewriter. This I/O typewriter is used for printout of prescriptions of radiation therapy as a result of treatment-planning, and for input and output of patient data.
(7) THERAC-II has two decks of cassette tape. One is used for

replacing job programs, the other for gathering data as well as retrieval and updating of each patient record.

Software Configuration

Programs provided for THERAC-II are:

(1) Dose-distribution planning for supervoltage X-ray therapy and gamma-ray therapy.
(2) Dose-distribution planning for electron beam therapy.
(3) Dose-distribution calculation for remote after-loading treatment.
(4) Dose-distribution calculation for interstitial therapy.
(5) Superposition of dose-distribution by different modalities or different energies.
(6) Treatment-scheduling.
(7) Tumor registry, including generation of master tapes and list tapes.
(8) Follow-up data-gathering.
(9) Statistical data analysis and output, etc.

Tumor Registry and Follow-Up Procedure

When a new patient visits a radiotherapy department, first of all his planning data for radiotherapy are stored in his cassette tape. These are data of his identification number, name, date of birth, strategy of tumor control including scheduled total dose and fractionation, data associated with diagnosis, etc. There are twenty-one separate items. If his dose-distribution planning has been made, that and his anatomical data are also stored in his cassette tape.

When treatment ends termination data are registered on his tape. These data are composed of eleven items.

Three kinds of file tapes can be generated for all patients by picking up correspondent data from each patient tape. A patient record of every item accumulated through the process is printed out. These printed tables are referred to if retrospective research is necessary. Essential data of each patient are condensed and transferred to a master tape. Tapes may be erased and re-used. Follow-up data for prognosis are added to a master tape and also used to obtain statistical data and for retrospective research afterward. Several kinds of list tapes can be generated, dealing with pathology code, site code, and location code. One of the most important lists is the follow-up—containing the names of patients who should be followed up after the treatment. Statistical data, such as five-years survival rate, or the number of cases in terms of location code, pathology code, and site code, are all obtainable by searching the master tape.

Retrospective search of resulting data in the radiotherapy department is possible by retrieving the master tapes, list tapes, and file tapes of the dose-distribution chart, prescription, and anatomical data, and by referring to printed lists or dose-distribution charts, prescriptions, and anatomical data.

Expansion to the Integrated System

A more integrated computer-aided radiotherapy system is currently under development. It will provide for almost total support in a department of radiotherapy. This system is composed of six subsystems:

(1) THERAC-III treatment-planning subsystem.
(2) THERAC-C4 4 MeV linear accelerator automation subsystem.
(3) THERAC-C18 18 MeV linear accelerator automation subsystem.
(4) Betatron treatment verification system.
(5) THERAC-III tumor registry, which covers processing of the treatment record, follow-up data-gathering, and statistical data analysis.
(6) THERAC-III also covers parameter readout from a simulator.

The system has three mini-computers. Each subsystem is connected by cassette tapes, which are assigned for all patients. The flow of patient tapes is such that, the main system picks up data from each subsystem and supplies these to other subsystems. It also compiles data from subsystems, which is then shifted to a master tape. The principle of the employment of patient cassette tapes is similar to that of THERAC-II mentioned before, but because each detail of the treatment record by the linear accelerators is added, retrospective retrieval of a patient's records can be more accurate and concrete. Moreover, interaction of cassette-taped data is possible between the subsystems—namely, picking up data from one subsystem and supplying them into other subsystems.

Weaknesses and Merits of Cassette Tape Based System

The weaknesses of this cassette-tape system compared with a disk system are as follows: the handling of cassette tape for each patient is somewhat troublesome. Updating of a cassett-taped record is not easy; it needs two passes of reading and writing. We however, believe, that the application of cassette tape is practical as far as large departments of radiotherapy are concerned—those which treat up to 2,000 patients per year. The capacity of a master cassette tape of 300 feet is 1,000 patients, two sets of tape are enough to contain all patients during a year. The merits of the system may be as follows:

(1) Extension or change of the subsystem is easy.
(2) Subsystems are easily added and removed, so that over all the system has flexibility.
(3) Low cost.

19. Information Storage and Retrieval for Tumor Registry Using a Mini-Computer

S. G. Prasad
R. M. Garces
R. A. Renn

In order to study the merit of various treatment techniques in cancer control, one has to store large numbers of patient information files and be able to retrieve the relevant ones for analysis. In the past, investigators (1, 2, 4, 6) had to search a library of patient files to recover the necessary information for analysis. Needless to say, this demanded considerable clerical time, and retrievals by such means were subject to human fatigue and error.

A large number of medium-sized radiotherapy departments in this country use mini-computers for treatment-planning. The manufacturers of these computers (3, 5) have each provided a tumor registry option that is easy to format and use. The user defines the fields and the number of possible selections in each field which he desires to store. With the aid of a teletype and/or a cathode ray tube terminal, the user enters patient information for subsequent retrieval and analysis. The information is usually stored on a magnetic tape or a disc. Retrieval is done with considerable ease and at the speed the computer allows.

At Evanston Hospital we have found these predesigned tumor registry programs inadequate for our needs because of the following reasons:

1. The number of selections that can be stored in each field is limited to one.
2. Numerical selection is restricted to a positive integer below a certain predesigned number.
3. One tape must be set up for each site of interest.
4. A search cannot be made in all fields.

To overcome these major drawbacks we developed a tumor registry system that can be easily adapted and operated by other oncology departments. The information can be stored on a magnetic disc or tape, and we have chosen the latter. The system can be broadly classified into three information groups entered in a total of 61 fields.

1. Administrative data: name, social security number, register number, and the magnetic tape identification number where patient information is stored.
2. Common tumor data: fields 1 to 14 are used for storing common tumor and follow-up information.
3. Specific tumor data: fields 15 through 61 are used for specific tumor information referable to each site. In the case of multiple primaries these fields must be repeated for each site.

Information is entered in a coded form into the computer via a teletype. Alternatively, one can choose to enter the data via a CRT terminal.

Our tumor registry system offers six choices: (1) Create, (2) Find, (3) Search, (4) Fast Search, (5) Modify, (6) Delete.

In the Create option, one enters the administrative data followed by the common tumor information. Administrative data is filed separately and is used for indexing indentification of the magnetic tape where patient information is stored. After the common tumor information is entered, the number of tumor sites is requested, and entries in fields 15 through 61, specific tumor information, are repeated for each tumor site. In each field we can store up to ten selections, and these selections can be in the range of 0.000001 to 999999.

In the Find option the user has a choice of social security number or register number as an index to locate the patient data file. One can add additional tumor sites or alter the information in existing ones.

In the Search option one can search up to ten selections per field but no more than twenty fields per search. When a match is found, the computer prints out the patient's social security number, register number, radiation therapy number, cumulative number of total sites, and the number of patients matched. At the end of the search of the entire library of magnetic tapes, the computer prints out the number of patients and the number of sites matched plus the total number of patients searched.

Each field represents a category of information pertaining to the patient or his disease, being broadly inclusive of history, specific findings, variables of therapy and follow-up. Scattered randomly throughout are a few blank fields for future use if categories arise which are not presently needed. Within each category a list of selections is available which represents all possible interpretations of the category. This allows us to store only that information pertinent to the case at hand and still be able to select individualized information for any specific category. Within each category there is provision to increase the number of selections to match the expansion of knowledge or need of information.

In the Modify option one can modify the existing information in any particular field without having to find information files on the patient. This option was created anew by ourselves to alleviate an inherent weakness in the predesigned tumor registry systems supplied by the manufacturers. In these systems it was necessary to retrieve each individual patient file before one could replace an old entry with an updated one. Our Modify option allows us to accomplish this replacement in a much simpler and faster way. This option will request the field number, old selection and the new one. This information is requested only once for the entire library and the computer will then make the appropriate replacement in the specified field for the entire library of patient information. The necessity of retrieval of individual patient files is thus eliminated.

In the Delete option the user can selectively delete patient information files from the library. Individual information entries within any one patient file cannot be deleted in this option.

This tumor registry system is composed of a number of programs written in FORTRAN. We find this system superior to manufacturers' predesigned systems. It is currently being used at our institution.

ACKNOWLEDGMENT

The authors gratefully acknowledge the help rendered by Mrs. Laura Patt Balin in preparing this paper.

REFERENCES

1. Alper, T., and Moore, J.L., *Brit. J. Radiol.*, *40*, 843 (1967)
2. Bagshaw, M. A., *Amer J. Roentgen*, *85*, 822 (1961).
3. Artronix correspondence.
4. Boag, J. W., *Acta Radiol.*, *54*, 289 (1960)
5. Digital Equipment Company correspondence.
6. Ellis, F., et al., *Brit J. Radiol.*, *36*, 153 (1963)

20. Some Comments on Automation and the Developing Center

P. V. Houdek
H. Turnier

A great deal of time has been spent at different conferences discussing the possible role of computers in the developing centers—and no simple conclusion has been reached. It seems that the problem is in the personal understanding of basic issues, i.e. (i) what role the computer can really play in the daily routine radiotherapy, and (ii) which centers are the developing centers? The individual opinion or image of the developing center varies from a stand-alone old cobalt irradiator to a fully equipped new center just built by the local health authority. The role of computers is seen in the same wide range. Apparently, it is very difficult to reach any agreement under these circumstances—in fact, any further discussion can hardly be fruitful unless the attempt is first made to establish common ground for the discussion by answering two questions.

Developed versus Developing Centers

The classification of centers into the above two categories is confusing, since, in regard to computerization of routine radiotherapy, there are no fully developed centers to date. In this respect different centers are only in different stages of development; hence, classification of centers as computerized or noncomputerized appears to be more logical. Experience shows that the progress made by the centers in this field depends primarily on their desire and need for computerization and their financial possibilities. The actual geographical location of the center is of small importance because computer technology as well as modern radiotherapy are more or less unified and generally available.

There is no apparent reason why the noncomputerized center that has the desire, the need, and the funds should not be successful in this type of project and, if necessary, should not be fully supported. On the other hand, there are several obvious reasons why the center that is lacking the desire and, especially, need can hardly benefit from computerization that would be achieved through varying sources of professional and financial assistance.

Automation and/or Computerization

The final goal of the majority of the activities performed at any radiotherapy department is to deliver the best treatment to the patient by achieving the best possible agreement between treatment strategy and the treatment actually given. To carry out individualized and accurate radiotherapy by means of human-assisted methods is very difficult, because it is too time-consuming when performed on a routine daily basis. By utilizing the computer as well as other technology, however, the majority of routine activities can be automated, and the desired goal may be reached.

Thus automation in radiotherapy is not synonymous with utilization of computers only, but covers the use of any technology that increases the overall accuracy and rapidity of procedures performed at a radiotherapy center. A typical involvement of noncomputer technology is, for example, use of the transverse axial layergraph for specification of patient-related data, or use of the isodose plotter for generation of dosimetric data.

Planning the Automation of a Noncomputerized Center

In reference to centers that comply with the necessary assumptions discussed above, a planning scheme may be outlined as follows:

(i) Specification of the center's needs and determination of its priorities.
(ii) Selection of the appropriate technology.
(iii) Establishment of a professional environment at the center which is adequate to the degree of the proposed automation.

The requirements of automation vary among centers, since they depend to a great extent on the routine and research activities carried out, as well as on the technology already available at a particular center. The future needs of centers that are planning automation today, however, are most likely different from those common several years ago, because of recent developments in radiotherapy and treatment hardware, e.g. linear accelerators with two beam modalities and variable beam energies (3). Optimal utilization of these new treatment units requires the performance of a large number of measurements on a frequent basis and, thus, the need to automate the generation of beam data may arise even before the first patient is treated. Similarly, the current concern with fulfillment of treatment strategy implies (2) that automation of the acquisition of the patient-related data (1, 4) may have higher priority than computation of elaborate treatment plans. In the future, large-scale automation may be needed, rather than isolated involvement of the computer for one particular activity (5).

Advances in the development of computer, radiotherapy, and dosimetric hardware, and especially in the design of the computer peripherals, make the task of the selection of the appropriate technology relatively simple but also expensive. It should be noted, however, that the cost of automation is small in comparison with the funds needed for the purchasing and servicing of the modern unit, e.g. the cost of a small computer is 10–20 percent of the price of the linac. Since automation can and should increase the quality of treatments provided by radiotherapy centers as well as permitting full and optimal use of the main therapy hardware, it appears that the expenses connected with this project should not be considered luxurious but necessary.

At a center the existence of logical systems for acquisition of different types of data, their processing, and also for the utilization of results obtained is of great importance to the actual process of automation. The computer and other forms of technological assistance should be employed in already functioning systems. In the hospital environment, however, it is more common that systems are being developed around already existing technology. This may result in an inadequate use of the hardware involved, as well as in overall disillusionment with automation. In the appropriate environment automation can relieve the involved professionals of time-consuming and nonattractive duties, as well as provide the information which is required but was not before available.

In the past, the limiting factor for adequate automation was the technology itself. In the future, however, the abilities of the professionals may pose the limits. Perhaps, it is one of the principal roles of the educational process to avoid this possibility.

REFERENCES

[1] Ambrose, J., Hounsfield, G., *British Journal of Radiology*, *46*, 148 (1973).

[2] Golden, R., Cundiff, J.H., Grant, W. H. III, et al., *Cancer*, *29*, 1468 (1972).

[3] Houdek, P.V., Charyulu, K. K. Sundarsanam, A., and Rao, A., *Radiology*, *110*, 203 (1974).

[4] Houdek, P., Turnier, Charyulu, K. K. Sudarsanam, A., Gargano, F., and Turnier, H., *Radiology 112*, 409 (1974)

[5] Houdek, P., Turnier, H., Sudarsanam, A., and Charyulu, K. K., "The Relative Importance of Different Procedures Involved in the Treatment Planning Process" (submitted to IAEA, 1973)

21. The IAEA Program on Computer Systems in Dosimetry

R. Abedin-Zadeh
H. H. Eisenlohr
I. A. Lerch

Since its establishment, the International Atomic Energy Agency has undertaken, as an important part of its program, the collection and dissemination of information on radioisotopes and radiation sources, to assist member states in acquiring the necessary knowledge and skills in their application. In the field of radiation therapy, the Agency has given its attention to provision, on a wide scale, of physical data and methods used for dose calculation. The goal of the Agency's program is to facilitate the introduction and assess the efficacy of suitable radiation dosimetry data and computer systems for use in developing radiotherapy centers with the cooperation of advanced institutions. This program consists of the following items:

1. Computer Applications in Radiotherapy

The application of computers has become routine in many advanced radiotherapy centers around the world. Advanced radiotherapy departments with substantial patient loads had to acquire an automated treatment-planning system in order to increase the efficacy of their therapy. It has been proved that the computer as a tool has served quite well both radiotherapists and medical physicists in their treatment-planning for cancer patients.

There are few disciplines in which such advanced cooperation has been established between scientific equals such as radiotherapists, physicists, and information scientists. The results are that with the help of such tools, the production of composite isodose curves for very complex plans and treatment strategies has been accomplished routinely. This, unfortunately, is true only in the case of advanced centers, mostly in advanced countries. Many developing radiotherapy centers are still using manual techniques which are retarding the progress promised by new information and technical advance. A question has therefore arisen: Can less developed therapy centers successfully incorporate the automated treatment-planning systems developed at advanced radiotherapy institutions? At first sight it cannot be disputed that developing centers will benefit from an affirmative reply, but in order to answer the question intelligently, we must carefully examine both the concept and the feasibility of such a program. At the same time, it must be recognized that the extent to which a given center can utilize and benefit from computer application depends on the stage of development of that center and on the overall environment in which it finds itself. A survey of high-energy radiotherapy centers all over the world has shown that there are still many therapy centers which have

a) a heavy patient load.
b) relatively few trained staff (therapists, physicists, radiographers, etc.).
c) a shortage of equipment.

It is evident that the acquisition of basic equipment and recruitment of competent staff should have a higher priority than adaptation of computer systems. The use of computers does not permit any reduction in the training and technical quality of therapists, hospital radiological physicists, and other professional staff. Considering these facts, one can classify existing developing radiotherapy centers into different categories, only the first of which will contain centers that have reached a high enough standard in radiotherapy and staff to qualify them for computerized services.

In order to create conditions for cooperation between disciplines and to try to coordinate different center all over the world, the IAEA, within the past decade, has organized three panels. The first panel, in October 1965 (1), perhaps for the first time brought together radiotherapists, computer specialists, and physicists in a programmed way. The second IAEA meeting on this subject (2) was held in July 1967. That panel conscientiously attempted to identify various radiotherapy activities in which the computer could be used to serve the needs of an existing radiotherapy center. The last panel, held in Vienna in October 1973 (3), was particularly aimed at finding ways in which the Agency and other scientific-medical communities could assist the developing radiotherapy centers in establishing and adapting computerized systems. This panel provided the Agency with specific guidance on means of assisting developing radiotherapy centers.

In order to define the needs and capability of automated treatment-planning systems, a questionnaire was distributed to radiotherapy centers derived from the 1970 edition of the Agency's Directory of High Energy Radiotherapy Centers. Thus only those centers which might conceivably have need of an automated treatment-planning service were contacted. To date, 242 questionnaires have been returned from all over the world—and that total constitutes roughly 40 percent of those distributed. The geographic distribution of the returned questionnaires has shown that liaison with regions which would require the greatest assistance is poor. This is due to the variety of reasons not all attributable to the fact that there is a smaller number of high-energy therapy centers in the developing regions as compared to Europe and North America. The differences in terminology as well as a lack of information played a significant role in limiting the responses from Asia and Latin America.

The survey has shown that many developing centers wish to use automation and are seeking assistance. The recommendations of the last panel of the Agency in this field form the basis for action in the development and institution of the Agency program. These recommendations are mainly based on technical aid provided by an "assisting" center, which might be an existing advanced radiotherapy center, or a regional computing center specially set up or a combination of the two. At the same time, the panel recommended that the Agency prepare various publications, which are now under consideration.

Within the framework of this project a coordinated research program on computer applications in clinical dosimetry has been initiated by the Agency. The objective of this coordinated program is:

To encourage and facilitate the use of computerized treatment-planning systems in the developing radiotherapy centers with the cooperation of the advanced centers;

To test the utilization of established computer techniques under local conditions. To achieve these objectives, the program would seek the following studies:

(a) development of a computer program for direct, accurate, and flexible calculation of the dose at any point in an irradiated volume adopted for individual sources and types of machines,

(b) study on optimization of treatment plans,

(c) study and recommendations on input data and preparation of manuals,

(d) study on means of long distance communications for computer input and output data exchange, and

(e) preparation of local atlases.

Up to now, nine institutions from eight countries have participated in this program, and a meeting with the chief investigators of this coordinated research program is expected to be held in 1976.

2. Radiation Dosimetry Data

In order to collect and disseminate information on radioisotopes and radiation sources with a view to assisting member states of the Agency, an agreement was signed in 1963 between the IAEA and the Hospital Physicists Association (UK), whereby the HPA Diagram and Data Scheme was transferred to the IAEA. The Agency published its first *Radiation Dosimetry Data Catalogue* in 1964 (4). A revision by M. Mauderli appeared in 1970 (5). Within the last decade the Agency has provided desired data to institutions from many countries. This service was on a nonprofit basis and received appreciation from many developing radiotherapy centers. After we had reviewed the requests for data within the last four years it appeared necessary to update and complete the catalogue, and therefore the Agency awarded a technical contract to Mr. D. E. A. Jones, who was closely associated with the initial HPA data collection, for a comprehensive updating and extension of the catalogue's contents. Mr. Jones has already contacted many of the contributors of the 1970 issue and announced the Agency's intention in many scientific journals. All members of the scientific communities are requested to submit any new information suitable for inclusion—expecialy such data as depth dose charts for X ray; electron and neutron beams, particularly from the newer machines; attenuation data for higher energy photon and particle radiation; and, especially, broad-beam coefficients.

Apart from this, the Agency has published four volumes of the *Atlas of Radiation Dose Distributions* (6). The first volume presents a selection of single-field isodose charts of Cobalt-60 and Caesium-137 gamma rays and of a wide range of high energy X-ray and electron beams currently used in radiotherapy. Volumes II and III present isodose charts and graphs for multiple fields and moving fields, respectively, together with analytical studies. Volume IV is devoted to brachytherapy isodose charts, illustrating dose distributions obtained in interstitial, intercavitary, and surface application of sealed radioisotope sources. Volumes V and VI currently under preparation will be devoted to nonradium sources (as a complement to Atlas IV), and Atlas VI to typical treatment plans. It is hoped that these Atlases will be useful for both reference in treatment-planning and practice for teaching.

Since 1959 the International Atomic Energy Agency has maintained a register of the known isotope and supervoltage teletherapy installations. The first edition of the *Directory of High-Energy Radiotherapy Centers*, published in 1968 (7), was well received, and the stock was sold out. The second edition was published in 1970 (8). In 1973 it was found necessary to compile and publish an updated edition. To this end, with the cooperation of the World Health Organization, a questionnaire was sent to all centers throughout the world. It is hoped that the completed register will constitute a valuable source of information on facilities for high-energy radiotherapy in many countries. It will assist the Agency, WHO, and other international bodies to develop their program in the field in question and utilize their valuable resources in the most appropriate manner. It will assist workers with related interests to establish and maintain contact with one another. The new edition is expected to be published at the beginning of 1975.

ACKNOWLEDGMENTS

We take the opportunity to express our gratitude to all the participating institutes for their cooperation and for valuable comments. It is a pleasure to record that this project and all the activities expressed in this report owe their inception to former IAEA staff members, Drs. M. Cohen, K. C. Tsien, M. Stovall, P. Pfalzner, H. Lanzl, W. Moos, M. Mauderli, V. Balamutov, and all others. The views expressed in this report are those of the authors and not necessarily those of the International Atomic Energy Agency.

REFERENCES

1. International Atomic Energy Agency, *Computer Calculation of Dose Distributions in Radiotherapy*, TRS no. 57 (IAEA, Vienna, 1966).

2. International Atomic Energy Agency, *Role of Computers in Radiotherapy*, STI/PUB/203 (IAEA, Vienna, 1968).

3. International Atomic Energy Agency, *Dose Computation and Computerized Treatment Planning in Radiotherapy* (to be published).
4. International Atomic Energy Agency, *Radiation Data for Medical Use*, MDS/CAT/1/1964 (IAEA, Vienna, 1964).
5. International Atomic Energy Agency, *Radiation Dosimetry Data Catalogue*, MDS/CAT/1970 (IAEA, Vienna, 1970).
6. International Atomic Energy Agency, *Atlas of Radiation Dose Distributions* (IAEA, Vienna, 1965, 1966, 1967, 1972), Vols. I - V.
7. International Atomic Energy Agency, *Directory of High-Energy Radiotherapy Centres*, STI/PUB/117 (IAEA, Vienna, 1968).
8. International Atomic Energy Agency, *Directory of High-Energy Radiotherapy Centres*, STI/PUB/251, (IAEA, Vienna, 1970), 1970 ed.

22. Documentation of Computer Programs

J. Rothmeier

Introduction

There are many factors to be considered before documenting a computer program:

1. The state of the computer project
2. The nature of the project
3. The programming language used
4. The person for whom the documentation is intended
5. The amount of use of the program

Before the inception of a computer project, it is desirable, though unfortunately not often done, to do a feasibility study. The most important aspect of this study should be to develop guidelines to determine the basis for evaluation of the project as it progresses. If it is expected that the project will become operational in a clinical environment, all members of the environment should participate in this study, and cost and time estimates should be made.

The next level should be a specification of the application. This should include a verbal description of the function of each program module and considerable detail on file design. It is often appropriate at this state to provide a flow chart on the overall system design and/or data flow.

Source code documentation, the next stage in the documentation spectrum, can require considerable programming energy and is highly dependent on the computer language used. The amount of energy spent on it should clearly be related to the value of the program. Two more useful documentation specifications are test data specification and results, and a user manual.

Thus the documentation elements are:

1. feasibility study
2. application design
3. source code documentation
4. test data and results
5. user manual

It is possible to structure the approach to source code documentation. A detailed approach to this problem utilizing the MUMPS language, which has been specifically designed for medical applications, will be discussed later.

General Considerations

Documentation elements may appear somewhat different for different users. The source code specification and test data and results are almost entirely programmer-oriented documents. It is possible, however, that a radiation physicist would be interested in test data to determine the range of use of a dosimetry program. If test data are intended for this purpose, they must cover a considerably wider range of cases.

The feasibility study and application design are primarily management-related documents. A more detailed application design will be necessary in order to provide sufficient information for a programmer. In some cases this can be accomplished by continuous verbal interaction.

The user manual should be self-contained and written in such a way that it can be understood by nontechnical personnel. It may also serve to help describe a program to a potential user.

While a program is being written, it is difficult and perhaps unnecessary to maintain complete source code specification. It is, however, very useful to maintain an up-to-date list of variables together with their description. It is not necessary to comment every line of code, but intelligent commenting can improve programmer efficiency.

When a program is completed and has been shown to serve a useful function, it is time to develop a more detailed source-code specification and write a user's manual. Since good documentation is a difficult task, it is important that the value of the program be objectively established before this step is taken. In a developmental environment most programs are never used by anyone except the original programmer. In this case it would be inefficient to do extensive source code documentation.

If a project is concerned with complex algorithms or unique numerical techniques, they should be clearly described in the documentation. If the project is concerned with information management, the format of all input and examples of all reports generated should be provided.

Some languages have been described as self-documenting. It is true that those which read more like prose (COBAL, BASIC) than like mathematics textbooks (FORTRAN, ALGOL) may require less documentation. But it is still necessary to provide more documentation than the code itself in order to eliminate many hours of puzzle-solving by programmers who wish to use a program written by someone else (or by themselves a long time ago). In some respects MUMPS, like APL, is more difficult to read without additional documentation than most languages. It requires the total range of program documentation and is therefore a useful language to use as a specific example of an approach to source code documentaiton.

Source Code Documentation

The smallest element of a MUMPS program is that which can fit in core memory at one time. It is called a routine and generally consists of fewer than 2,000 characters. This element is visible to the programmer and can serve to modularize programming. A closed set of routines that perform a specific task is called a program, and a collection of programs that function together in an application is called a package. Documentating a routine is accomplished by completing a form that requests the purpose of the routine, description of variables used, name of routines related to the routine, and a description of the files (calles "globals" in MUMPS). An example of the form used is shown in Figure 1. The form has the added advantage that it serves as a reminder to a programmer of the documentation elements to be considered. Such fundamental items as listings and test data can be easily overlooked. An abstract is shown in Figure 2. The abstract is intended to provide data on the purpose of a routine, program, or package as well as sufficient technical detail to determine the difficulty of using it in a different computer environment.

A face sheet, shown in Figure 3, is intended to provide an overview of a program or package. It should be followed by flow charts and narrative describing the interrelation of routines and programs. This greatly contributes to the organization of what can be a considerable amount of information.

Since MUMPS is a language designed primarily for file management, documentation of files is very important. All files are sparsely allocated tree structures. In order to improve retrieval efficiency, programmers often design files that optimize disc usage. This may obscure the logical use of the file. A pictorial hierarchical description of the file from both a logical and physical point of view facilitates understanding.

Although some of the source program documentation described is specific to the MUMPS language, the general principle of organization and use of forms to guide a programmer's documentation style is applicable to a wide variety of languages and applications. Any program that has been documented with these principles in mind will be much easier to understand. This will contribute to the program's transferability and maintainability.

FORM FOR MUMPS ROUTINE DOCUMENTATION

(A routine is defined as a collection of MUMPS statements filed, called, and/or overlayed as a single unit.)

```
*DATE

*ROUTINE MNEMONIC

*GENERAL DATA
    purpose

   1author(s)

   1computer and MUMPS dialect

SIZE
   *partition currently used
    estimated minimum partition required
    number of characters in routine

ENTRY POINT(s)
---*description
--- variables required

LOCAL VARIABLES
---*name
---*use
---*type
--- function
--- cross-reference listing

*GLOBALS
---name

RELATED ROUTINES
--- routines which invoke this one
---*routines which are invoked by this one

DETAILED DESCRIPTION
--- narrative description
--- flow chart
---*listing

INTERACTION AT PERIPHERAL DEVICE(s)
--- principal input device
--- principal output device
--- 1/0 to other devices

TEST RUNS---
```

*Mandatory items.

[1]Unless this is a stand-alone routine, this item may be specified only once on the package/program face sheet.

Figure 1

MUMPS ABSTRACT

ROUTINE☐ PROGRAM☐ PACKAGE☐

APPLICATION AREA:

SHORT TITLE:

DATE LAST MODIFIED:
PURPOSE (up to 150 words; underline key words; continue on back if necessary):

AUTHOR(S)

CONTACT
NAME:
BUSINESS ADDRESS:

TELEPHONE:

DIALECT
AHS-11☐ DEC-11☐ DEC-15☐ ITA☐ MGH☐ MIIS☐ MUMPS-PC☐ OTHER______

MACHINE
NOVA☐ PC-12☐ PDP-9☐ PDP-11☐ PDP-15☐ SYSTEM/7☐ OTHER_______

PERIPHERALS
DISC☐ TAPE☐ PRINTER☐ CRT☐ A/D☐ OTHER_______

PARTITION SIZE (characters):

GLOBAL SIZE (number of blocks and block size):

RESTRICTIONS (continue on back if necessary):

NUMBER OF CHARACTERS OF CODE:

NUMBER OF ROUTINES:

SOURCE LISTING☐

COMMERCIAL SERVICE☐

DOCUMENTATION☐

Figure 2

MUMPS

PROGRAM/PACKAGE FACE SHEET

DATE:

PROGRAM/PACKAGE (delete one) NAME:

PURPOSE (continue on separate sheet if necessary):

AUTHOR'S NAME(S), MAILING ADDRESS & PHONE:

COMPUTER AND MUMPS DIALECT:

PARTITION SIZE CURRENTLY USED:

LIST OF GLOBALS USED:

GLOBAL DOCUMENTATION APPENDED Y/N:

TEST RUN DATA APPENDED Y/N:

TOTAL NUMBERS OF ROUTINES:

MNEMONIC(S) OF CALLING ROUTINE(S):

INTER-ROUTINE FLOW SHEET APPENDED Y/N:

ROUTINE INTERFACE SPECIFICATIONS APPENDED Y/N:

TOTAL NUMBER OF PROGRAMS:

INTER-PROGRAM FLOW SHEET APPENDED Y/N:

PROGRAM INTERFACE SPECIFICATIONS APPENDED Y/N:

Program: a closed set of routines used to perform a specific task.

Package: a collection of programs which function together in an application.

Figure 3

IX. Submitted Abstracts

Treatment Planning

A PILOT PROGRAM FOR TRUE 3-DIMENSIONAL DOSE CALCULATIONS IN EXTERNAL BEAM RADIOTHERAPY.

Harvey Frey, Dennis Chapman, Dennis Freida, Alan Miller, and Ranon Vokoff. University of Southern California Health Sciences, Los Angeles, California.

In order to determine the feasibility of defining the scatter contribution to a point by integrating over the entire irradiated volume, a pilot program has been written using a scatter function S(d, Δd, r), defined as the scatter contribution at point (d + Δd, r) for one rad of primary dose at (d,)). The methods of deriving this function from TAR tables and the accuracy and speed of the pilot program will be presented.

A SUPPORT AND DISSEMINATION CENTER FOR USERS OF DEDICATED COMPUTERS IN DEPARTMENTS OF RADIATION ONCOLOGY.

C. S. Chui, J. Hahn, S-N. Yu, Laboratory of Computer Science, Mount Sinai School of Medicine; L. J. Lidofsky, Nuclear Science and Engineering, Columbia University, New York.

In 1972 and 1973 the Laboratory of Computer Science of the Mount Sinai School of Medicine cosponsored a group of meetings to support the use of dedicated medium-sized computers in departments of radiotherapy. Such systems, costing in the neighborhood of $100,000 or less, can provide a range of computer support for a department of radiotherapy, including:

(a) Dose calculations
(b) Patient data base
(c) Therapy machine control, and
(d) Patient scheduling

To further this approach the American Cancer Society has provided the Laboratory of Computer Science with a grant to enable it to function in the calendar year 1974 as:

(a) A repository for computer programs and systems relating to the use of dedicated medium size computer systems in radiation oncology.
(b) A center for the development of computer programs and program modules not available from other sources.
(c) A dissemination center for the programs and information available through (a) and (b) above.

Since the beginning of the program we have contacted a number of users to begin task (a). We have adapted the programs received when necessary and have begun dissemination. Our experiences during the first six months of this program will be described.

THE FUTURE ROLE OF THE COMPUTER IN RADIOTHERAPY TREATMENT PLANNING.

J. M. Wilkinson. Regional Physics Department, Christie Hospital, Manchester, England.

Radiotherapy treatment-planning consists of (a) proposing a system of treatment, and (b) assessing that proposal. If it is satisfactory, the treatment can proceed; if not, the proposal is modified and reassessed. If we consider just external beam radiotherapy the proposal relates to the type and quality of the radiation, number of beams, their directions, field dimensions, beam-weightings, and beam-modifying filters. The assessment is based on the resulting dose-distribution. The dose levels required and a suitable fractionation scheme are assumed. Currently the computer's role is to provide information about the dose-distribution, and in the majority of cases it does this by producing an isodose display. But does the isodose display provide the information that is both necessary and sufficient to assess the proposed treatment? Systems that are restricted to producing isodose displays in a single plane may well not provide sufficient information, as nothing is learned about dose levels outside that plane, and one is forced to do additional point calculations or make the assumption that changes in patient cross-section do not result in significant changes in the isodose distribution. To be sure of having suf-

MPUTER GENERATION OF HIGH-ENERGY X-RAY DOSE STRIBUTIONS.

J. Schulz, F. McKiernan, and A. Agostinelli. Dept. of Therapeutic diology, Yale University, New Haven, Connecticut.

st external beam treatment-planning programs that are written large computers require a method for generating the dose distribu- n produced by a single field for specified geometrical and physical nditions. Treatment-planning programs for mini-computers often quire extensive libraries of dose distributions, and the most practi- way to acquire these libraries is by computer calculation. A beam neration program has been developed specifically for the genera- on of beam libraries for mini-computers, but which is also used to nerate dose distributions for unusual treatment plans, and could be ed in large-computer treatment-planning programs.

The program was designed to take account of the physical para- eters of each machine for which beams are to be generated. Input arameters include source diameter, collimator distance, treatment istance, wedge dimensions and location, zero-field-size tissue-air atios, and scatter-air ratios. Flattening filters, such as that on the linac 4, which produce unusual beam profiles are simulated by the rogram.

The operating principles of the program include the initial estab- shment of an X-ray beam profile for the field size, wedge, and lattening filter employed. This profile includes the penumbra that esults from the source diameter and collimator location. The dose o any point in the irradiated medium is calculated as a sum of doses rom primary and scattered radiations. The primary dose is obtained rom the zero-field-size TAR modified by the value of the beam pro- file for the specific ray under consideration. The dose from scattered radiation is obtained by summing the contributions from 1 cm wide scatter strips. Scatter-air ratios are calculated for each scatter strip, and these, too, are modified by the appropriate value of the beam profile. The scatter strip method is unique, and provides the beam generation program with great flexibility.

A FAST NEUTRON TREATMENT PLANNING SYSTEM BASED ON A REAL TIME MULTIPROGRAMMED MINI-COMPUTER.

R. E. Pengilley. Medical Research Council, Cyclotron Unit, Hammersmith Hospital, London, U.K.

A graphics-oriented radiotherapy treatment-planning system for use with cyclotron-produced fast neutrons in a multi-user mini-com- puter environment is described. The hardware and software of the basic computer system are dealt with briefly to give an indication of the advantages and limitations of such a system. The graphical

ficient information in all cases, the capability of
ated volume three-dimensionally must exist. If tl
take the form of isodose displays, we can have pl
parallel planes, or in three orthogonal planes, or lo
3-D imaging system. However, if we are sure that
sufficient information on which to assess the syst
dose displays at all? Can we not simply extend th
and ask it to give us an objective assessment? This
dose and dose-gradient calculations in specified re
the tumor volume, around critical organs, and nea
points. If the assessment resulted in a rejection of
puter could be programmed to indicate which para
treatment proposal were chiefly responsible for the
features of the dose distribution. If we can manage
displays, we obviate the need for dose calculations
the dose is not going to affect the assessment of the
posals, and, further, we avoid some of the problems
ated with the large amounts of data otherwise neces
planning with non-coplanar beams.

QUALITY CONTROL IN A REGIONAL MEDICAL PROGRAM.

Marilyn Stovall, Alfred R. Smith, Robert J. Shalek. T
of Texas System Cancer Center, Houston, Texas.

This paper reviews the efforts of center personnel in a
cal physics program to ensure quality control in radiot
metry systems by means of:

(1) On-site reviews of dosimetry methods. A physic
center visits the local hospital, at the invitation of the h
cist, and reviews all dosimetry techniques, such as mach
tion, beam alignment, beam characteristics, patient cha
Types of errors found during reviews are discussed.

(2) Mailed thermoluminescent dosimeters for check
output.

(3) Mailed films for check of light and radiation bean

(4) Check of the application of dose distributions cal
computer. Various methods, such as verification of treat
ensure that the dose distributions calculated by the cente
stood and used correctly.

Computer-generated data are viewed as one part of a c
metry system, involving both radiotherapist and physicist
requires various continuing checks in order to deliver the
dose in radiotherapy. Data presented are based on six yea
perience in providing medical physics services to outlying

hardware for the treatment-planning subsystem is then described. The software to control data input, calculation, and output of results is outlined and a separate section traces the development of the computational algorithm to its current state. Finally, the possibility of extending the system to include routine use with other sources of radiation is mentioned.

RADGRAF PROGRESS REPORT AND PROJECTIONS FOR THE FUTURE.

Carol M. Newton and Jerald W. Johnson, Health Sciences Computing Facility, Department of Biomathematics, and Department of Radiology, School of Medicine, University of California, Los Angeles, California, 90024, U.S.A.; Richard F. Nelson, Department of Radiological Physics, Cooper Hospital, Camden, New Jersey, 08103, U.S.A.

RADGRAF is a radiation treatment-planning system in which a low-cost remote interactive graphics terminal communicates with its host processor by way of ordinary dial-up telephone lines. At the time of our last meeting, the Cooper Hospital Terminal had been installed, but only preliminary information could be offered regarding operating statistics. We now can provide more definitive information on response times, costs, reliability, and experience with communications problems. We have focused our efforts more on improvements requested by our users or suggested by watching them at their work, than on the addition of major new components. Especial emphasis has been on facilitating treatment-specification procedures and providing more versatile outputs.

We shall attempt to apply what we have learned to consideration of alternatives for developing future computer support systems for radiation therapy. First, we shall contribute to the data required for such deliberations. Second, we shall seek to direct our recommendations both to the broad base of radiation therapy needs that has been suggested and to some issues, such as networking, that relate to medical computing considered as a whole.

A TREATMENT PLANNING SYSTEM.

Richard F. Nelson, Mary J. Lansu, Mary W. Denk. Department of Radiological Physics and Department of Radiation Therapy and Nuclear Medicine, Cooper Hospital, Camden, New Jersey.

The use of computers for radiation therapy treatment-planning is now commonly employed. Interactive graphics systems are now also being used by many institutions [1,2,3].

At Cooper Hospital all radiation therapy candidates go through the treatment-planning section of the Physics Department. The patient is first simulated with a Picker Simulator. Using these techniques, the treatment area of interest is determined. We then employ gray scale ultrasonography with modified transducers. This system is directly interfaced with our Imlac graphics computer and in this manner the external and internal contours are considered in the dose computations. Treatment plans with and without inhomogeneities being considered will be shown. Once the best treatment strategies have been determined, a hard copy is made for the patient's records. Using Xerox teleprocessing and a grafpen system, treatment strategies are computed for outside institutions both for external and for intracavity dose distributions. The applications of this system in different areas will be presented.

REFERENCES

1. Newton, C. M., "*Remote* Graphics Radiotherapy Treatment Planning," in *Afterloading in Radiotherapy: Proceedings of a Conference Held in New York City* (1971), pp. 139-145.
2. Mohan, R., et al., "Incorporation of a Minicomputer as an Intelligent Terminal in a Treatment Planning System," *Radiology*, *110*, 183-1 190 (1974).
3. Sternick, E. S., et al., "External-Beam Treatment Planning on a Time-Sharing Graphics Terminal System," *Radiology*, *110*, 467-472 (1974).

A METHOD FOR THE AUTOMATIC RECORDING OF PATIENT OUTLINE INFORMATION.

J. Milan, S. C. Lillicrap, Royal Marsden Hospital, Downs Road, Sutton, Surrey, England.

When computer systems are used for treatment-planning, a considerable amount of spatial information concerning patient outlines and internal structures must be digitized. The transfer of data from the patient to the computer generally involves two stages: first, some method is used to transfer the patient information to paper, then the information thus recorded is digitized. For minimum labor a recording system that would omit the intermediate stage and allow data to be transferred directly between the patient and the computer appears to be attractive. However, such a system is likely to have technical problems that would limit its usefulness and make its operation, when considered in relation to the overall planning process, inefficient.

An automatic recording device has been developed at the Royal Marsden Hospital which has been found to be accurate to within ±2 mm. This device is attached to a simulator and produces output in a form that is inherently suitable for direct input to a computer. When all factors were considered, however, it was concluded that the device could be most efficiently used to generate the conventional outline tracing on paper.

THE USE OF COMPUTERS IN A REGIONAL RADIOTHERAPY PHYSICS CENTER.

Douglas Jones, John Washington, Northwest Medical Physics Center, University of Washington RC-08, Seattle, Washington, 98195.

The Northwest Medical Physics Center provides physics support to 27 radiotherapy departments, at which some 7,600 cancer patients are treated annually. The growth of the Center from 1969 will be discussed and statistics given on the utilization of the services provided. The rationale for the development of a computer-based dose-calculation service for brachytherapy, irregular field therapy, and external beam therapy will be described. Plans for the introduction of a treatment-planning service and automatic processing of the patient therapy record will be given.

APPLICATION OF A LOW COST COMPUTER GRAPHICS TERMINAL TO RADIOTHERAPY TREATMENT PLANNING.

D. G. Jameson, P. Crossland, Middlesex Hospital Medical School, London; J. L. Haybittle, Addenbrooke Hospital, Cambridge, England.

The hardware is specified and the principles of operation discussed, e.g. vector format and communications procedures.

The software philosophy for the operating system is discussed and also the principles behind the design of the radiotherapy applications programs, e.g. the languages used and how the choice of the large host computer affects the system design.

The problems experienced during the work on this project are discussed, even though some might be peculiar to the United Kingdom.

Finally there is discussion on how a system such as discussed here would operate in centers other than where it was developed.

DIDOS, A MATRIX-BASED DOSE-PLANNING SYSTEM.

Thomas Gustafsson, Ulla-Brita Nordberg, Kurt Liden. Department of Radiation Physics, University of Lund, Sweden.

The two-dimensional computerized dose-planning system for external beam therapy, DIDOS, has been developed in Lund and used in clinical routine for one year. It is based on a library of measured absorbed dose-distribution matrices, stored on disc or tape. The system allows for plane as well as wedged fields for photons and electrons of different energy. Corrections for oblique incidence and all sorts of heterogeneities are performed. Calculations are made in a grid with 3 mm-spacing for the whole cross-section, with as many details as are desired, and in five colors. Great effort has been made to create a form of presentation meeting the needs of the users.

The dose-distribution matrices are recorded on film, having the advantage of collecting a lot of information simultaneously during a period of time corresponding to that normally used for patient irradiation. Wedged fields are recorded directly, avoiding the errors due to an analytic correction. The film is exposed in the principal plane of the beam, and its resulting density is scanned automatically, digitized in a matrix with a cell-size of 3 mm, and punched on paper tape. The film density is kept linear to dose by appropriate film-processing. The energy dependence of density is taken care of by calibration to absorbed dose along the central axis and in the absolute dose maximum. This is performed by a special program.

The cross-section of a patient with all details, up to seven regions of heterogeneity, and the planning suggestions are punched on paper tape by means of a sonic pen digitizer, consisting of two microphones 50 cm long, connected to a teletype.

One field at a time is read from the disc, containing about 600 field-matrices, and up to 50 can be added cumulatively. Corrections for oblique incidence and for heterogeneities are made along the field-matrix columns according to isodose-shift method.

The system is run in remote-batch mode on a Univac 1108 at the University Computer Center. The average computational time is 30 seconds for a three-field plan, almost independent of the amount of heterogeneity correction. The average cost is about nine dollars.

INTERACTIVE TREATMENT PLANNING IN RADIOTHERAPY.

G. Gell. Univ.-Klinik für Radiologie, Graz, Austria.

Our planning procedure consists of the following steps:

1. Input of patient contour with a grafpen (ultrasonic digitizer) with immediate display and correction possibility.
2. Input of field configuration on the keyboard.

3. Calculation of dose distribution (following the formulae of Richter and Schirrmeister).
4. Display of the dose distribution on the video-screen with isodose lines.
5. If other field configurations are to be tested, a screen-size hard copy of the isodose picture can be produced in less than 10 seconds. Then the cycle restarts with step 2.
6. The final distribution is plotted in life size on the Calcomp plotter.

A three-dimensional representation of the dose distribution is available for special cases. The system handles coplanar fixed and rotational external beams as well as radioactive implants.

The complete procedure (steps 1 through 6) takes about 8–15 minutes (depending on the number of fields and the size of the contour). One planning cycle (steps 2 through 5) takes about 2–5 minutes.

The dose calculation is done routinely for every radiotherapy patient. Interactive planning is necessary for 5–10 percent of the patients.

The hardware consists of a PDP15 with 16K, DECtapes, fixed head disk, grafpen, TTY, Tektronix display with hard copy, and a Calcomp plotter.

INTEGRATION OF TREATMENT PLANNING WITH TUMOR REGISTRY BY MEANS OF A CASSETTE TAPE FOR EACH PATIENT.

K. Inamura, S. Otani, A. Matsuoka, Y. Ueda, N. Furushima, Y. Kubo. Nippon Electric Co. Ltd., Fuehu City, Tokyo, Japan.

A cassette magnetic tape for each patient in a radiotherapy department was adopted as a memory medium in order to combine the treatment planning with the tumor registry by THERAC-II system (1). Treatment-scheduling data, dose-distribution chart, anatomical data, and treatment prescription are stored in a cassette tape that is assigned for each patient. When the treatment is terminated, each patient record is condensed and transferred to a master tape and list tapes. Second-handed tapes are again used for new patients. Follow-up data are added to master-tape data, and they are used to get statistical data afterward.

THERAC-II system has two decks of cassette tape. The one is used for replacing job programs. The other is for data collection as well as retrieval of each patient record. Programs that are provided for THERAC-II are: (1) Dose-distribution planning for supervoltage X-ray and gamma-ray therapy, (2) Dose-distribution planning for electron beam therapy, (3) Dose-distribution calculation for remote after-loading treatment, (4) Dose-distribution calculation for interstitial therapy, (5) Superposition of dose-distributions by different modalities, (6) Treatment-scheduling, (7) Tumor registry, (8) Generation of master tapes and list tapes, (9) Follow-up data gathering, (10) Statistical data analysis, and so on.

Retrospective search of resulting data in radiotherapy is possible by retrieving list tapes and file tapes of the dose-distribution chart and anatomical data. Key words are patient number, location code, pathology code, and site code.

System components of THERAC-II are a mini-computer, NEAC-M4 with 24 KB/8 bits, a grafpen anatomical data input and source position data input device for both external beam therapy and brachytherapy, a function keyboard with numerical tenkeys, a CRT graphic display, two decks of cassette magnetic tape, a digital plotter, and a high-speed input/output typewriter.

Automation and verification for linear accelerator treatment will be integrated to our system in the near future.

REFERENCE

(1) S. Otani et al., "Treatment-Planning Computer System THERAC-II System Description, Fourth International Conference on the Use of Computers in Radiation Therapy, Uppsala, Sweden (August 7-11, 1972).

CALCULATION OF DOSE DISTRIBUTIONS FOR ELECTRON DEPTH THERAPY WITH ATTENTION TO INHOMOGENEITIES.

Dieter Fehrentz. Universitats-Strahlenklinik, 69 Heidelberg, Vobstrabe 3, FR Germany.

A semi-analytical method for description of dose-distribution in electron beams is proposed, using an approximation for attention to body inhomogeneities. This approximation is a modification of the method announced by Laughlin. The accuracy is discussed in terms of measured dose-distributions in inhomogeneous phantoms. In lungs and cavities or bones in greater depth no important variations of dose arise by scattering electrons. Therefore scattering effects can be neglected. Above all, dose-distributions are influenced by the different densities of tissue. Single inhomogeneities with small diameters, like ribs, can be neglected without a greater mistake. Lungs and stomach with many small inhomogeneities can be handled as areas with suitable chosen homogeneous densities.

The accuracy of calculated dose-distributions compared with real ones in the body depends on knowledge of form, position, size, and density of voluminous inhomogeneities, especially of the lungs. Mistakes are estimated which can be made in spite of using transmission measurements and ultrasonography.

RADIATION TREATMENT PLANNING ON A MULTITASKING SYSTEM.

J. S. Clifton, A. Todd-Pokropek, D. Ingram. University College Hospital, London WC1E 6AU, England.

A PDP 11/45 configuration comprising 56 K of core store and appropriate peripherals has been designed and installed to support simultaneously a number of different clinical areas, notable radiotherapy, nuclear medicine, and neonatal intensive care. A novel video disc system also has been developed capable of supporting up to 60 separate displays.

The D.E.C.-supplied real-time operating system RSX-11D is used. The U.C.H. radiation treatment-planning package, preexisting as a batch-orientated suite of programs on an IBM 360/65, has been converted to run under this system. Because of the multitasking commitment, programs have been heavily overlain and (excluding system libraries, file, and input-output routines) require only 8 K of memory. Particular attention has been paid to making the system suitably interactive. The benefits (and constraints) of using the system will be described.

For radiotherapy the treatment-planning terminal has three independent displays, one color, two black and white. Interaction is by either keyboard or joystick. Dose-distributions, patient outlines, and related information may be directed to and held on any display. Direct visual comparison of different plans is thus provided. The advantages of using color, grey scale, black and white, and multiple displays will be discussed.

SOURCE VIGNETTING AND SCATTER-AIR RATIO DOSE CALCULATIONS IN TELETHERAPY.

J. F. Drew, J. C. F. MacDonald, D. J. Dawson. Ontario Cancer Treatment and Research Foundation London Clinic, Victoria Hospital, London, Ontario, Canada.

Significant errors arise in the calculation of large beam-dose distributions using scatter-air ratios in Cobalt-60 teletherapy. Analysis of the primary component shows that source-vignetting by the collimator is significant for large beams. A modifying function is determined to describe the primary component, and a method is shown of using this function to calculate the dose-distribution produced by large regular or irregular beams. The possibility is discussed that present values of scatter-air ratios for large radii are in error.

COMPUTER AUTOMATION OF COMPENSATING FILTER DESIGN.

J. Clemens, Mass. General Hospital; B. Bjarngard, Joint Center for Radiation Therapy; A. L. Boyer, Mass. General Hospital; M. Goitein, Mass. General Hospital; R. Larsen, Joint Center for Radiation Therapy; G. Svenssen, Joint Center for Radiation Therapy, Boston, Massachusetts.

The aim of delivering a uniform dose to a tissue volume is thwarted by the natural surface irregularities of the human body. An effective and clinically practical tissue-compensation system has long been sought after. This paper describes an approach that utilizes a computer to translate a description of a particular surface into a specification of a compensator for that surface. A program has been written for the PC-12 which designs filters. One of two input formats can be selected to enter surface data automatically and interactively. The program allows for rotation of the beam to any angle around the surface. One of two types of compensators can then be specified on previously stored data about the therapy machine and the filter elements.

This paper describes the system, physical measurements, and clinical experience.

TREATMENT PLANNING IN THE BRITISH NATIONAL HEALTH SERVICE.

Montague Cohen. The London Hospital, London, E.1., England.

In 1972 the British Institute of Radiology, jointly with the Faculty of Radiologists, set up a Working Party to study the use of computers in treatment-planning in British hospitals in the context of a wider study on "Modern Technology in Radiotherapy." The group commissioned (with funding by the Department of Health) an operational research specialist, Dr. B. Barber, to undertake a detailed survey of the existing practice of treatment-planning, both manual and computer assisted, in relation to the organization of radiotherapy and medical physics in the National Health Service, and with particular reference to the cost-effectiveness of available systems.

Radiotherapy in the U.K. is carried out in approximately 70 centers, assisted by about 150 diagnostic and follow-up clinics. Every treatment center has at least one full-time radiation physicist. The amount and quality of dose computation varies widely, and it is certainly not yet true that every patient is individually planned, with or without a computer. Computing in this field is mainly on a batch-processing or time-sharing basis, with alphanumeric I/O. Comparatively few centers have a free-standing real time system of the "RAD-8" type, and the interactive terminal system with graphical I/O is still under development.

The situation in British hospitals is discussed in the light of (i) Dr. Barber's report, (ii) the BIR Working Party's report and (iii) known Department of Health policy on computers in hospitals. An attempt is made to assess the likely impact of these reports on the development of computing in British radiotherapy departments.

A TECHNIQUE FOR SUPERIMPOSING CROSS SECTIONS OF THE PELVIC BONE STRUCTURE ON CALCULATED RADIATION ISODOSE CURVES FOR GYNECOLOGICAL CURIETHERAPY.

Roger Mampey, Henri Regis, Leon Bousquet. Center d'Etudes et de Recherches de Toulouse, France.

Several programs for calculating radiation isodose lines for gynecological curietherapy are now in existence. None of these programs, however, associates the isodose contours to the anatomical structure of the patient under treatment. The work presented in this paper is a preliminary approach to this problem; it concerns a representation which associates each isodose contour in a given plane with the corresponding cross-section of the pelvic bone structure.

CLASSIFICATION OF SYSTEMS FOR COMPUTERIZED TREATMENT PLANNING.

Bengt A. Olsen. Uppsala University Datacenter, Uppsala, Sweden.

The purpose of this paper is to give a brief review of existing computer configurations for computerized treatment-planning in radiotherapy. It includes a figure that shows the cost per year vs. the number of calculated isodose curves per year, and a table that summarizes the relative merits of the various solutions. In principle there are at least seven main kinds of configurations employed in radiotherapy, allowing for different kinds of operation:

1. Manual
2. Batch computers

3. Time-sharing terminals
4. Small dedicated computers
5. Medium-sized, multipurpose computers
6. Remote-batch terminals
7. Intelligent remote-batch terminals

Variants with chip computers and multiple local computers will be only mentioned briefly.

In my opinion the intelligent remote job-entry terminal is the most general and attractive solution to the problem of introducing computers into radiotherapy.

A COMPUTER ASSISTED METHOD FOR COMPUTING MACHINE TIME FOR SQUARE AND RECTANGULAR FIELDS ON A CO-60 TELETHERAPY MACHINE.

W. D. Renner. West Virginia University Medical Center, Morgantown, West Virginia.

A computer program was written to produce a printout booklet that greatly simplifies the task of computing machine time for square and rectangular fields on a Co-60 teletherapy machine. A direct relationship between field-size correction in air and area divided by perimeter of the field was experimentally verified and used in the method. The printout incorporates the machine output, field-size air correction factor, backscatter factor and percentage of depth dose into a single number that can be read off for any particular depth and any given area divided by perimeter ratio. The need of interpolation between columns and rows of a table is thus eliminated.

COMPUTER MODELING OF NEUTRON DOSE AT VARIOUS LOCATIONS WITHIN THE BODY DURING PION RADIOTHERAPY.

Mario E. Schillaci, Dennis L. Roeder. Los Alamos Scientific Laboratory, Los Alamos, New Mexico.

The dose due to neutrons produced by nuclear capture of negative pions during radiotherapy is calculated at various locations within the body for each of several treatment volumes and positions. These calculations are a continuation of work reported earlier (Schillaci and Roeder, 1973) on neutron whole-body dose using a spherical tissue model and utilizing the same Monte Carlo transport code, ANDY. Here we model the head, neck, and torso using combinations of spheres and cylinders, and we include the spinal column, rib cage, and skull for bone, and the brain, lungs, and heart for specific organs. Otherwise, the chemical composition of soft tissue is approximated throughout the model. The source of the neutrons is taken as the region of stopped pions (treatment volume)—any neutrons produced in flight along the entrance path being safely ignored. The results are presented for typical treatment doses.

REFERENCE

Schillaci, M. E., and Roeder, D. L., "Dose Distribution Due to Neutrons and Photons Resulting from Negative Pion Capture in Tissue," *Phys. Med. Biol.*, *18*, 821 (1973).

RUSH RADIATION ONCOLOGY COMPUTER SYSTEM.

Thomas Wachtor, Anthony Chung-Bin. Section of Medical Physics, Rush–Presbyterian–St. Luke's Medical Center, Chicago, Illinois.

Radiation Oncology at Rush Medical College and Presbyterian–St. Luke's Hospital has a computer system that meets virtually all the requirements of a busy clinical department. The system hardware is built around a PDP-11/45 computer having as its main features 28 K of core memory and two 1.2 million-word disk drives. The system software is a modified disk-operating system allowing up to 8 users on a time-sharing basis.

The functions performed by this computer system are as follows: (1) External beam treatment-planning—scope and graphic output; (2) Implant dosimetry—graphic output; (3) Multiple treatment machines monitoring and verification; (4) On-line sampling of transit dose information for arcing and rotation therapy; (5) Patient information (demographic, treatment and pathology)—storage and retrieval; (6) Dose related computation—TAR, SAR, NSD, etc.; (7) Radiobiological modeling and parameter fitting; (8) Special clinical study project; and (9) Teaching.

Future developments include the addition of components and software for greater reliability and a dual-processor configuration to allow therapy machine control in a time-sharing environment.

A COORDINATE SYSTEM FOR COMPUTER BEAM ANGLES AND DETERMINATION OF INDICATOR ANGLES FOR PATIENT SETUP IN RADIATION THERAPY.

Suresh M. Brahmavar. Departments of Pathology-Radiology, Springfield Hospital Medical Center, Springfield, Massachusetts.

The increasing use of computers in radiation treatment-planning has resulted in use of different coordinate systems to relate the radiation beam angles that describe the beam positions used in radiation treatments. The computer beam angles need to be translated into actual gantry beam positions and the indicator angle readings of the therapy unit before the patient is set up for treatment. The relationships between the radiation beam angles and the indicator angle readings differ from one therapy unit to another because of the different orientations of the gantry rotation scales. At this time there is a need to standardize all the parameters used in patient treatment and the treatment-planning.

A standard system of coordinates for computer beam angles is proposed. Such a standard system of rotation coordinates will specify:

(a) all rotations shall be scaled from 0 to 359 degrees irrespective of the range of rotation desired,
(b) the rotation scale shall read zero when the radiation beam is directly vertically downward, and
(c) viewed from the point on the axis of rotation on the patient contour, the rotation scales shall increase from 0 to 359 degrees in anticlockwise direction.

In addition, the formulae to obtain the Indicator Angle (IA) from the Computer Beam Angle (CBA) are given for two widely used rotational therapy units with vertical gantry rotation indicators. With the above systems of coordinates for computer beam angles, these formulae are:

(1) Theratron 780 (AECL)	:	Cobalt-60 unit
	:	IA = 360 – CBA
(2) Clinac-4 (Varian)	:	Linear Accelerator
	:	If CBA is less than 180°, then IA = CBA + 180°
	:	If CBA is greater than 180°, then IA = CBA – 180°

These formulae will be valid for all other therapy units that use the identical gantry rotation scales. The routine use of these formulae has helped to minimize the confusion between the medical physicist, dosimetrist, radiation therapist, and technologists.

THE ROUTINE APPLICATION OF DIAGNOSTIC ULTRASOUND IN COMPUTERIZED RADIATION TREATMENT PLANNING.

Donn J. Brascho, Associate Professor, Department of Radiation Oncology, University of Alabama School of Medicine, Brimingham, Alabama.

Diagnostic ultrasound provides the radiation therapist a very practical method of acquiring anatomical information for developing optimized radiation therapy plans. With ultrasound it is possible to record simultaneously the contour of the patient and the location and size of tumors and normal structures. This information can easily be incorporated into current methods of computerized treatment-planning. In this paper the specific applications of ultrasound examination in routine therapy-planning will be demonstrated. Methods of incorporation of the ultrasound information into radiation dosimetry will be described, including a unique system in whioh the ultrasound equipment is interfaced directly to a digital computer.

MEDICAL COMPUTER NETWORK—A PREREQUISITE FOR FASTER PROGRESS IN COMPUTERIZED RADIATION THERAPY.

J. Cederlund (1), H. Dahlin (2), S. Graffman (1), I. Hesselius (1), B. Olsen (2), W. Schneider (2), J. E. Snell (3).
(1) Uppsala University Hospital, S-750 14 Uppsala, Sweden.
(2) Uppsala University Datacenter, Box 2103, S-750 02 Uppsala, Sweden
Siemens-Elema MD, Rontgenvagen 2, S-171 95 Solna, Sweden.

It was more than a decade after the introduction of computers into radiation therapy before it was recognized that in order to take full advantage of the gains offered by the computer technique, the use of computers must be integrated to a very large extent with the ordinary working procedures of the department. The central problem is to find a strategy that allows a balanced distribution of data-processing power. In order to facilitate the introduction and use of data techniques into different medical areas in an economically realistic way, a long-range strategy was developed in Uppsala in 1965. This strategy was called the MSS (Multisatellite Strategy) and permits a gradual development with respect to any area's suitability for data treatment and economic resources. The MSS is based upon a well-balanced use of large-sized, medium-sized, mini, and micro computers. The problems of hardware and software compatibility, data transmission etc. introduced by this approach have been treated and solved for present needs. Thus a number of satellite systems in the medical field as well as regional application systems have been introduced during the last eight years. In this paper the application of the MSS to radiation therapy is discussed.

complete hospital-wide summaries for planning and review purposes, i.e. categorizing patients by services, physicians, diagnoses, treatment modalities, survival, and follow-up rates.

Details of the system, its integration within existing hospital information activities, and its costs, as well as possible linkage of several hospital registries into a network, will be discussed.

INFORMATION STORAGE AND RETRIEVAL FOR A TUMOR REGISTRY USING A MINI-COMPUTER.

S. G. Prasad, R. M. Garces. Department of Radiation Therapy, Evanston Hospital, Evanston, Illinois.

Mini-computers are used in medium-sized radiotherapy centers for treatment-planning and tumor registry. The manufacturers have developed programs for tumor registry. In using the above program, the centers usually define a format that meets their needs. We have found that the above programs are inadequate for our needs: (1) the number of selections that can be stored in each field is limited to one; (2) when a numerical selection is made, the numbers have to be integers; (3) a search cannot be made in all fields. We have developed a program that overcomes the above drawbacks: (a) ten selections per field can be stored; (b) the acceptable range of numerical selection is .000001 to 999999; (c) all fields can be searched. This program can be adapted by other radiotherapy centers with very minor modifications. The program is written in FORTRAN.

CLINICAL MOTIVATIONS FOR AN INTERNATIONAL RADIOTHERAPY DATA BASE.

Judith M. S. Prewitt. National Institutes of Health, U.S.A.

Computer usage in radiotherapy is well-accepted for compiling archives, scheduling patients and facilities, and constructing empirically reasonable treatment plans. Attention is turning next toward prospects for improving therapy end-results by utilizing computer-based, radiobiologically motivated, and clinically validated treatment models of optimum therapy regimes which enhance the likelihood of oncologic cure or control at acceptable risk to the patient. Pilot studies by several radiotherapists and biomathematicians indicate that this is both feasible and worthwhile.

A radiotherapy data base of varified integrity, representing collective clinical experience, and a companion radiobiological research data base are of utmost importance for this endeavor. First, if coverage is broad, a retrospective data base can partially substitute for prospective clinical trials designed to assess protocols and optimization criteria. Second, retrospective data are likely to contain information on extreme dosages, data unobtainable now because of nonconformance with current legal restraints. Third, these data are valuable for testing sensitivity and robustness of models to controllable clinical parameters, especially fractionation schemes, and hopefully can lead to parsimonious yet reliable models. Lastly, they can help determine if present differences in techniques are major or inconsequential, and whether any meaningful gain can be expected from introducing the "fine detail" of cell and tissue kinetics models.

My survey of Western country tumor registries after the Fourth International Congress showed substantial agreement on minimal information requirements for adequate statistical evaluation of current practices and design of improved protocols. A preliminary proposal to UICC for an International Cancer Radiotherapy Data Base, encouraged by NCI-USA, was enthusiastically received, but no international support or cooperation under their auspices was offered. This Fifth International Congress is perhaps the best forum for specifying contents and formats and selecting a repository. Alternatively, a network of autonomous but cross-referencing data bases might be more practical. After initial grant support or user contributions, it could ultimately operate on a fee-for-service basis. It seems timely and appropriate that this Working Cadre lay the foundations for such a cooperative and beneficial endeavor.

CORADS (COMPUTERIZED ONCOLOGY RADIATION AND DATA SYSTEM).

Melvin L. Griem, Lawrence H. Lanzl, Martin Rozenfeld, University of Chicago; Patricia Z. Clarke, Case Western Reserve University Hospitals, Cleveland, Ohio.

The CORADS project is an attempt to develop in radiation oncology a computer system for medical record-keeping patterned after the University of Vermont's PROMIS Laboratory medical record-keeping system. We plan to develop question and answer techniques to gather medical information concerning the oncology patient to create a medical record not only for improved patient care but as a historical data base for research use. Our plan is to use the PLATO interactive terminal and a mini-computer as the data-gathering system. There would be interaction with the Institute for Computer Research and a large computer as the backup and data-analysis system. Individual aspects of this system will be discussed.

IMPLICATIONS OF DEPARTMENT SCHEDULING ON THE OPERATION OF A TUMOR REGISTRY.

Don. P. Ragan, Mallinckrodt Institute of Radiology.

The accumulation of research data for radiation therapy (cancer?) is costly in terms of physician effort and computer expense. In an effort to make these two areas more cost effective we have integrated our tumor registry efforts with other department-computing functions (previous paper). The information in our present registry is the union of (1) our highly codified summary information (back to 1950, previously on a time-shared campus computer), (2) the results of daily patient scheduling, and (3) the information from chart dosimetry-checking. No extensive tumor registry forms are needed. Redundant information is often available which enhances data validity. The computer hardware is available as a result of performing the ancillary department functions. The computer–medical personnel interface is also facilitated by the system's multifunction nature.

In order to accommodate the needs of our department, the operating system (MUMPS, MIIS dialect) was expanded in three areas, (1) disk storage, (2) arithmetic capability, and (3) large-file searching speed. This was done in cooperating with the manufacturer, and all improvements are available as standard features and are supported by the manufacturer. The added capability alters many of the design restrictions usually associated with MUMPS.

A DEPARTMENTAL TUMOR REGISTRY ON THE PDP-8/I 8K COMPUTER.

Prakash N. Shrivastava, Division of Radiation/Oncology, Allegheny General Hospital, 320 East North Avenue, Pittsburgh, Pennsylvania.

A project has been undertaken to test the feasibility of effectively utilizing a small PDP-8/I Computer with 8 K word memory for collection, storage, and retrieval of data for patients receiving radiotherapy. Two original features not available in the Patient Index Program supplied by the Digital Equipment Company have been included. One, our program allows the possibility of data input via paper tape which can be prepared at the clinic without using the computer memory. Two, the program operates using the interrupt facility so that it can allow several different jobs to run simultaneously on the computer. A third feature, which will allow use of a "Grafatran" device or a light pen for data input from standard information sheets, is being considered. This will result in greater convenience compared to teletype input and is also expected to reduce errors.

The system described is a general purpose record-keeping program. The peripherals utilized are: the KV8-I oscilloscope, teletype, analog to Digital converter, light pen, "Grafatran," and two DECtapes. The program will accept digital or alphanumeric data for patients' files.

The input and retrieval data are displayed on the scope for verification before a hard copy is made either on the DECtape or on paper.

The system being tested is expected to result in more accurate and complete data collection compared to the present methods. The possibility of quick retrieval of information will benefit the analysis of specific treatment techniques, training of residents, and control of patient flow in the department.

Role in Developing Centers

THE IAEA PROGRAM ON COMPUTER SYSTEMS IN DOSIMETRY.
R. Abedin-Zadeh, H. Eisenlohr, I. A. Lerch. International Atomic Energy Agency, Vienna, Austria.

The International Atomic Energy Agency has organized different activities in the field of computer application within the last decade with the objective of assisting developing radiotherapy centers.

The goal of this program is to facilitate the introduction and to assess the efficacy of suitable radiation dosimetry data and computer systems for use in developing radiotherapy centers with the cooperation of advanced institutions. This program consists of the following two components: (1) Computer application in radiotherapy, and (2) Data collection, evaluation and distribution.

Within the framework of the first component three panels have been organized during the last nine years. The last panel, held in Vienna on 22–25 October 1973, entitled "Dose Computation and Computerized Treatment Planning in Radiotherapy," provided guidance for the Agency on means of assisting developing radiotherapy centers to establish automated treatment-planning systems.

In order to define the need and capability of these systems, a questionnaire was distributed to over 1,000 centers in the IAEA member states. The result of a survey of the returned questionnaires has demonstrated that there is a strong demand and need for assistance in this field in most centers.

Because of this need for radiation dosimetry data in many developing radiotherapy centers, it is the intention of the Agency to prepare atlases of radiation dose-distributions and to update and complete the existing radiation dosimetry data catalogue.

PLANNING THE AUTOMATION AT THE DEVELOPING CENTER.

Pavel Houdek, Herbert Turnier. University of Miami and Jackson Memorial Hospital, Miami, U.S.A.

Planning the computerization for a future center, which is the theme of this Conference, can be outlined in the following manner: (i) the specification of the Center's needs in regards to automation, (ii) the determination of their priorities, (iii) the selection of an appropriate computer system, and (iv) the development and/or implementation of existing software. It is the purpose of this communication to discuss the need for a fifth—the establishment of an adequate computer environment in addition to the above scheme. The discussion is focused on centers that are in the process of developing automation. Examples of different computer applications in such developing centers are presented, to demonstrate that computer phenomena, e.g. rapidity, accuracy, and memory capacity, are developing a constant pressure on involved professionals to generage more data than ever before, as well as to absorb and utilize large amounts of computer-produced information never before available. It appears that more advanced technology will only increase this impact of the computer on its environment—all of which seems to indicate that the ability to utilize computer technology fully may be the limiting factor for future automation, rather than the technology itself as it existed in the past. It is, therefore, a main concern of this contribution to point out the necessity to create an adequate environment at the developing center which will allow the optimal use of computer technology. The role of education in this process is emphasized.

DOCUMENTATION OF COMPUTER PROGRAMS.

Jeffrey Rothmeier. University of Massachusetts Medical School, Worcester, Massachusetts.

It is very difficult to transfer computer software from one place to another. This is often true even if the same computer language is used and the programs appear to be very useful in a new environment. Small differences in hardware or systems software can cause considerable programming problems.

Good documentation cannot only be a major factor in helping a new environment to assess the usefulness of a program, but it can also be a significant aid in getting a program to run. Documentation does, however, require programmer time. It is important to realize that this time is not wasted. Most programmers find documentation valuable and time saving even when maintaining their own code. This is especially true if considerable time has passed since a program was originally written.

Fundamental to documenting a program is a concise meaningful description and purpose for each module and carefully thought-out comments within the code. Further aids, such as variable descriptions and detailed information on file structure, are also extremely valuable.

The nature of precise documentation techniques is often dependent on the computer language.

Computer Systems in Current Use

AN INTELLIGENT REMOTE BATCH TERMINAL "SIDOS-U" FOR USE IN RADIATION THERAPY.

J. Cederlund, Dept. of Radiation Physics, Uppsala University Hospital, S-750 14 Uppsala, Sweden; M. Dade, Siemens UB Med., Henkestrasse 127, 8250 Erlangen, Fed. Republic of Germany; H. Dahlin, Uppsala University Datacenter, Box 2103, S-750 02 Uppsala, Sweden; and J. E. Snell, Siemens-Elema MD, Rontgenvagen 2, S-171 95 Solna, Sweden.

Since 1969 the use of computers in radiophysics and radiotherapy has been studied in a joint project between Uppsala University Hospital, Uppsala Datacenter, and Siemens-Elema. One of the results of this project is a new radiotherapy system, SIDOS-U, that will be presented in this paper. The system consists of a local terminal (PDP-11 series) for interactive input and manual optimization of data for dose-calculation in external and intracavitary radiation therapy. Curve digitizer and keyboard are used for input of data, and typewriter, plotter, and graphic display for output. The optimization is performed by interactively displaying point doses and/or isodose levels and by changing beam parameters. A remote batch computer is used via transmission (1200–4800 baud) for heavy calculations and large data-base handling, e.g. 3-dimensional dose calculations and follow-up. When developing the SIDOS-U system, a great flexibility in the choice of hardware and software was kept in mind. It is possible for a user to choose an initial system that suits his economy and applications. When his economy allows and his needs increase, it is possible to add more peripherals and software.

A COMPARATIVE ANALYSIS OF SYNECTIC SYSTEMS FOR COMPUTER-ASSISTED RADIOTHERAPY OPTIMIZATION.

Frederick W. George, III, National Cancer Institute, National Institutes of Health, Bethesda, Maryland.

Descriptions of central-processing units and peripherals for several radiotherapy systems emphasizing cost-benefit factors in the context of commercially available software support, as well as software availability from noncommercial sources (e.g., other investigators developing and utilizing such systems). A description of the specific functions of the hardware and software components of the systems is included for the benefit of noncomputer scientists. Listings of application programs, subroutines, and operating systems are tabulated to permit easy comparison between systems and the current status of their development. Data in the form of video-terminal displays, hard copy printouts, performance characteristics, down-time and maintenance records, and other useful parameters are also incorporated in this report. Finally, recommendations are made for the several environments and varying needs of typical radiotherapy programs. Systems based on the Varian 620/I, 620/F, V73, V80, PDP-8, PDP-11, Artronics, and NEC Therac systems, as well as time-sharing systems, will be compared.

THE ROLE OF THE DARTMOUTH TIME-SHARING COMPUTER SYSTEM IN RADIATION ONCOLOGY.

M. Hughes, B. Curran, J. Lester, J. Ting, E. Sternick, Department of Therapeutic Radiology, Dartmouth-Hitchcock Medical Center, Hanover, New Hampshire.

The Dartmouth Time-Sharing computer system has proved to be an effective tool in many tasks fundamental to radiation oncology. The configuration and operation of this system in conjunction with an on-site, intelligent terminal system is described.

Programs now in use support the following activities: (1) treatment-planning for external regular and irregular fields and implanted sources—the programs allow input and output from a broad range of terminal arrangements; (2) a tumor registry capturing cases occurring in a multihospital, geographically large area; (3) radiation physics—data acquisition via a scanning water tank and a film densitometer—density measurements of internal structures based on an automated transmission scan system—computer-aided design of wedge filters—treatment machine calibration checks. Since time-sharing computer costs relate directly to usage, processing costs for the above activities can be presented.

THE THOMAS JEFFERSON UNIVERSITY HOSPITAL RADIATION THERAPY DEPARTMENTAL COMPUTER SYSTEM.

J. Steben, R. Wu, N. Suntharalingam, and C. Mansfield. Thomas Jefferson University Hospital, Philadelphia, Pennsylvania, U.S.A.

A PDP 11/45 midi-computer with 16 K core is presently in use for treatment-planning and patient records. The radiation dose distribution calculations are performed under DOS using a modified version of Cunningham's software with a DECwriter, P-O device, scope, and plotter as peripherals. Patient data-retrieval studies are carried out under two-user MUMPS. Other departmental activities of immediate interest are monitoring of treatment machines by dedicated minicomputers, which will be linked to the central computer as fast ascii communications terminals; on-line measurements of radiation beam characteristics using isodose plotter and film densitometer; graphic data entry of ultrasonic patient surface and internal structure measurements; and patient flow and billing.

Considerations are under way to combine all these activities into a real-time multitask system. This will require expansion of the central PDP 11/45 computer both in core size and in disc storage. Different approaches to the problem will be discussed.

Biological Models

DOSE-VOLUME RELATIONSHIPS.

Manfred Busch and Ulf Rosenow. Medizinische Universitäts-Poliklinik, Röntgenabteilung, D-355 Marburg/GFR. Universitats-Frauenklinik, Strahlenabteilung, D-34 Gottingen/GFR.

The intention of the present investigation is to apply a mathematical model to the dose-volume relationships in radiotherapy of tumors. Cure probabilities as well as normal tissue damage depend on dose in a similar way and may be described in the same model.

The suppositions of the model are:

(1) equally small parts of a lesion are equally sensitive to the same dose,
(2) different parts of a lesion react independently to irradiation,
(3) a certain cure or damage probability observed in a large volume as effect of a dose D will be observed in a similar volume as effect of a dose f.D, where f is greater than 1.

Formulas are derived which give the well-known S-shaped dose dependency of the radiation effect. The application to clinical data allows the determination of the constants of the model.

The model is then used on a computer to investigate the influence of different parameters on the treatment result and to derive conclusions in respect to an optimization of dose distributions. It is understood that such a model can be only a first approximation to the clinical situation, as in the above supposition, and applicable only to a restricted range of cases. Neither homeostatic control of the tumor nor the presence of anoxic cells or necrosis in the center of the tumor is taken into account. A variety of further factors may influence radiation effect too. These should be subject to later extensions of the model.

Nevertheless, the results obtained are in agreement with a number of clinical observations, as the decrease of cure probability and the increase of damage with volume at a certain dose. Furthermore, some important conclusions can be drawn:

A change in the treated volume will influence the probability of local control and of normal tissue damage in different modes.

A more homogeneous dose distribution across the tumor will increase the cure probability, while tissue damage is hardly influenced. A higher selectivity of the treatment results.

Dose "hot-spots" should be carefully considered in normal tissue, as the radiation effect increases unproportionally with dose. Correspondingly, the usual treatment of carcinoma of the cervix, with high dose levels in the center of the tumor where normal tissue tolerance is no limitation, and a dose distribution as homogenous.

BIOLOGICAL PARAMETERS REQUIRED FOR OPTIMIZATION OF THE TREATMENT SCHEDULE.

Lionel Cohen. Michael Reese Medical Center, Chicago, Illinois.

The clinical response expected with various dosage schedules can be evaluated and standardized by using (1) graphical plots relating dosage to treatment time (Strandqvist iso-effect lines); (2) regression equations for estimating position and slope of empirical lines fitted to clinical dose-time-volume data; or (3) the NSD formula with three parameters relating dosage to the number of fractions and over-all time.

Cell population kinetic models also yield realistic iso-effect curves which are nonlinear and differ in origin, slope, and shape for different tissues and tumors. Well-defined optima, or fractionation schemes giving the maximal differential response between a given tumor and the associated normal tissue, can sometimes be identified. Parameters required are the single- and multi-target radiosensitivity constants, extrapolation number, and repopulation rate. Logistic or Gompertzian growth-limiting factors, hypoxic fraction and re-oxygenation potential, and factors for cycle-linked variation in response may be included.

Several algorithms for deriving best-fitting values of the parameters from available clinical data have been studied. These include programs for maximizing the coefficient of separation (between reactors and nonreactors or "cures" and "failures"), or for minimizing the chi-square value derived by multiple probit analysis of individually computed cellular surviving fractions. Search patterns explored include systematic "grid" surveys of the entire multidimensional parameter space, a sequential "ridge" search for following trends to their peak positions, and computation of gradients so as to converge iteratively on an approximate solution set. The sequential ridge search proved the most efficient and widely applicable procedure and has yielded plausible, though probably not ideal, solutions for the response of a number of human tissues and tumors.

A MATHEMATICAL MODEL FOR TIME OPTIMIZATION OF TREATMENT REGIMES IN CLINICAL RADIOTHERAPY.

J. Kirk, T. E. Wheldon. West of Scotland Health Boards, Department of Clinical Physics and Bio-Engineering, 11 West Graham Street, Glasgow, G4; 9LF., Scotland. (Communications to Dr. J. Kirk.)

The biological damage generated in normal connective tissue by radiation therapy can be measured on a scale of accumulated subtolerance radiation damage, the Cumulative Radiation Effect (CRE). By using the CRE system, the effects on normal tissue of a variety of treatment regimes can be assessed and compared. However, regimes that have equivalent effects on normal tissue will in general have different effects on neoplastic tissue.

Using a simple mathematical model, in which the effects on normal tissue are assessed as a CRE and those for tumor tissue as a fractional cell survival, many treatment regimes are examined for tumors having a wide range of doubling times. Preliminary results suggest that:

(a) regimes that assessed on the CRE system as having equivalent normal tissue effects can have tumor tissue effects differing by several orders of magnitude, and
(b) regimes that have optimal curative effect may involve treatment over considerable longer periods of time is the current practice and may not be simple or regular schedules.

The model gives rise to suggestions for animal experiements which may assist in determining the schedule that is optimal for the cure of a tumor for which the kinetic properties are known.

Automation and Verification

DYNAMIC TREATMENT.

D. L. Neblett, J. W. Schaeflein, H. R. Haymond, F. W. George, III, E. R. Ahten, J. G. Mackinney. University of Southern California Medical Center, Los Angeles, California.

The phrase "dynamic treatment" is used to describe radiation therapy treatment delivered while the radiotherapy unit and patient move simultaneously. A small computer connected to an isometrically mounted 4 MeV linear accelerator has been used to coordinate the simultaneous movement of the patient-support mechanism (holding the patient) and the beam-defining jaws of the linear accelerator. A wedge-shaped dose distribution is produced in a treatment volume by synchronizing the closure of the jaws of the collimator with the appropriate movement of the patient.

The rate of this closure and rate of patient movement are determined by the computer from the following inputs: desired isodose wedge angle, dose rate, total dose delivered at a given point, and position of the treatment-unit axis. Film dosimetry techniques were used to determine the dose-distributions from the treatment beam in a phantom. Dynamic wedge dose-distributions have been produced for a variety of field sizes and wedge angles.

THE HARDWARE AND SOFTWARE USED IN THE AUTOMATION OF A THERATRON 80 COBALT MACHINE.

Peter W. Neurath, Richard M. Seymour. Dept. of Therapeutic Radiology, Tufts–New England Medical Center, 171 Harrison Avenue, Boston, Massachusetts.

A minicomputer, used for maintenance of a MUMPS 11 medical history system, operates in a closed-loop fashion with the machine. The system performs simultaneous positioning of ten axes, pauses for operator verification and adjustment, and then directs the treatment delivery. Upon completion of treatment, a printout is provided for insertion into the patient's records, and similar data are stored on line by the computer. Goals of the system are to provide higher patient through-put by minimizing motion time, to improve treatment quality by minimizing the chance for operator error during field set-up, to improve accuracy in record-keeping, and to provide capability to perform complex motion patterns to produce irregularly shaped fields. Obstacles to completion include avoidance of intramachine collision, allowance for deviation from planned motion paths, and hardware reliability. Efforts to guarantee patient safety are also detailed.

ON THE POTENTIAL OF COMPUTER CONTROL TO IMPROVE DOSE DISTRIBUTIONS IN RADIATION THERAPY.

Bengt Bjarngard, Peter Kijewski. Joint Center for Radiation Therapy, 50 Binney Street, Boston, Massachusetts.

In current clinical practice, all parameters of the therapy machine with the exception of the gantry angle are fixed during the setup and remain unchanged during the treatment. While this approach is adequate for many treatments, more difficult cases require dose-distributions that cannot readily be obtained with these limitations. At present, sophisticated treatment-planning is the most common method to solve complex dose-distribution problems. The restrictions imposed by the fact that machine parameters are changed only between treatments limit the flexibility of the planning procedure. A variety of mechanical devices have been invented to enhance the capabilities to obtain more optimal dose-distributions during treatment. Some of these methods have not been accepted, since the execution of the treatment, as is the case with complex plans in general, time-consuming, error-prone, and cumbersome.

A whole new approach to these problems is possible with the advent of inexpensive control computers. Control technology developed for the machine tool industry is applicable to the control of the therapy machines. Gantry angle, field size, field angle, field shape, couch position, turntable angle, dose rate, and energy are all adjustable parameters on the modern radiation therapy machine. Under computer control, these parameters can be varied while treatment is in progress, and execution of more complex treatment schemes could become practicable. With computer costs steadily decreasing, the computer control function will not add unreasonably to the cost of present therapy equipment. A high initial investment is required to adapt existing hardware and write the appropriate software. Additionally, much work needs to be done on safety related aspects of computer control. Both radiation accidents and collision accidents should be impossible in the event of hardware failure, software failure, or improper operation by personnel.

It seems very likely that more optimal dose-distributions, characterized by a higher tumor dose and less dose to surrounding tissue, will be possible under computer control. The success or failure of computer control in radiation therapy will be based on the clinical significance of the improvements in dose distribution.

AN INTEGRATED APPROACH TO SIMULATOR AND TREATMENT UNIT AUTOMATION.

C. J. Karzmark, D. C. Rust. Stanford University School of Medicine, Stanford, California.

The automation of radiotherapy treatment units using digital minicomputers has proceeded via treatment prescription verification, since this is most easily implemented. Prescription verification can reduce treatment-delivery error but in itself is likely to increase costs. In justifying automation of the treatment unit from economic considerations, therefore, one usually cites higher utilization factors along with higher dose-delivery rate. The chances for error increase under these high treatment-rate conditions, taxing contemporary treatment-surveillance practice. This burden should logically be assumed by the mini-computer. It is our contention, however, that treatment-unit automation with interactive simulation as an integrated part of the system is more readily justified on economic grounds (Karzmark and Rust, 1972).

For improved space utilization, we find that an orthovoltage treatment unit can be efficiently combined with a megavoltage simulator. To this end we have constructed and recently installed a simulator closely duplicating the Varian Clinac 4 treatment unit. The simulator will provide the initial input for an automated Clinac 4 system. It has been installed in a room together with an overhead mounted orthovoltage treatment unit so as to conserve space and accommodate two functions: simulation of patients for megavoltage therapy and orthovoltage treatment. The Clinac 4 treatment couch incorporated in the system is shared for these functions. The orthovoltage treatment unit is positioned overhead in a remote corner of the room when not in use.

REFERENCE

Karzmark, C. J., and Rust, D. C., "Radiotherapy Treatment Simulators and Automation: A Case for Their Provision from a Cost Viewpoint," *Radiology*, *105*, 157-161 (1972).

COMPUTER OPERATIONS FOR SUPPORT OF PION RADIOTHERAPY AT LOS ALAMOS.

Arvid Lundy, Michael Minor, Sally Shlaer. Los Alamos Scientific Laboratory, Los Alamos, New Mexico.

Some minicomputers offer expansion capabilities such that an expanded system has the computing power and storage capacity of a medium-sized system but considerably lower hardware cost. The capabilities of such a system using a commercial real time, multitasking software operating system are described.

At present the system does automated set-up, control, and data-logging on the LAMPF pion radiation therapy beam line. This involves over 400 control and data channels, all interfaced via a CAMAC system. In addition, high speed experimental data-logging is done through CAMAC. Positioning of the patient treatment couch will be controlled, and the beam scanning parameters set by the system.

An interactive treatment-planning code is being implemented and the system will eventually include automatic logging of patient contours, data-logging from a simulator, and medical record-keeping. Finally, the system is used for biological and physical modeling problems.

All tasks run simultaneously on a rapid time-share basis and four operator terminals are in use.

While the pion treatment facility at LAMPF is peculiar, many of the problems correspond to those in conventional radiation therapy.

A DEDICATED COMPUTER FOR THE CHECKING OF FIELD SETTINGS AND THE MAINTENANCE OF RECORDS FOR TREATMENTS GIVEN ON A LINEAR ACCELERATOR.

M. E. Rosenbloom, R. E. Bentley. Physics Department, The Royal Marsden Hospital, Downs Road, Sutton, Surrey, England.

A PDP 8 computer has been interfaced directly to an SL 75 medical linear accelerator for the checking and recording of treatments. The system compares set-up parameters (field size, wedge angle and sense, orientation of treatment head, gantry, and patient couch) against data entered on a punched tape. An error message is typed when any quantity set differs from its expected value by more than a preset tolerance, and treatment is inhibited. Records are automatically maintained of the dose given to each patient, and can be reproduced on demand.

The system has been run for a trial period with a limited number of patients under clinical conditions.

A brief description is given of the hardware and the programs used.

The overall objectives of the system and its integration into a clinical environment are discussed.

COMPUTER ASSISTED ENTRY, VERIFICATION, AND RECORDING OF TREATMENT PARAMETERS FOR A 45 MeV BETATRON.

J. Steben, N. Suntharalingam. Thomas Jefferson University Hospital, Philadelphia, Pennsylvania, U.S.A.

A computer system for entry, examination, editing, verification, and recording of patient treatment parameters is under investigation for the Brown Boveri 45 MeV Asklopitron. A mini-computer (GT 40) with 8 K core and DECtapes will be interfaced for the direct monitoring of treatment setups. Data entry will be interactive via keyboard-generated "snapshots" of initial setup. All motions for patient set-up are to be manually executed by a technician with computer examination of correctness within preestablished tolerances prior to commencing radiation. A BBC-furnished combination of digital and analog signals for 5 rotational and 7 general coordinates and 10 additional treatment parameters will be monitored. A live digital scope display of current and initial set-up parameters will be used. Capability of patient pooling for daily treatments will be available. Software will be developed largely in a higher level language, probably RT-11 FORTRAN IV. The mini-computer will be tied into the departmental central PDP 11/45 computer for retrieval and updating of patient records, and scheduling functions.

THE CART SYSTEM: AUTOMATED VERIFICATION, RECORDING, AND CONTROLLED ACCELERATOR SET-UP.

D. Kipping, R. Potenza, Varian Associates, Palo Alto, California.

The CART (Computer Assisted Radiation Therapy) system integrates automation-support functions into the normal procedures of a radiotherapy department treating patients with a medical linear accelerator. This paper describes the design philosophy and choice of components which has resulted in the current CART System.

CART operates with either a Varian Clinac 4, 12, or 18, and is designed in two system configurations: CART-D and CART-DC. The CART-D configuration assists the technologist in verifying and recording a prescribed treatment with the accelerator. Prior to each treatment, the CART-D system displays data describing patient diagnosis, current status of the treatment course and details of the next treatment. The system prevents the commencement of a treatment until the technologist has set the machine parameters to correspond with the prescribed treatment parameters. The CART-DC configuration provides the additional function of controlling accelerator and couch motions during patient set-up.

These clinical functions and experience with an earlier version of CART lead to a new overall design philosophy, and specific hardware and software systems. Since CART interfaces with both the accelerator/couch system and the daily procedures of a radiotherapy department, hardware and software design must incorporate such factors as safety, reliability, operator convenience, effective patient-record maintenance, and economy. The system includes a disk-based software system that is modular and designed for convenient maintenance and expansion.

AN ATTEMPT TO CHECK RADIATION TREATMENT PARAMETERS WITH A MINI-COMPUTER.

J. Cederlund, P-O Lofroth, S. Zetterlund. Radiation Physics Department, Akademiska Sjukhuset, S-750 14 Uppsala, Sweden.

In order to check parameters in patient radiation treatment we have used an available interface between our medical linear accelerator, type SL 75, and a Siemens 305 computer which the department has access to for development work. A small computer has been simulated by the 305 computer using only about 1 K (24 bits) of the core store. The program guides the reading of accelerator parameters. The readings are converted to actual values, such as MM, degree, etc. The data from each treatment—both set-up and given values— are printed out on a teletype and on punched tape. Besides such parameters as kind of radiation, energy, dose, time, wedge angle, orientation of treatment head, gantry angle, etc., readings were made from micro-ionization chambers for monitoring of the reference dose on the skin of the patient.

Information on the tape had to be transfered to a disk before the treatment data for each patient could be edited and printed out in tables to provide a good survey of the given treatment. The check of parameters was limited to approximately one month, during which time about 240 treatments were registered. At least twice a week, three to five different settings for each parameter was read and stored in a special program which checked the calibration values to convert the readings.

The material does not allow statistical analysis, but some observations can be made. No obvious errors were discovered during the test period. Set-up values for dose and time were correct, as well as wedge angle and sense. The gantry angle was set up with a precision of better than one degree. Treatment-field dimensions were set up with deviations in the interval 1–3 mm and on some occasions up to 5 mm. Angles for the treatment head have shown considerable deviation during treatment period ±3–4°. At small field sizes the corresponding deviation amounted to maximum ±5°. The size of the angle deviation is quite reasonable when considering the lack of special attachments for patients on the treatment table.

From this trial we conclude that with a fairly simple computer it is possible to build, check, and confirm systems without (or maybe with) possibilities to store the parameters for each treatment.

DEVELOPMENT AND EXPERIENCE IN COMPUTER MONITORING AND THE VERIFICATION OF DAILY PATIENT TREATMENT PARAMETERS.

Anthony Chung-Bin, Ponnunni Kartha, Thomas Wachtor, Frank Hendrickson. Rush-Presbyterian-St. Luke's Medical Center, Chicago, Illinois.

The department of Radiation Oncology has developed and implemented monitoring, recording, and verification of treatment parameters since November 1972 with the PDP-11 computer. Accidental errors (collimator rotation greater than 15°, gantry angle greater than 15°, treatment time greater than (one half minute) in daily set-up of treatment parameters have been studied for several hundred set-ups and have been found to be about 2 percent per parameter and 14 percent per treatment. The need for verification of treatment is justified, since the error may influence the outcome of the patient's survival. The presentation will include: (1) analysis of human error in treatment execution; (2) procedure for verification of treatment; (3) difficulty and problems in its routine implementation and the necessity of computer to have the capability of time sharing; (4) time and cost factors, and (5) conclusion and future development.

Control of Patient Flow and Records

COMPUTER-BASED PATIENT RECORD AND FOLLOW-UP SYSTEM FOR RADIOTHERAPY.

Torgil R. Moller, John-Erik Johnsson, Arne Sundstrom, Thomas Gustafsson, Department of Radiotherapy, University Hospital & Lund University Computer Centre, S-221 85 Lund, Sweden.

A computer system with automatic acquisition of medical data from patient records, a detailed documentation of external-beam treatment, and a follow-up system for patients is described. It has been in use at a radiotherapy clinic since 1972 and contains up to now about 10,000 patient records. The information collected is part of the data base for a future regional cancer register.

The medical records are written on a special typewriter, IBM MT 72, equipped with two small magtape cassettes, one master tape, and one slave tape. The information is dictated in a structured way and written according to a special layout. The headings and subheadings to be used are transferred from the master tape (together with an internal code number), and these headings as well as the typewritten text are simultaneously recorded on the slave tape. The information is then converted to computer-compatible magtape. Decoding of the text and formation of transactions are performed, and these transactions update the register, stored on disk or magtape. Record-linking is based on the civic registration number. The register is a variable-length format, and in addition a special file in fixed format is generated for statistical purpose. A direct-access facility has been developed for easy correction and search in the main register.

A special record form for documentation of external-beam treatment has been designed. At the conclusion of treatment a large number of variables are punched on cards, forming the input to a separate register of external-beam treatments, from which treatment reports and statistics are generated. Data may be transferred between this system, the record system, and the dose-planning system.

Usually after five years of recurrence-free personal observation, further follow-up of many patients is performed by a mailing routine. Special questionnaires, based on the type of disease for which the patient was treated, are sent to the patient at certain time intervals. The patient's answer is recorded on the MT 72. If the patient describes new symptoms, he is called for a personal check-up; if not, he will receive an anknowledgment. Formulas can also be sent to other clinics or to the registrar's office at the patient's location.

SCHEDULING IN EXTERNAL BEAM RADIOTHERAPY.

H. Dahlin (1), B. Jung (2), P. O. Karlsson (1), A. M. Thelin (2).
(1) Uppsala University Datacenter, Box 2103, S-750 02 Uppsala, Sweden; (2) Uppsala University Hospital, S-750 14 Uppsala, Sweden.

For some years an automatic system for record-keeping in external-beam radiotherapy has been running at Uppsala. The program schedules the whole treatment series from the treatment dose. The printout simulates the manual record and lists the dates of treatment, and the corresponding field numbers, reference doses, accumulated maximum, mean, and minimum doses in the target area, as well as accumulated doses in up to three critical organs. The treatment-scheduling is based on our field per day for multiple-field techniques and a weekly mean target dose. Currently, the program is being run as a remote-batch job, but intelligent-terminal remote-batch operation was recently implemented. The program automatically takes Saturdays, Sundays, and other holidays into account and allows for automatic contraction of the treatment series should the preliminary schedule and immediately after a long holiday (Christmas, Easter, etc.). In-course changes in the schedule due to radiation equipment failure and patient's absence from a scheduled treatment, or altered weekly or total dose prescriptions, are easily carried out, and results in the print-out of an updated treatment schedule.

A TIME AND MOTION STUDY DATA COLLECTION SYSTEM USING A SMALL DEPARTMENT COMPUTER.

D. L. Neblett, E. Webb, P. Apeles, D. P. Anderson, F. W. George, III.
University of Southern California Medical Center, Los Angeles, California.

This study involves the use of a computer to collect data for evaluation of the utilization of radiation therapy treatment facilities. The computer is used as a stop watch, scratch pad, and automation recording device for an observer. Two CRT terminals, one inside the treatment room and one outside, are used to display a list of sixteen treatment events. The observer selects one of these events, and the computer records the time and any other pertinent treatment parameters: monitor units, treatment time, or treatment-unit positional parameters. Limited patient identification, mobility, diagnosis, number of fields, and treatment site are also added to the record. The collected data are then reorganized and merged with the previously collected data and saved on magnetic tape.

DIVERSIFIED RADIOTHERAPY DEPARTMENT COMPUTER SUPPORT.

Don P. Ragan, Mallinckrodt Institute of Radiology.

A radiotherapy department information system has been implemented at Mallinckrodt Institute of Radiology on a PC 12/7 computer. The design criteria for this system were to perform as many functions for the medical and paramedical staff as possible in a worksheet or schedule form and therby to improve patient care, enhance department efficiency, accession research data effortlessly, and boost computer credibility within the department.

The functions performed include:

1. Bookkeeping and financial management
2. Automatic generation of patient charges
3. Daily therapy machine scheduling
4. Notification of hospital nursing stations of in-patient treatment times
5. Rapid retrieval of individual patient information
6. Administrative summaries
7. A queue of patients currently in the department
8. Chart library
9. General table and text editing
10. Keypunch simulation and communication to the Campus IBM 360
11. Tumor registry service
12. Therapy machine verification
13. Dosimetry checking and other physics aids

A flexible framework is included to facilitate the addition of more functions. The system is currently serving two hospitals and is capable of supporting several hospitals on the same main frame.

The initial phases of system implementation have centered on enhancing department operations. Three areas where the computer system has been most helpful are patient billing, the patient queue, and chart dosimetry checking.

FLOW OF PATIENT INFORMATION IN A DEPARTMENT OF RADIATION ONCOLOGY WITH THE AID OF A DEDICATED PDP 11/45 TIME-SHARING COMPUTER.

Thomas Wachtor, Anthony Chung-Bin, Frank Hendrickson. Rush–Presbyterian–St. Luke's Medical Center, Chicago, Illinois.

A PDP 11/45 computer has been installed to perform all of the routine computer needs of a radiation oncology department. Hardware and software have been developed and perform the following functions concurrently in a time-sharing mode: (1) Initial patient registration; (2) Treatment-planning and associated dose-computation; (3) Recording the definition of disease and the physician's prescription of the treatment; (4) Daily automatic recording of treatment-parameters; (5) Recording the patient's response to the treatment; (6) Recording follow-up information.

Since the information is available randomly in time and at different stations in the Department, a time-sharing, multiterminal computer is a necessity in the procurement of all this information. The presentation will include: (1) Problems in the reliability of the computer; (2) Problems related to human interaction with the computer in a clinical environment; (3) Success and failure of procurement of information under the current system; (4) Usage of procured information; and (5) Requirements for future development.

RADIATION THERAPY SYSTEM USED AT SAHLGRENSKA SJUKHUSET IN GOTEBORG.

B. Lindskoug, K-A. Johansson, G. Notter, I. Ragnhult, L. Fridh. Radiation Therapy and Physics Departments, Sahlgrenska Sjukhuset, Goteborg, Sweden.

This paper will briefly describe the organization and work at the Radiation Therapy and Physics Departments, Sahlgrenska Sjukhuset. The routines currently in use together with planned developemnts for the next two years are presented. The complete radiation therapy system will have facilities for the following tasks:

1. Determination of position and shape of tumor and internal structures.
2. Patient outlines in several sections (SCOPE).
3. Compensation and blocking.
4. Calculation of 2-dimensional dose-distributions in several sections and selection of the best set of plans.
5. Routine dosimetry checks during treatment (semiconductors).

6. Dosimetry checks using automated TLD system.
7. a. checks in phantoms
   b. checks in vivo
7. Fractionation regimes and scheduling of treatments.
8. Patient record and follow-up.

All calculations (except number 8) are made on a PDP 8/e minicomputer (12 K) with two discs, plotter, display, and high-speed reader/punch. The TLD system is automated and adapted to computer-handling of data.

The concept of cumulative radiation effect (CRE) is used in clinical routine for the calculation of doses to be given in order to achieve a specific biological effect. Fractionation regimes of various types are used, including dynamic fractionation.

Author Index

Includes participants in discussions. Numerals in bold face refer to the first page of a paper or an abstract.)